Encountering Treatment Resistance

Solutions Through Reconceptualization

Encountering Treatment Resistance

Solutions Through Reconceptualization

H. Paul Putman III, M.D.

*Distinguished Life Fellow, American Psychiatric Association, and
Fellow, the American College of Psychiatrists*

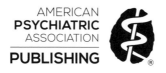

AMERICAN
PSYCHIATRIC
ASSOCIATION
PUBLISHING

If you wish to buy 50 or more copies of the same title, please go to www.appi.org/specialdiscounts for more information.

Copyright © 2024 American Psychiatric Association Publishing

ALL RIGHTS RESERVED

First Edition

Manufactured in the United States of America on acid-free paper
28 27 26 25 24   5 4 3 2 1

American Psychiatric Association Publishing 800 Maine Avenue SW, Suite 900 Washington, DC 20024–2812 www.appi.org

Library of Congress Cataloging-in-Publication Data

Names: Putman, H. Paul, III, author. | American Psychiatric Association Publishing, publisher.
Title: Encountering treatment resistance: solutions through reconceptualization / H. Paul Putman III.
Description: First edition. | Washington, DC : American Psychiatric Association Publishing, [2024] | Includes bibliographical references and index.
Identifiers: LCCN 2023051581 (print) | LCCN 2023051582 (ebook) | ISBN 9781615375158 (paperback ; alk. paper) | ISBN 9781615375165 (ebook)
Subjects: MESH: Mental Disorders—therapy | Treatment Failure | Problem Solving | Concept Formation | Therapeutic Alliance
Classification: LCC RC480.5 (print) | LCC RC480.5 (ebook) | NLM WM 100 | DDC 616.89/1—dc23/eng/20240202
LC record available at https://lccn.loc.gov/2023051581
LC ebook record available at https://lccn.loc.gov/2023051582

British Library Cataloguing in Publication Data

A CIP record is available from the British Library.

Dedication

I dedicate this book to my children,
Alex, Bonnie, Charlotte, and Houston,
who have brought me so much love and joy
and have made me so proud.

Contents

Acknowledgments

Laura Roberts, M.D., M.A., Editor-in-Chief of American Psychiatric Association (APA) Publishing, first deserves my thanks and gratitude, not only because of her support of my work with APA Publishing and the American College of Psychiatrists, but also for suggesting I write this book. Following our discussion about *Rational Psychopharmacology: A Book of Clinical Skills* on her podcast "Psychiatry Unbound," Dr. Roberts suggested my next volume include examples of how the metacognitive methods I write about have reversed treatment failures, and this book was born.

My appreciation also extends to John McDuffie, then Publisher, and Erika Parker, Acquisitions Editor, for embracing and approving the project. Both have been steadfastly supportive and helpful throughout my work with APA Publishing. I also thank Timothy Marney, Director of Digital Publishing and producer of "Psychiatry Unbound," for his enthusiastic and helpful support, and Annie Birge, Acquisitions Coordinator, for helping to shepherd this work to completion. Thanks also to Carrie Y. Farnham, Senior Editor, Books, and Margaret May, Marketing Associate. Much gratitude also goes to Catherine F. Brown, Executive Editor of *Psychiatric News*, who has been extremely generous in accepting my articles for publication.

I am also quite grateful to my valued colleagues who contributed their own clinical examples of treatment failures reversed by reconceptualization: Giuseppe Guaiana, M.D., M.Sc., Ph.D., FRCPC; Melvin J. Thomas, M.D. (a fellow former Chief Resident at the Medical University of South Carolina); and Jesse L. Hite, M.D. It is a pleasure to work with all of you. Appreciation additionally goes to Scott Aaronson, M.D., for allowing me to include his wonderful phrase emphasizing how anecdotes are not evidence.

Thanks also to my local colleagues of many years, Simone Scumpia, M.D.; James Kreisle, M.D.; and Rex Wier, M.D., for supporting my proposals.

My deep love and appreciation go to my wife, "Meg" Putman, for her support and patience during this yearlong project, and to my children, to whom I also dedicate this book. Special thanks to my son, Houston Putman, and daughter-in-law, Mona Chang, for their generous ongoing assistance with my online presence at drpaulputman.com.

I am grateful for the many teachers, professors, and clinicians who imparted a firmly scholarly approach during my education and training. Finally, as always, I continue to be grateful to my patients, who over 35 years, allowed me to work with them and do my best to help resolve their problems.

Introduction

In clinical practice today, 20%–60% of psychiatric diagnoses eventually become labeled *treatment resistant* (Howes et al. 2022). Even more disconcerting is a lack of consensus on a definition or clear criteria for this unrecognized diagnosis (American Psychiatric Association 2022), leading to communication and interrater reliability problems as we attempt to address and understand this phenomenon. Because second opinions identify additional treatment options in more than two-thirds of these cases (Nirodi et al. 2003), this poorly defined category likely includes errors in cognition, incomplete assessments, inadequate treatment planning, poor compliance, and faulty therapeutic alliances.

Because we know that hope is essential for recovery (Langlands et al. 2008), this rush to therapeutic nihilism can lead to malignant psychodynamics that limit clinical success as additional treatment attempts proceed (Shepherd et al. 2009). Rather than identify treatment resistance as an end point diagnosis, or as an entity at all, clinicians may better serve their patients by considering this situation a phase of treatment, still expecting and looking forward to eventual remission. The treatment attempts themselves, but neither the patient nor the diagnosis, may be labeled *treatment failures*, and a case may be described as *pending remission* rather than treatment resistant because it is likely that many treatment options remain.

The actions we clinicians take to solve problems are determined by our conceptualizations of them. Our conceptualizations, in turn, are based on our brain structure, knowledge, observations, and professional traditions. We must therefore be quite circumspect regarding our assumptions, definitions, and labels during treatment. We must strive to make these as conscious and examined as possible, relying only on the most reliable science and evidence and remaining value-free.

While we wait for better definitions and criteria, new models and explanations, we can begin to address so-called treatment resistant, or rather pending remission, cases by confirming our diagnostic validity and accuracy, the thoroughness of our evaluations and monitoring efforts, the clarity of our therapeutic instructions, and the quality of our therapeutic alliances. Rather than asking "What kind of problem is this?" our thought must become "What data am I missing that would solve this clinical dilemma?"

I open this book with the processes underlying conceptualization and how inaccurate or misleading concepts may be developed. I proceed to describe the best practices for problem-solving and the consequences for relying on less effective methods. Evidence-based medicine will be explored, with guidelines for adoption. The usefulness and validity of treatment resistance as a concept will be further examined; examples of misconceptions based on limited data and the clinical risks to patients labeled "treatment resistant" will be discussed.

Methods to ensure that a clinician consistently achieves a thorough evaluation at each patient contact will be outlined, and the concept and utility of Bayesian inference will be reviewed. Anonymous, but actual, case vignettes from psychiatric practice will be presented, illustrating how reexamination and additional data can lead to reconceptualization, then progression from treatment failure(s) to satisfactory clinical results.

Common but underappreciated medical causes of treatment resistance and examples of impaired therapeutic alliances interfering with diagnosis, treatment selection, and compliance will be highlighted. I include proactive steps that will help clinicians self-check and self-correct initial assessments, diagnostic formulations, and ongoing monitoring and reassessment. Readers wishing to deepen these skills further may also wish to (re)read my previous book *Rational Psychopharmacology: A Book of Clinical Skills*, especially Chapters 2–5 (Putman 2020, pp. 13–102). I conclude this work with examples of how to work with and support patients experiencing extended periods of treatment resistance while pending remission.

Each chapter of *Encountering Treatment Resistance: Solutions Through Reconceptualization* includes a summary and list of key points, self-assessment questions, discussion questions for seminars and journal clubs, recommendations for additional reading, and references.

Practicing clinicians: There is still abundant hope when early treatment attempts are disappointing. Your attitude must embody this hope, and you should share it generously with your patients as you continue to work with them and your colleagues until answers are found. Not only is this sharing the truth; it is an essential factor in their recovery.

References

American Psychiatric Association: Diagnostic and Statistical Manual of Mental Disorders, Fifth Edition, Text Revision. Washington, DC, American Psychiatric Association Publishing, 2022

Howes OD, Thase ME, Pillinger T: Treatment resistance in psychiatry: state of the art and new directions. Mol Psychiatry 27(1):58–72, 2022 34257409

Langlands RL, Jorm AF, Kelly CM, Kitchener BA: First aid for depression: a Delphi consensus study with consumers, carers and clinicians. J Affect Disord 105(1–3):157–165, 2008 17574684

Nirodi P, Mitchell AJ, Mindham RHS: Survey of expert second opinions in a tertiary psychiatric outpatient clinic in the Yorkshire region between 1988 and 2000. Psychiatr Bull 27:416–420, 2003

Putman HP: Rational Psychopharmacology: A Book of Clinical Skills. Washington, DC, American Psychiatric Association Publishing, 2020

Shepherd D, Insole L, McAllister-Williams R, Ferrier I: Are specialised affective disorder services useful? Psychiatr Bull 33(2):41–43, 2009

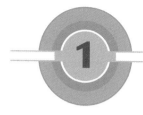

Conceptualization (and Failed Concepts)

The notion of treatment resistance is a conceptualization, so let's begin by looking at concepts and how we form them. Awareness of this process, and how it may create and sustain errors, is quite useful in clinical practice.

Theories of Concept Formation

You no doubt recall from your undergraduate studies that there are many theories of cognition. At one time, scientists believed the human mind was a "blank slate" on which teaching, experience, and socialization would write such concepts as customs, stereotypes, and behavioral choices (Pinker 2002). There is now compelling evidence that our minds are created with a predetermined conceptual structure that links mental representations to linguistic expressions, a process that can be inferred by observing infants acquire and learn language. This is the *conceptual structure* hypothesis (Gobet and Lane 2012; Jackendoff 1983, 1987; Pinker 2011; Zwarts and Verkuyl 1994).

Language can be a window into this innate human conceptual structure, which guides, bundles, and measures our experience. Neologisms (newly created words, such as webinar, malware, selfie, and mansplain) become necessary when the words existing in our language do not match the preexisting conceptual structures in our brains (Pinker 2011). Through linguistics, Steven Pinker described our conceptual structure as categorical, binary (all or nothing), and composed of abstract frameworks, rather than sensory, motor, or motivational features. This system abstracts *space* and *intentionality* but, even more, *time* and *causality*, linking language and grammar with inference and reasoning (Pinker 2007, pp. 153–233; Pinker 2011).

If we can accept that the brain has an underlying structure for forming concepts, how does it function? Conceptualization has been described as the construction of theoretical ideas from experience or incorporated information, employing innate cognitive processes and verbalization (Sam 2013). *Dual process* theory describes two types of cognitive processes that combine in various ways to provide concepts for us to employ (Croskerry 2009a; Evans 1984; Wason and Evans 1974). Type (or System) 1 processing is basically pattern recognition. Type 2 processing involves the conscious use of logic and science, including Bayesian inference (see section "Essential Value of Bayesian Inference" in Chapter 5, "Essential Assessment and Reevaluation").

The cognitive structure theory mentioned earlier refers to the hardwired modules in Type 1, a type of processing that is less appropriate for modern times. It is very influenced by context, especially a current one, copying diagnostic traditions and the assessments of distinguished individuals. This may be one explanation for how the concept of treatment resistance has blossomed. Errors in conceptualization are more likely to occur in Type 1 processing because of this contextual distortion, lack of objectivity, and innate *heuristics* contained within our basic brain structure (see section "Errors in Conceptualization"). These heuristics are rules of thumb, shortcuts that conserve cognitive function by performing automatic estimates for us. This is one way our brains reduce complexity to save time and processing effort (another way is by chunking; see section "Chunking Theory and Expertise").

Type 2 processing is usually error-free unless some element is not functioning properly, such as a reliance on incorrect data, as we saw with the blank slate theory. It also takes more time. An error in Type 2 conceptualization may have a greater impact than a Type 1 error, however, because Type 2 processing is, justifiably, more trusted. The two types of processing can complement each other overall if the advantages of each (speed of Type 1, complex analysis of Type 2) are used appropriately for the situation (Tay et al. 2016).

Chunking Theory and Expertise

Because of a phenomenon known as the *cognitive miser* function, humans default to the least cognitive effort in conceptualization and problem-solving (Croskerry 2009a). This is evident from studies of how chess grand masters develop their expertise, which led to the realization of chunking theory. First proposed in 1946 (De Groot 1946/1978) and formalized in 1973 (Chase and Simon 1973), *chunking* gives a correct measurement of the amount of information that can be processed in human cognition (Miller 1956). It also describes the ways experts eventually employ great variability in responses because the cognitive effort becomes more efficient.

It has been established that human short-term memory is limited to the retention of 7 ± 2 items (Miller 1956), although there is individual variation in capacity for short-term memory and learning rates, leading to differences in individual performance. When items are joined together, however, our short-term memory can hold three to five of these larger packets of information, expanding memory and processing power (Gobet and Lane 2012; Mathy and Feldman 2012).

Pieces of data gleaned from the environment are collated into one entity, that is, a chunk. An example is how we remember phone numbers: 123-456-7890, rather than 1234567890. The elements in a chunk have strong associations with each other but weak associations with the elements comprising other chunks (Gobet and Lane 2012). It should come as no surprise that chunking plays an important role in the development of vocabulary and syntactic structures (Gobet and Lane 2012; Pinker 2014a, pp. 67–69).

When this process is constant, automatic, and unconscious, such as with speech processing, it is labeled *perceptual* chunking (Chase and Simon 1973; De Groot 1946/1978; Gilbert et al. 2014). Perceptual chunks (and templates; see below) appear to be stored in the parahippocampal gyrus and fusiform gyrus of our temporal lobes (Campitelli et al. 2007; Gobet and Lane 2012; Guida et al. 2012). Conscious efforts to use chunking to improve memory are labeled *goal directed*: dividing large amounts of data into smaller chunks to commit to working memory, a process that activates the prefrontal and parietal areas (Guida et al. 2012; Miller 1956).

Acquiring information in a domain (an area of inquiry) with practice and study leads not only to a greater number of chunks but also to chunks of larger size. Learning is slow because information is moved from short-term to long-term memory by this process. However, the recognition of information *within* chunks (e.g., potentially useful moves in chess, diagnostic and treatment options in medicine) is rapid and measurably faster than accessing data *across* chunks (Chase and Simon 1973; Guida et al. 2012). Some incidences of Type 2 processing may eventually be converted to Type 1 chunks as experience and expertise develop; the complex, rational analysis becomes pattern recognition in some cases, improving the speed of processing (Tay et al. 2016).

Experts use even higher level structures called *templates* (or schema) made up of frequently used chunks (Gobet and Simon 1996). Templates consist of a core of constant information and slots that store variable information, further extending memory capacity. For example, whereas chunks are simpler patterns, templates can accommodate different but related positions of competing chess pieces (Guida et al. 2012). Chess grand masters quickly realize potentially helpful moves without having to think through every possibility. Clinicians with more than a decade of practice may also recognize this phenomenon: for them, diagnostic probabilities readily come to mind rather than having to sort through the entire *Diagnostic and Statistical Manual of Mental Disorders*, Fifth Edition, Text Revision (DSM-5-TR; American Psychiatric Association 2022). The minimum amount of time required to complete the brain's reorganization into expert function appears to be 6 years, but ultimately, this is only a measure of retained significant knowledge in a domain rather than competence (Guida et al. 2012).

The advantages of chunks and templates are that we humans can work around the limits of our short-term memory and cognitive-processing ability to increase our potential number of responses to a complex environment. Downsides of chunks are that they are created by individuals (i.e., they are not universal), represent (in most cases) Type 1 processing, and are not easily transmitted to another person. One individual may assume their chunks are the same as another's, resulting in miscommunication and conceptual error (Pinker 2014b). We must never forget that conceptualization requires agreed-on definitions; with many dimensions, a concept may include many definitions. Furthermore, the process of conceptualization must be open to revision as science proceeds (De Carlo 2018) lest it lead to many of the errors that are described later in this chapter.

It is essential to remember that although conceptual knowledge is built on perceptual skills anchored in concrete examples (Gobet and Lane 2012), the concepts themselves do not exist beyond abstract ideas in our heads (De Carlo 2018). Although science may temporarily use concepts as constructs to better understand the physical world (e.g., gravitational fields), science must also proceed to establish external validity of the abstraction through empirical research. The examples on which a concept is based may be concrete, but our conceptualization of it is not tangible. Treatment resistance is but an idea in the minds of some people.

Classification of Concepts

Concepts may be organized into hierarchies or groups to accomplish different intellectual tasks. To understand such taxonomy requires appreciating the differences between a domain, a dimension, and a category.

The word *domain* has many disparate meanings; the concept is fluidly applied to almost any area of study and is redefined frequently. Psychology defines the term *domain* as a class of entities or events constituting the subject matter of a science or discipline (American Psychological Association 2022). For example, five perspectives or viewpoints in psychology have been identified by some authors as domains: biological, cognitive, developmental, social and personality, and mental and physical health (Lumen 2022).

Conceptualization and conceptual learning are often divided into three domains: the cognitive, the affective, and the psychomotor. Within each of these domains, areas of function, from normal to abnormal, are described as psychological or biological *dimensions*, sometimes also called *constructs* (National Institute of Mental Health 2022a). Psychologists' terms for dimensions are often uncommon and confusing for the standard medical clinician. In the National Institute of Mental Health's Research Domain Criteria (RDoC) initiative, the domains under study are defined as areas of neurobehavioral functioning: arousal/regulatory, positive valence, negative valence, sensorimotor, cognitive, and social processes.

In psychiatry, our current focus is predominantly on categorizing symptoms, using this effort to compile diagnoses and choose and monitor treatment. *Categories* are lists of objects with many similarities, such as books, cars, and clothing. Although they may still have many differences, they can also be treated as equal in some way: desks, chairs, tables, and lamps may all be categorized as furniture. Mental representations of these categories are also *concepts* (Murphy 2022).

DSM-III (American Psychiatric Association 1980) significantly altered psychiatric diagnosis by changing from the presumed etiology of disease to nosological descriptions. This effort retained the focus on disease definitions instead of describing and measuring function (or dimensions), a choice repeated in DSM-IV (American Psychiatric Association 1994); DSM-5 did evolve to describe syndromes (American Psychiatric Association 2013). These views of humans and their problems are described as *categorical* approaches, in that we are grouping our observations into categories we constantly work to refine. The current clinical language of psychiatry remains geared toward this categorization.

Much current effort is going into researching how domains may become more clinically useful and even eventually integrated into psychiatric diagnosis (Casey et al. 2013; Fluyau 2018). This might allow greater specificity and granularity in diagnosis, targeting subgroups of our current categories that have been identified with genetic and treatment outcome data. RDoC is a major effort to make progress in this area (National Institute of Mental Health 2022a).

Concepts in Medical Education

Concepts may also be organized to describe the process of knowledge acquisition and how the information learned is used to draw the best conclusions. A framework for categorizing our cognitive processes according to educational objectives has evolved, including its own development of domains: cognitive, psychomotor, and affective (Adams 2015; Anderson et al. 2001, pp. xxi, xxvi).

The cognitive domain, known as Bloom's taxonomy of educational objectives, originally consisted of knowledge, comprehension, application, analysis, synthesis, and evaluation (Table 1–1) (Bloom 1949, 1956). Synthesis involves the emergence of a new result in a specific situation, such as formulating a new and helpful clinical question after identifying information gaps (which will become crucial in our discussion of solving treatment "resistant" cases; see Chapter 5 and Chapter 8, "Reducing Treatment Failure"). An example of evaluation is assessing the quality of published medical research (Adams 2015). Bloom and colleagues later also described the affective domain that includes awareness, attention, and responses according to prioritized and internalized values, influencing empathy and responses to patients (Krathwohl et al. 1956).

Bloom's original cognitive terms were eventually relabeled as verbs, such that the cognitive domain in this effort now consists of six dimensions (or functions): remembering, understanding, applying, analyzing, evaluating, and creating (see Table 1–1) (Anderson et al. 2001, p. 265). Note that the original final two stages have also been reversed to place evaluating before creating (synthesis) (Adams 2015; Anderson et al. 2001, p. 268).

The current version of this taxonomy also describes a new dimension: the four types of knowledge being addressed during clinical assessment

Table 1–1.   Bloom's taxonomy of educational objectives

1956 (nouns)	2001 (verbs)
Knowledge	Remembering
Comprehension	Understanding
Application	Applying
Analysis	Analyzing
Synthesis	Evaluating
Evaluation	Creating

Note.   A framework for categorizing our cognitive processes according to educational objectives was developed by Bloom et al., utilizing nouns (Bloom 1956, pp. 18, 201–207). It was revised to a verb form by Anderson et al. (2001).

of a patient (Figure 1–1): factual (terminology, individual facts), conceptual (categories, theories, principles, models), procedural (technique, process, methodology), and metacognitive (self-assessment, conscious learning skills and techniques) (Adams 2015; Anderson et al. 2001).

Notably, examination of primary and continuing medical education reveals that curricula overfocus on the lower levels of this cognitive taxonomy: 96% of objectives target the two lowest levels, knowledge (remembering) and comprehension (understanding), insufficiently developing the higher thinking skills of critical thinking and evaluative judgments (Adams 2015; Blanco et al. 2014; Légaré et al. 2015). In one study, half of medical students tested relied fully or partially on Type 1 reasoning to solve analytical questions best suited to Type 2 processing (Tay et al. 2016). Forced metacognition is therefore recommended, in which the clinician consciously identifies the system they are using to determine its fit and whether they should change processing type from Type 1 to Type 2, as previously described (Croskerry 2009a; Tay et al. 2016).

Errors in Conceptualization

The mechanisms of thought allow for broad recombination: we can conceive of many different conclusions and solutions rather than recreating the same ones over and over. The trade-off is the limitation on accuracy, however. Because we can frame events in multiple ways, we distort our understanding on the basis of the syntax of the language: we prefer seeking a *gain* to risking a *loss*, for example, even though the odds are objectively the same. We also erroneously extend statistical difference into

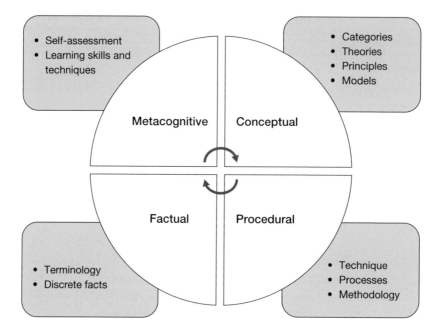

Figure 1–1. Knowledge dimensions used in the clinical assessment of patients.

The four types of knowledge being addressed during clinical assessment of a patient, as described by Adams (2015). The emphasis of this book is metacognitive knowledge.

binary assessments—one choice is clearly better than the other—ignoring shades of gray (Pinker 2007, pp. 85–86).

It may be difficult to extend our understanding of space, time, substance, and causality enough to grasp quantum mechanics because we all prefer teleological explanations in scales we can observe. This extends to the extreme difficulty all humans, even scientists, have in conceptualizing statistics (Weber et al. 2018). We all have a few favorite theories, simple ones that are based on observable scales (e.g., simple mechanics rather than relativity). These pet theories also align with prior known observations, leading to a probability bias.

As we grow more sophisticated with scientific thinking, we often make significant errors in reasoning across scales, not accounting for the emergence of multilevel processes that cannot be explained by lower levels of complexity (such as *mind* from neurons). We turn, instead, to generalized narrative explanations, including teleology: describing phenomena in terms of purpose rather than cause (e.g., attributing an ultimate goal to natural processes, such as that giraffes developed long necks in order to reach food on trees rather than that creatures with long necks reproduced well in an environment where most food was at the top of trees) (Barnes et al. 2017; Chi et al. 2012; Scott et al. 2018).

As we collate and absorb new biomedical information, we incorporate misconceptions along with the correct concepts (Badenhorst et al. 2015). Additionally, the learning of new, correct scientific theories does not simply replace original naive and inaccurate theories. Rather, the new information is deposited alongside the outdated information, the latter of which must be continually repressed for many years in order to recognize the new. The time this suppression requires is even measurable (Foisy et al. 2015; Shtulman and Valcarcel 2012). Further, as discussed earlier, effort-reducing heuristics encoded into our Type 1 processing carry biases that can lead to diagnostic error; more than 40 cognitive and affective biases have been identified that may misdirect clinical reasoning (Croskerry 2008; Croskerry et al. 2008).

Amos Tversky and Daniel Kahneman led the study of heuristics a half century ago (Tversky and Kahneman 1973), although the concept had been identified two decades earlier by Herbert Simon, who characterized *bounded rationality* or *satisficing* as our acceptance of the satisfactory over the optimal (Simon 1956). The *availability* bias describes how we base estimates of the probability of an event on how similar it is to one we can readily recall rather than on statistical factors; for example, seeing a movie about shark attacks will lead us to overestimate the risk the next time we are at the beach. *Anchoring* occurs when we limit our estimates to sparse initial data; for example, we accept a high price for an item if, rather than surveying prices from many stores, we are shown that it is discounted.

Because of the *representativeness* heuristic, we are likely to judge a person or situation by our preconceived mental prototypes: a patient with symptoms similar to those in a difficult-to-treat case will also be expected to be difficult to treat (Croskerry 2009b; Lovett and Anderson 1996). When employing the *base rate* fallacy, all relevant data are not considered in estimating frequency; for example, on seeing one blue car, we overestimate the probability of the next car we see also being that color, unless we take into account that only 20% of all cars are blue. *Functional fixedness* (Pinker 2014a, pp. 70–72) demonstrates our difficulty using an object or concept in more ways than our original use—a failure to "think outside the box" and find novel applications and solutions, such as those necessary for solving so-called treatment resistance.

The *illusion of validity* leads to overconfidence about the predictions and estimates we make about data sets (Einhorn and Hogarth 1978). Because of the *salience bias*, we pay more attention to prominent and emotionally laden information than other data that are possibly more important, such as eating foods that look, smell, and taste better, despite a lack of nutritional value. Using the *ambiguity effect*, we avoid unclear or missing information, such as choosing to view a movie with a mediocre rating over one with no rating or ignoring an article with methods or conclusions we don't understand. With the *framing effect*, choices are influenced by the way information is presented; compare a 20% chance of having a side effect versus an 80% chance of not having the same side effect. With the famous *gambler's fallacy*, we believe, irrationally, that the probability of an event is influenced by its previous occurrence; after flipping a coin heads up five times in a row, we see a higher probability of tails coming up next even though the correct probability is always 50%. And the *bandwagon effect* is particularly germane to our discussion of treatment resistance: we adopt behaviors and beliefs because we observe many others do the same. These are just a few of our inborn heuristics, also known as *fallacies* for their frequent incorrectness (Table 1–2).

Implications for Clinical Practice

We must never forget that all concepts do not exist beyond abstract ideas in our heads—we must never think a concept is concrete or tangible (the mistake of reification) (De Carlo 2018). This leads us to the realization that although our brains contain structures for gathering and packaging information into memories and concepts, the nature of this structure allows not only for myriad conclusions but for many errors of assessment. Concepts will be generated that cannot be supported empirically with observation or experience. The implications for the practice of psychiatry range from diagnosis to treatment planning. We see this as we struggle every few years to reconcile our diagnostic categories with clinical observations and outcome studies.

Diagnostic errors occur in all specialties at an estimated rate of 10%–15% (Berner and Graber 2008; Elstein 1995, pp. 49–59); three-quarters of these errors are cognitive in nature (Graber 2013; Graber et al. 2005). We also know from studies of second opinions in psychiatry that the original diagnosis may be overturned 33%–50% of the time (Nirodi et al. 2003; Wallace and Rayner 2015). Overall error rates in diagnosing severe psychiatric illness have been measured in some specialized tertiary care

Table 1–2. Examples of heuristic bias

Bias	Result	References
Availability	Probability estimate distorted by recall of recent events	Tversky and Kahneman 1973, 1974
Anchoring	Estimate skewed by sparse initial data	Furnham and Boo 2011; Tversky and Kahneman 1974
Representativeness	Judgment skewed by preconceived mental prototypes	Croskerry 2009b; Lovett and Anderson 1996
Base rate	Probability estimate distorted by small samples	Bar-Hillel 1980
Functional fixedness	Limited application of object or concept outside original use	Pinker 2014a, pp. 70–72
Illusion of validity	Overconfidence about predictions and estimates formed from data	Einhorn and Hogarth 1978
Salience	More attention given to prominent and emotionally laden information	Bordalo et al. 2022
Ambiguity	Avoidance of missing or unclear data	Heath and Tversky 1991
Framing effect	Choice influenced by how information was presented	Gong et al. 2013; Tversky and Kahneman 1981
Gambler's fallacy	Estimate of probability distorted by previous occurrences	Roney and Trick 2003
Bandwagon	Beliefs or behaviors adopted because many others have adopted them	Blumenthal-Barby 2016; Cohen and Rothschild 1979

Note. This is a partial list of effort-reducing heuristics, encoded into our Type 1 processing, that carry biases that can misdirect our clinical reasoning, based on the work of Simon (1956).

facilities at greater than 39%: 75% in patients with schizoaffective disorder, 54.72% in major depressive disorder, 23.71% in schizophrenia, and 17.78% in bipolar disorder (Ayano et al. 2021). The problem is even worse in primary care, where misdiagnosis rates have been observed at 65.9% for major depressive disorder, 92.7% for bipolar disorder, 85.8% for panic disorder, 71.0% for generalized anxiety disorder, and 97.8% for social anxiety disorder (Vermani et al. 2011).

The fact that so many cases are labeled treatment resistant when valid therapeutic options remain gives us the opportunity and mandate to examine factors complicating and misdirecting diagnosis. Even the high rate of misdiagnosis is not as egregious as proceeding to relabel the original diagnosis *treatment resistant* when 66% of cases referred for second opinion find ready therapeutic alternatives (Nirodi et al. 2003). This is a prime example of reification—believing that our concept of treatment resistance matches a concrete reality.

As we see from Type 1 processing errors, concepts generated by some people, especially those in authority, influence the conclusions of others. As more and more practitioners make a Type 1 error, the problem expands as the influence is disseminated, and soon a large portion of our field is comfortable with a concept that does not match observed outcomes, as with treatment resistance.

The concept of treatment resistance in clinical practice implies treatment failure in a single patient who originally carried a diagnosis expected to respond to or remit with standard treatment. Recall that by response, we mean a partial reduction in symptoms as measured by peer-reviewed clinical scales (Marshall et al. 2000), although there is still no fully agreed-on threshold (see section "Inconsistent Criteria" in Chapter 4, "The Myth of Treatment Resistance?"). By remission, we mean complete symptom resolution, with full functioning restored. There will be patients who have what may be termed a partial response, with some improvement, yet do not meet the criteria for response and require additional treatment (Nierenberg and DeCecco 2001).

The many conceptions and definitions of treatment failure include the National Institute of Mental Health contract study Sequenced Treatment Alternatives to Relieve Depression (STAR*D; National Institute of Mental Health 2022b), which used failure to achieve remission as the definition for treatment failure. This seems a reasonable definition when we consider that our hopes, and those of our patients, are for a return to full recovery. Despite significant improvement, we are leaving patients with residual symptoms and functional deficits.

The conceptual error we make is confusing treatment *failure* with treatment *resistance*. Failure implies many possible causes: poor assessment, poor judgment, poor treatment planning, poor compliance, treatments of poor quality, and so on. Failure can be a result of the practitioner, the patient, an intermediary, or the situation. Resistance, however, refers only to the diagnosis. Rather than continuing to search for the cause of failure, embracing the concept of resistance directs us to rediagnose a syndrome that should be treatable to remission, replacing it with a diagnosis that implies it cannot be treated to the point of full recovery.

The faulty logic in these steps involves heuristics as well as other Type 1 errors. Because of the representativeness heuristic, our preconceived mental prototypes direct any observation of residual symptoms toward a judgment of treatment resistance. Because of the base rate fallacy, observing one case labeled treatment resistant may lead us to overestimate the true rate of treatment failure, accepting treatment resistance as a final assessment rather than searching for alternative explanations or solutions. Because of the availability bias, the more we see the term *treatment resistant* in the literature and poster sessions and hear it in lectures and clinical discussions, the more we overestimate the probability that such a problem will occur. Plus, once treatment resistance is accepted as a concept, our functional fixedness makes it hard to let go and revise it to find new definitions of and solutions for treatment failure.

With treatment resistance, we have created a meme in the original, evolutionary sense—a system of behavior that is passed from person to person by imitation (Dawkins 1976). In this case, it is a chimera of no clinical utility that does not communicate consistent and useful information to other providers, does not clarify the nature of the failure, is too vague and nonspecific to predict prognosis, and certainly offers no direction for treatment. One has to question the wisdom and utility of this pseudo rediagnosis (see Chapter 4). A diagnosis should contain specific information, and treatment resistance contains essentially none.

Even long clinical experience, without reflection or feedback, can reinforce conceptual error and lower clinical performance (Tay et al. 2016). Employing metacognition, then, lets us consciously examine how Type 1 errors have led us to the misconception of treatment resistance and choose Type 2 processing to reconceptualize, not on the basis of the crowd and recent professional fashion but on the basis of logic and science, as we tirelessly search for clues and methods to reverse the many possible causes of failure in the treatments of our patients.

Summary

Our brains have a predetermined conceptual structure that is illustrated through linguistics. Dual process theory describes two systems of thought processing. Type 1 is pattern matching: rapid, but prone to error through context, influence, and inborn heuristics designed to preserve processing effort. Type 2 is slow; uses science and logic in complex, rational analysis; and is usually error-free if the data relied on are correct. Chunking theory describes the development of expertise through the linking of frequently associated elements in memory, naturally or consciously. Experts also make use of templates, frequently used chunks with fixed and variable information.

Concepts may be organized into domains, dimensions (constructs), or categories to accomplish different intellectual tasks. Psychiatric diagnosis uses categories, but in the future it may evolve to incorporate dimensions (or functions) for greater discrimination. Medical education focuses mostly on remembering and understanding rather than critical thinking, evaluation, and the creation of new questions to address information gaps. Forced metacognition (thinking about how we think) is encouraged to assess processing and help with choosing the better method.

Practitioners must remember that concepts are abstract ideas and are never tangible. Errors in cognition are common for multiple reasons, including syntax, heuristics, multiscale processes, and teleology; incorrect concepts must continue to be suppressed even after correction. Diagnostic error in psychiatry occurs in at least a third of cases; in two-thirds of cases labeled treatment resistant, therapeutic options are still available. Treatment failure must not be routinely relabeled as treatment resistance.

Key Points

- Our brains form concepts from experience and information through two methods.
- Type 1 processing is fast but often inaccurate.
- Type 2 processing is slow, rational, and preferred.
- Consciously assess your processing to choose the best method for the task, reducing error.
- Concepts exist only in our heads, not matching concrete reality until science confirms them.
- Strive for levels of critical thinking beyond remembering and understanding.
- Evaluate your data and create new clinical questions to address missing information.
- Never equate treatment failure with treatment resistance.
- Never stop searching for the causes of treatment failures.

Self-Assessment Questions

1.   Which of the following statements is illustrated by linguistics?

   A. Our minds contain a predetermined conceptual structure.
   B. The mind is a blank slate.
   C. The mind contain links from mental representations to linguistic expressions.
   D. A and C

   Correct answer: D. A and C.

   These two statements are elements of the structural hypothesis theory.

2.   Which of the following is true about chunking?

   A. It expands short-term memory and processing power.
   B. It can be goal-directed.
   C. It can be perceptual.
   D. All of the above.

   Correct answer: D. All of the above.

   Chunking collates data gleaned from the environment into one entity with strong association among its elements and, along with templates, is a mechanism for developing expertise. It can be automatic (perceptual) or conscious (goal-directed).

3.   Which of the following statements about heuristics is correct?

   A. Heuristics are part of Type 2 processing.
   B. Heuristics provide accurate statistical estimates.
   C. Heuristics are innate "rules of thumb" that guide our judgment.
   D. Heuristics seldom lead to errors in cognition.

   Correct answer: C. Heuristics are innate "rules of thumb" that guide our judgment.

   Heuristics are innate estimates encoded in Type 1 processing that accelerate the pace of decision-making. However, they may be responsible for many errors in conceptualization because they are not statistically sound.

4.   Which of the following statements about dual process theory is *false*?

A. Type 1 processing is faster than Type 2.
B. Type 2 processing is less likely to be accurate.
C. Metacognition can allow us to choose our method of processing.
D. Type 1 processing is very influenced by context.

Correct answer: B. Type 2 processing is less likely to be accurate.

Type 2 processing relies on logic and science for complex rational analysis and is more trusted, as long as the data used are correct. The two types may complement each other if they are chosen appropriately for the situation.

5.   Which of the following is true of concepts?

A. They are tangible.
B. They are free from influence.
C. They are abstract.
D. They are valid across scales

Correct answer: C. They are abstract.

Concepts are abstract ideas in our heads, never concrete or tangible. Those formed from Type 1 processing are often influenced by context and the assessments of experts. We often make errors of judgment conceptualizing across scales, not taking emergent properties into account.

Discussion Topics

1. Identify cases in which you were influenced by the assessments of others, especially those considered experts. Employing metacognition, assess your processing of the data and evaluate your choices and accuracy. Discuss opportunities to reduce conceptual errors in your practice.

2. Consider ways in which you can improve your clinical skills by moving beyond remembering and understanding and on to analyzing, creating, and evaluating. Discuss how you can better evaluate treatment failure by identifying information gaps, then formulating new clinical questions to answer.

Additional Readings

Azarian B: The Mind Is More Than a Machine. Los Angeles, CA, Noema Magazine, June 9, 2022. Available at: www.noemamag.com/the-mind-is-more-than-a-machine. Accessed June 13, 2022. *Current theories of how mind and consciousness may emerge from neuronal activity*

Bassett DS, Gazzaniga MS: Understanding complexity in the human brain. Trends Cogn Science 15(5):200–209, 2011: *A refreshingly accessible synthesis of the structure, function, and multilevel processes of our brains, using complex network theory*

Jackendoff R: Patterns in the Mind: Language and Human Nature. New York, Harvester Wheatsheaf, 1993: *A seminal argument for innate conceptual structure*

Kahneman D: Thinking Fast and Slow. New York, Farrar, Straus and Giroux, 2011: *Heuristics discussed by the master himself*

Lewis M: The Undoing Project: A Friendship That Changed Our Minds. New York, WW Norton, 2016: *An engaging historical account of Amos Tversky and Daniel Kahneman and their research into heuristics*

Pinker S: The Stuff of Thought: Language as a Window Into Human Nature. New York, Viking, 2007: *An explication of how language can demonstrate the innate cognitive structuring of our brains*

Putman HP: Rational Psychopharmacology: A Book of Clinical Skills, Washington, DC, American Psychiatric Association Publishing, 2020: *History of rational thought (Chapter 1), critical assessment of data (Chapter 2), rational treatment planning (Chapter 4), and abductive reasoning in medical practice and how errors are generated by extrapolating across scales (Chapter 5)*

References

Adams NE: Bloom's taxonomy of cognitive learning objectives. J Med Libr Assoc 103(3):152–153, 2015 26213509

American Psychiatric Association: Diagnosis and Statistical Manual of Mental Disorders, 3rd Edition. Washington, DC, American Psychiatric Association, 1980

American Psychiatric Association: Diagnosis and Statistical Manual of Mental Disorders, 4th Edition. Washington, DC, American Psychiatric Association, 1994

American Psychiatric Association: Diagnosis and Statistical Manual of Mental Disorders, 5th Edition. Washington, DC, American Psychiatric Association, 2013

American Psychiatric Association: Diagnosis and Statistical Manual of Mental Disorders, 5th Edition, Text Revision. Washington, DC, American Psychiatric Association, 2022

American Psychological Association: Dictionary of Psychology. Washington, DC, American Psychological Association, 2022. Available at: https://dictionary.apa.org/domains. Accessed June 9, 2022.

Anderson LW, Krathwohl DR, Airasian PW, et al (eds): A Taxonomy for Learning, Teaching and Assessing: A Revision of Bloom's Taxonomy of Educational Objectives, Abridged Edition. New York, Longman, 2001

Ayano G, Demelash S, Yohannes Z, et al: Misdiagnosis, detection rate, and associated factors of severe psychiatric disorders in specialized psychiatry centers in Ethiopia. Ann Gen Psychiatry 20(1):10, 2021 33531016

Badenhorst E, Mamede S, Hartman N, Schmidt HG: Exploring lecturers' views of first-year health science students' misconceptions in biomedical domains. Adv Health Sci Educ Theory Pract 20(2):403–420, 2015 25099944

Bar-Hillel M: The base-rate fallacy in probability judgments. Acta Psychol 44(3):211–233, 1980

Barnes ME, Evans EM, Hazel A, et al: Teleological reasoning, not acceptance of evolution, impacts students' ability to learn natural selection. Evolution (NY) 10:1–12, 2017

Berner E, Graber M: Overconfidence as a cause of diagnostic error in medicine. Am J Med 121(Suppl 5):S2–S23, 200818440350

Blanco MA, Capello CF, Dorsch JL, et al: A survey study of evidence-based medicine training in US and Canadian medical schools. J Med Libr Assoc 102(3):160–168, 2014 25031556

Bloom BS: A taxonomy of educational objectives. Paper presented at the Meeting of Examiners, Monticello, IL, November 27, 1949

Bloom BS (ed): Taxonomy of Educational Objectives: Handbook I: Cognitive Domain. New York, David McKay, 1956

Blumenthal-Barby JS: Biases and heuristics in decision making and their impact on autonomy. Am J Bioeth 16(5):5–15, 2016 27111357

Bordalo P, Gennaioli N, Shleifer A: Salience. Annual Review of Economics 14:521–544, 2022

Campitelli G, Gobet F, Head K, et al: Brain localization of memory chunks in chessplayers. Int J Neurosci 117(12):1641–1659, 2007 17987468

Casey BJ, Craddock N, Cuthbert BN, et al: DSM-5 and RDoC: progress in psychiatry research? Nat Rev Neurosci 14(11):810–814, 2013 24135697

Chase WG, Simon HA: Perception in chess. Cogn Psychol 4:55–81, 1973

Chi MT, Roscoe RD, Slotta JD, et al: Misconceived causal explanations for emergent processes. Cogn Sci 36(1):1–61, 2012 22050726

Cohen L, Rothschild H: The bandwagons of medicine. Perspect Biol Med 22(4):531–538, 1979 226929

Croskerry P: Cognitive and affective dispositions to respond, in Patient Safety in Emergency Medicine. Edited by Croskerry P, Cosby K, Schenkel S, et al. Philadelphia, PA, Lippincott, Williams and Wilkins, 2008, pp 219–227

Croskerry P: Clinical cognition and diagnostic error: applications of a dual process model of reasoning. Adv Health Sci Educ Theory Pract 14(Suppl 1):27–35, 2009a 19669918

Croskerry P: Context is everything, or: how could I have been that stupid? Healthc Q 12:167–173, 2009b 19667765

Croskerry P, Abbass AA, Wu AW: How doctors feel: affective issues in patients' safety. Lancet 372(9645):1205–1206, 2008 19094942

Dawkins R: The Selfish Gene. New York, Oxford University Press, 1976

De Carlo M: Conceptualization, in Scientific Inquiry in Social Work. Pressbooks, 2018, Updated March 2019. Available at https://scientificinquiryinsocialwork. pressbooks.com/chapter/9-2-conceptualization. Accessed June 8, 2022.

De Groot AD: Thought and Choice in Chess. The Hague, Netherlands, Mouton, 1946/1978

Einhorn HJ, Hogarth RM: Confidence in judgment: persistence of the illusion of validity. Psychol Rev 85(5):395–416, 1978

Evans J: Heuristic and analytic processes in reasoning. Br J Psychol 75:451–468, 1984

Elstein A: Clinical reasoning in medicine, in Clinical Reasoning in the Health Professions. Edited by Higgs J. Oxford, UK, Butterworth-Heinemann, 1995, pp 223–234

Fluyau D: Integrating DSM/ICD, research domain criteria, and descriptive psychopathology in teaching and practice of psychiatry. Front Psychiatry 9:484, 2018 30344498

Foisy LB, Potvin P, Riopel M, et al: Is inhibition involved in overcoming a common physics misconception in mechanics? Trends Neurosci Educ 4(1–2):26–36, 2015

Furnham A, Boo HC: A literature review of the anchoring effect. J Socio Econ 40(1):35–42, 2011

Gilbert AC, Boucher VJ, Jemel B: Perceptual chunking and its effect on memory in speech processing: ERP and behavioral evidence. Front Psychol 5:220, 2014 24678304

Gobet F, Lane PCR: Chunking mechanisms and learning, in Encyclopedia of the Sciences of Learning. Edited by Seel NM. New York, Springer, 2012, pp 544–541

Gobet F, Simon HA: Templates in chess memory: a mechanism for recalling several boards. Cognit Psychol 31(1):1–40, 1996 8812020

Gong J, Zhang Y, Yang Z, et al: The framing effect in medical decision-making: a review of the literature. Psychol Health Med 18(6):645–653, 2013 23387993

Graber ML: The incidence of diagnostic error in medicine. BMJ Qual Saf 22(Suppl 2):ii21–ii27, 2013 23771902

Graber ML, Franklin N, Gordon R: Diagnostic error in internal medicine. Arch Intern Med 165(13):1493–1499, 2005 16009864

Guida A, Gobet F, Tardieu H, Nicolas S: How chunks, long-term working memory and templates offer a cognitive explanation for neuroimaging data on expertise acquisition: a two-stage framework. Brain Cogn 79(3):221–244, 2012 22546731

Heath C, Tversky A: Preference and belief: ambiguity and competence in choice under uncertainty. J Risk Uncertain 4(1):5–28, 1991

Jackendoff R: Semantics and Cognition (Current Studies in Linguistics, Vol 8). Cambridge, MA, MIT Press, 1983, pp 17–19

Jackendoff R: Consciousness and the Computational Mind (Explorations in Cognitive Science Series). Cambridge, MA, MIT Press, 1987

Krathwohl DR, Bloom BS, Masia BB: Taxonomy of Educational Objectives, Handbook II: Affective Domain. New York, David McKay, 1956

Légaré F, Freitas A, Thompson-Leduc P, et al: The majority of accredited continuing professional development activities do not target clinical behavior change. Acad Med 90(2):197–202, 2015 25354076

Lovett MC, Anderson JR: History of success and current context in problem solving: combined influences on operator selection. Cogn Psychol 31(2):168–217, 1996

Lumen. The five psychological domains. Lumen Learning, 2022. Available at: https://courses.lumenlearning.com/waymaker-psychology/chapter/psychological-perspectives. Accessed June 9, 2022.

Marshall M, Lockwood A, Bradley C, et al: Unpublished rating scales: a major source of bias in randomised controlled trials of treatments for schizophrenia. Br J Psychiatry 176:249–252, 2000 10755072

Mathy F, Feldman J: What's magic about magic numbers? Chunking and data compression in short-term memory. Cognition 122(3):346–362, 2012 22176752

Miller GA: The magical number seven plus or minus two: some limits on our capacity for processing information. Psychol Rev 63(2):81–97, 1956 13310704

Murphy G: Categories and concepts, in Psychology. Edited by Biswas-Diener R, Diener E. Champaign, IL, Diener Education Fund Publishing, 2022. Available at: http://noba.to/6vu4cpkt. Accessed June 9, 2022.

National Institute of Mental Health: Research Domain Criteria (RDoC). Bethesda, MD, National Institute of Mental Health, 2022a. Available at www.nimh.nih.gov/research/research-funded-by-nimh/rdoc. Accessed May 25, 2022.

National Institute of Mental Health: Sequenced Treatment Alternatives to Relieve Depression (STAR*D) Study. Bethesda, MD, National Institute of Mental

Health, 2022b. Available at www.nimh.nih.gov/funding/clinical-research/practical/stard. Accessed June 14, 2022.

Nierenberg AA, DeCecco LM: Definitions of antidepressant treatment response, remission, nonresponse, partial response, and other relevant outcomes: a focus on treatment-resistant depression. J Clin Psychiatry 62(Suppl 16):5–9, 2001 11480882

Nirodi P, Mitchell AJ, Mindham RHS: Survey of expert second opinions in a tertiary psychiatric out-patient clinic in the Yorkshire region between 1988 and 2000. Psychiatr Bull 27:416–420, 2003

Pinker S: The Blank Slate: The Modern Denial of Human Nature. New York, Viking, 2002

Pinker S: The Stuff of Thought: Language as a Window Into Human Nature. New York, Penguin, 2007

Pinker S: Language as a window into conceptual structure [video]. Presentation at the Shalem Center's Psycho-ontology Conference, December 2011. Available at: www.youtube.com/watch?v=d02BbdFZJrs. Accessed June 7, 2022.

Pinker S: The Sense of Style: The Thinking Person's Guide to Writing in the 21st Century. New York, Viking, 2014a

Pinker S: Why academics stink at writing. Chron High Educ 61(5):1–23, 2014b

Roney CJR, Trick LM: Grouping and gambling: a Gestalt approach to understanding the gambler's fallacy. Can J Exp Psychol 57(2):69–75, 2003 12822837

Sam N: Conceptualization. Psychology Dictionary, April 7, 2013. Available at: https://psychologydictionary.org/conceptualization. Accessed June 8, 2022.

Scott EE, Anderson CW, Mashood KK, et al: Developing an analytical framework to characterize student reasoning about complex processes. CBE Life Sci Educ 17(3):ar49, 2018 30183566

Shtulman A, Valcarcel J: Scientific knowledge suppresses but does not supplant earlier intuitions. Cognition 124(2):209–215, 2012 22595144

Simon HA: Rational choice and the structure of the environment. Psychol Rev 63(2):129–138, 1956 13310708

Tay SW, Ryan P, Ryan CA: Systems 1 and 2 thinking processes and cognitive reflection testing in medical students. Can Med Educ J 7(2):e97–e103, 2016 28344696

Tversky A, Kahneman D: Availability: a heuristic for judging frequency and probability. Cogn Psychol 5(2):207–232, 1973

Tversky A, Kahneman D: Judgment under uncertainty: heuristics and biases. Science 185(4157):1124–1131, 1974 17835457

Tversky A, Kahneman D: The framing of decisions and the psychology of choice. Science 211(4481):453–458, 1981 7455683

Vermani M, Marcus M, Katzman MA: Rates of detection of mood and anxiety disorders in primary care: a descriptive, cross-sectional study. Prim Car Companion CNS Disord 13(2):PCC.10m01013, 2011 21977354

Wallace D, Rayner S: A military second opinion mental health clinic. J Mil Veterans Health 23(3):12–17, 2015

Wason PC, Evans J: Dual processes in reasoning? Cognition 3(2):141–154, 1974

Weber P, Binder K, Krauss S: Why can only 24% solve Bayesian reasoning problems in natural frequencies: frequency phobia in spite of probability blindness. Front Psychol 9:1833, 2018 30369891

Zwarts J, Verkuyl HJ: An algebra of conceptual structure; an investigation into Jackendoff's conceptual semantics. Linguist Philos 17(1):1–28, 1994

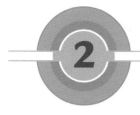

Keys to Problem-Solving

Now that we understand more about how concepts are formed, consciously and unconsciously, correctly and incorrectly, let's consider how we can best use these concepts to help our patients solve more of the problems they bring to us, rather than labeling too many of them treatment resistant. This requires examination of the nature of problems, the mechanisms of expertise, common errors in problem-solving, and the best practices for achieving clinical solutions and avoiding treatment failure.

General Nature of Problems

As clinicians, our goal is to provide solutions to patients who present us with problematic situations. When seeking valid parameters to describe this task, consider a problem to be the relation between human will and reality: when these do not coincide, the resolution of the gap between them is the solution of the problem. Problems imply a desired outcome coupled with an apparent deficiency or inconsistency preventing its realization—a puzzling circumstance that has to be resolved (see www.definitions.net/definition/Problem) and contains the embedded concept of solvability (Agre 1982; Borasi 1986). By these definitions, treatment failure is a problem with a discoverable solution, and treatment resistance is not. To become better problem-solvers, we need to be exposed to many different problems, as well as a variety of conceptions about them. Problems with different structural characteristics may carry different expectations of possible solutions, requiring different skills and strategies (Borasi 1986).

In medicine, clinicians clarify and recognize (formulate) problems as diagnoses, seeking to supply appropriately matched therapy, be it treatment, reassurance, or palliation. Many decisions must be made about the collection, validity, and interpretation of data. These data are compared with our expectations, which may be inaccurate, indiscriminant, or incomplete (Connelly and Johnson 1980). Once described as using hypothetico-deductive reasoning, the practice of modern medicine and psychiatry is now seen more broadly to employ abductive reasoning—forming hypotheses, testing them, reformulating a new hypothesis based on fresh data, then repeating this process (Connelly and Johnson 1980; Fann 1970; Upmeier zu Belzen et al. 2021); see section "Defining Evidence" in Chapter 3, "The Goal of Evidence-Based Practice." However, because of human adaptability to different problem contexts and structures, we are likely to employ a range of reasoning strategies to solve problems, particularly in medicine, given its complexity and dense knowledge base (Patel et al. 2005, pp. 727–750).

We must remember that problem-solving skill is the value we practitioners offer to patients, not just our proficiency at remembering facts. Treatment failure resulting in the relabeling of a diagnosis as treatment resistant actually represents a failure of problem-solving, which should be as unsatisfying to most clinicians as it is to our patients. Learning and improving clinical problem-solving skills represents a challenge for practitioners, in both primary and continuing medical education (Barrows and Tamblyn 1980), but it leads to greater professional satisfaction and better outcomes for our patients.

Expertise

Our goal is always to become expert practitioners and to retain and improve our expertise. The cognitive processes of expert problem-solving have been described across professional fields, including psychiatry and psychotherapy. The theory of *knowledge restructuring through case processing* suggests that, even early in training, professionals approach and recognize cases as formulations of highly specific situations, expressing their previous experience and the requirements of professional activity. Examples include a case of schizophrenia, a case of alcohol withdrawal, a case of sexual abuse, and a case of depression. Expertise develops as practitioners generalize across increasingly complex cases, learning from both expected and novel outcomes (Boshuizen et al. 2020; Hoffman 1998; Shanteau and Phelps 1977).

This advancement in problem-solving involves the restructuring of knowledge into *macro concepts* and *scripts* (or, in our case, *illness scripts*). Experts remember cases as these scripts: knowledge structures linking conditions for a disease (e.g., age, lifestyle, individual and family history) to the consequences of a disease (symptoms, prognosis). Biomedical knowledge is increasingly integrated with clinical case processing into a macro concept—not forgotten, but not consciously accessed unless used as a fallback tool with more difficult problems (Boshuizen et al. 2020).

This encapsulation of knowledge is an example of the chunking and template development discussed in Chapter 1, "Conceptualization (and Failed Concepts)" (see section "Chunking Theory and Expertise"). Curiously, whereas in chess there is a linear relationship between case recall (i.e., chunks) and expertise, in medicine the relationship appears to be curvilinear: there is an increase in case recall performance for the first 6 years of training, followed by a decrease with further experience as knowledge is restructured into macro concepts (i.e., templates, schema, diagnoses) and scripts are refined. Experts use more complex and restructured case formulations, based on more complete concepts, than do novices (Arkes and Harkness 1980; Boshuizen et al. 2020; Schmidt and Boshuizen 1992). Differences in diagnostic accuracy and reasoning have been measured between experts and novices in psychiatry (Gabriel and Violato 2013; Patel et al. 2005).

Obstacles to Problem-Solving

Despite this advanced cognitive restructuring, and often because of it, practitioners at all levels of expertise make errors in problem-solving (Frensch and Sternberg 1989, 2014). Conceptualization is inadequate when not fully developed, as with novices. Flawed chunks, containing poor solutions, repeatedly lead to poor outcomes (Campitelli and Speelman 2014). Even when honed with experience and restructured, as by experts, important information is still likely to be ignored if it is unexpected or atypical; experts do not appear to weigh multidimensional information similarly (Einhorn 1974) and are prone to subjective errors such as lack of attention or sensitivity to rare facts (see section "Implications for Medical Practice" below).

As with conceptualization, our structures for solving problems allow errors. Type 1 processing (see section "Theories of Concept Formation" in Chapter 1) makes us unconsciously susceptible to *groupthink* as we conform to the opinions and solutions of authorities and peers, especially in difficult cases, following failures, and when time pressured (Janis 1972; 't Hart 1991). The Einstellung effect, applied to psychology, describes the *long-term mental set*, often defined as expertise in a field (or domain), in which knowledge may lead to confirmation bias through un-necessary constraints on creative thinking (Lovett and Anderson 1996; Öllinger et al. 2008; Wiley 1998). Because of this, our brains tend to stay with the most familiar solution and steadfastly ignore alternatives, as with the functional fixedness heuristic discussed in Chapter 1, section "Implications for Clinical Practice" (Ellis and Reingold 2014; Huang et al. 2018; Ricks et al. 2007; Schultz and Searleman 2002; Wiley 1998). Proto-typical information (that which matches with existing chunks) is pro-cessed faster than atypical and incompatible information by both medical students and full-time practitioners (Gagnon et al. 2006). This inflexibil-ity of thought induced by prior knowledge and similar problem situations adds bias to our assessments (Bilalić et al. 2008; Lovett and Anderson 1996), as does the representativeness heuristic (see section "Implications for Clinical Practice" in Chapter 1).

The contraction in focus is only strengthened by repetition. Expertise over time, without sufficient feedback, narrows and becomes routine (Huang et al. 2018; Ohlsson 1992; Öllinger et al. 2008). A long tenure of practice without reflection can result in reinforced conceptual error, poor problem-solving, and disappointing clinical outcomes(Tay et al. 2016); see section "Ways to Receive and Give Feedback in Practice" in this chapter and section "Implications for Clinical Practice" in Chapter 1. Further, we progressively underestimate our mistakes, reducing the opportunity for useful feedback—the same illusion of validity mentioned in Chapter 1, "Errors in Conceptualization" (Einhorn and Hogarth 1978; Hetmański 2020; Ryback 1967). Overall, the quality of a practitioner's performance depends on the amount of time spent practicing relevant skills, as well as the quality of that practice (Guest et al. 2001).

Best Practices for Problem-Solving

Practitioners are unlikely to be aware of errors in their problem-solving until treatment failure is evident. However, the use of ongoing feedback, called *real-world problem-solving,* can alert the clinician to reversible er-rors more quickly; continuous interaction between the solver and the en-vironment reduces the chance of failure (Sarathy 2018). This process begins with representing the problem in short-term working memory (with activation of the prefrontal cortex, default mode network, and dor-sal anterior cingulate). Then a search for solutions begins, with analytical problem-solving: heuristic searches, hill climbing, and progress moni-toring (Öllinger et al. 2014, 2017; Sarathy 2018). Treatment resistance may be one heuristic prototype that resonates with the practitioner, especially in our current clinical environment (see section "Errors in Conceptualization" in Chapter 1).

During these initial phases, attention is directed inwardly to free up processing effort. Although this practice is associated with creativity and may enhance problem-solving (Salvi and Bowden 2016; Sarathy 2018), this also is when atypical and inconsistent data may be ignored (see section "Implications for Medical Practice" below). This is why feedback (real-world interaction) must be available to alert the practitioner early in problem-solving that an impasse has been reached—that is, that the routine solution to the problem is not successful because the solution is not reachable from the initial problem representation (Ohlsson 1992). Carrying it to further conclusion is neither helpful nor necessary.

According to Bellman's principle of optimality, just breaking problems into subproblems and solving each does not always lead to the optimal solution of the original problem (Egidi 2006). What does work is breaking familiar *patterns* into components to be regrouped into newly meaningful configurations (Huang et al. 2018; Knoblich et al. 1999). Once an impasse is detected and consciously acknowledged, the anterior cingulate cortex switches from analytic planning to creative search and discovery. The problem representation must then be restructured by elaboration (detecting new features of the problem), reencoding (repairing mistaken or incomplete representations of problems), relaxing constraints (from narrowing), and decomposing existing chunks (Öllinger et al. 2014; Sarathy 2018). Because chunks may introduce inaccurate restraints on thinking creatively in problem-solving, their deconstruction at an impasse is essential for success (Knoblich et al. 1999, 2001; Sarathy 2018).

This reduction of routine patterns can be into elements that each has a separate meaning (loose decomposition) and into components with no meaning as separate elements (tight decomposition) (Huang et al. 2018). The tighter decomposition (of atypical, seemingly irrelevant data) is more difficult but, when reorganized, may lead to more creative insights and solutions (Huang et al. 2018; Knoblich et al. 1999). This opportunity to reform associations, leading to novel solutions, requires conscious effort through metacognition (our awareness of the necessity). Top-down cognitive control must be initiated, and previous representations of the problem must be inhibited. Therefore, there must be conscious awareness of this change in context (Tang et al. 2016).

During this reconstruction, we revert back from a focused mode to a defocused one, in which we consider new associations (Sowden et al.

2015). Once we are again defocused, previously unnoticed partial clues in the environment link to long-term memories in the medial temporal lobe (Yoruk and Runco 2014), and we consider subcues such as atypical symptoms and mild expressions of feeling (Zabelina et al. 2016); see section "Implications for Medical Practice" below. Context and applications may be shifted as we reflect on these new memories. Heuristic prototyping may then be retriggered in the dorsolateral prefrontal cortex.

Hopefully, regular feedback will lead to the resolution of problem-solving errors as they occur. However, should the problem still reach the point where a practitioner is poised to relabel a condition as treatment resistant, the provider should always be alerted to the fact that what has actually developed is an impasse in problem-solving. Relabeling as treatment resistant should be delayed while these additional steps in solving the problem are implemented. At this point, the clinician is unaware of their error(s) but should now be aware that their initial solution is incorrect, rather than thinking that they have uncovered a chimera. To recognize an impasse, of course, goal completion must be very clear from the outset of problem-solving.

Implications for Medical Practice

The errors physicians most commonly make in problem-solving come from a propensity for making rapid assessments and conclusions based on our previous experience. We make quick diagnoses and then search for supporting evidence while missing, or considering irrelevant, important data for making a correct initial diagnosis (Huang et al. 2018). We can be misled by information as we struggle to define what is irrelevant and what is not (Einhorn 1974; Scordo 2014). The act of forming a diagnosis results in our later differential recognition of symptoms, including false ones. We do not encode (i.e., remember in long-term memory or long-term working memory) a patient's original symptoms but rather encode our diagnosis (prototype, schema, template, or macro concept) (Arkes and Harkness 1980; Zoudji et al. 2010). Unstructured, random case information not supporting that diagnosis is poorly remembered (Boshuizen et al. 2020). Once we make a diagnosis, we recognize new symptoms that appear (or we become aware of them) by their proximity to this prototype, so even important ones may not be recognized at all.

Further, as has been demonstrated under experimental conditions, once a diagnosis is made, we "remember" newly disclosed symptoms that relate to it as being part of the original presentation, even though they had not actually been mentioned before. New symptoms unrelated to our diagnosis are more confidently rejected, however, because they do not match the schema—both a loss and a gain in accuracy (Arkes and Harkness 1980; Borasi 1986). Distortions due to this false recognition (or inferential reconstruction) may increase over longer intervals (Spiro 1977; Sulin and Dooling 1974). Therefore, when inconsistent symptoms appear in an initial presentation, clinicians who proceed to make a diagnosis perform more poorly than do those who delay diagnosis (Arkes and Harkness 1980). All diagnoses (chunks, templates, or schema) may introduce inaccurate restraints on creative thinking during problem-solving, as discussed earlier (see section "Obstacles to Problem-Solving"). Although it eventually takes less time to problem-solve with reinforced solutions (ones repeatedly employed without contradiction), it also becomes increasingly difficult to seek alternative solutions when outcomes disappoint (Neroni et al. 2017).

Gather data on your conclusions. Expect, don't underestimate, errors in your solutions—actively search for them. Treatment failure, reaching the impasse, tells you errors are there, even when early feedback does not. Practitioners who have achieved a level of expertise midway through their practice do not automatically continue to enhance or even maintain their clinical skills through the routine treatment of patients. What is required is seeing a large number of patients with similar symptoms and receiving feedback so that one can develop methods for distinguishing among diagnoses requiring different treatments. As specialists, we are more likely to see patients with similar symptoms but must receive and consider feedback to improve our diagnoses and treatment recommendations (Ericsson 2004).

Ways to Receive and Give Feedback in Practice

We must always, then, be seeking information about the quality and effectiveness of our individual skills. Feedback to practitioners from various outcome measurements has been demonstrated to improve clinical outcomes, especially in cases that are not proceeding as planned (Carlier et al. 2012; Gondek et al. 2016; Knaup et al. 2009; Lambert et al. 2003). Surgeons and internists once regularly reviewed autopsy reports to obtain feedback and improve their skills, although the rate of autopsies in the United States has fallen significantly over the last half-century (Allen 2011; Hoyert 2011). Hospital committees review deaths to reduce mortality rates (Vargas-Rosendo et al. 1992). Using this method, one system reduced its mortality index by half over a 6-year period while also cutting the morbidity of delirium in its hospital by half (Barbieri et al. 2013).

Two methods for obtaining feedback on your practice and problem-solving skills are to *listen* for it and to *ask* for it. This openness will help you avoid diagnostic and treatment problems as you use the information to test your conceptualizations and solutions. Once we complete our formal medical education and begin practicing, usually unsupervised, our opportunities for formal, formative, or summative feedback are greatly reduced. Teaching or supervising commonly stimulates a process of self-evaluation, and continuing medical education (CME) courses, of course, may enhance a caregiver's database (Lockyer et al. 2011). Preparing for and seeking specialty board certification and recertification also provides some feedback, but it is easier to assess knowledge acquisition and retention than problem-solving skills.

Informal feedback, however, is frequently available to us verbally and behaviorally from patients and any member of a treatment team, even when it is unexpected (Hardavella et al. 2017). Obtaining such feedback from patients, directly or indirectly, is potentially useful for improvement, although many have struggled to determine the best method for obtaining it; issues of transference and countertransference, along with fears of harming, rather than improving, the therapeutic alliance and outcomes, may complicate asking for direct feedback (David et al. 2022; Solstad et al. 2019). Standardized forms seeking patient feedback may also be influenced by factors other than the provider's performance, such as impatience with practical and therapeutic limits in distressed patients with depression (Romanowicz et al. 2022). However, patients provide this informal feedback indirectly, prompting self-assessment, when features of their presentation or outcome are unexpected and when they ask questions or introduce information from the internet. Patients leaving treatment unexpectedly or without explanation often provoke self-assessment in clinicians, who also may find themselves reassured, deservedly or not, when receiving little challenge from patients (Lockyer et al. 2011).

Although patient satisfaction has been linked to successful clinical outcomes (Shipley et al. 2000), tools that actually measure provider competencies from patient feedback, rather than simply customer preferences, have been developed and are establishing validity (Baines et al. 2019; Hansen et al. 2010; Reese et al. 2013; Violato et al. 2008). Feedback from patients to providers during psychotherapy has been found to improve clinical outcomes, especially in cases where treatment failure was predicted (David et al. 2022; Hawkins et al. 2004; Lambert et al. 2001).

The Royal College of Psychiatrists has developed ACP 360, a tool for psychiatrists that provides feedback from patients and colleagues (Royal College of Psychiatrists 2022). In the United Kingdom, a majority of physicians receiving formal feedback from patients found it to be the most helpful type of information in supporting reflection on their practice: 37.3% found it moderately helpful and 21.5% found it extensively helpful (Archer et al. 2016).

Ideally, informal feedback also occurs daily, on a reciprocal basis, with team members and peers. This feedback should be considered (and offered) reflectively and nonjudgmentally, with mutual respect, so that you and your colleagues can all improve. In other words, you should offer *and* seek feedback, asking for it when it is not offered to you. It is generally best to receive and provide timely feedback privately, one-on-one. You can most effectively receive feedback by listening completely, framing it positively as a learning situation, and asking for clarification as needed (see Hardavella et al. 2017). Processing this feedback reflectively, especially when it is unexpected or negative, is most likely to result in behavioral change and advancement in your skills. If your emotional reaction to the feedback is strong, another professional, such as a peer or supervisor, may be able to help facilitate your reflection (Sargeant et al. 2009).

More formally, practitioners should readily ask for a second opinion from a trusted colleague at any impasse. This is often attempted informally through conversation, sharing sanitized details of a case and asking for ideas. Unfortunately, the results of such an effort are based on what you tell the consultant (i.e., your conceptualizations that have resulted in disappointing results), not on reevaluation of the raw data by a new set of eyes. Peers and supervisors should have the opportunity to provide truly useful information and correct any errors in conceptualization and problem-solving that practitioners have made. We must formally provide peers and supervisors with all of our data and an opportunity to interview and assess the patient themselves.

Our profession is strengthened and patients benefit when we support their care with sound second and, if necessary, third or more opinions. Therefore, in addition to requesting these opinions often, we must also expect to provide them frequently to others. When a colleague or mentee begins an informal attempt at consultation, respectfully request that they make a formal request before proceeding. There will be ample opportunity to discuss the case at length after proper and thorough evaluation.

To minimize bias when providing a second opinion, it is often preferable to interview the patient prior to reviewing the chart, then thoroughly review the complete record. The second clinician should generate new questions to ask the patient and the referring provider, then offer impressions and suggestions verbally to the patient and in writing (plus, hopefully, verbally) to the requesting practitioner to discuss with their patient and to keep in their record. This full reevaluation is then available for the provider to review at any time. The consultant should remain available for further discussion or reevaluation of the case as it progresses.

Chat groups for the practice of psychiatry, psychotherapy, and psychopharmacology exist online and through social media. It is amazing how frequently practitioners ask for advice and give only a few details of the problem. Even more astoundingly, people offer ready answers, rarely asking for additional information. It is not helpful to anyone, especially our patients, to participate in informal discussions based on incomplete data, which can so easily misdirect diagnosis and treatment. If you do participate, encourage the authors to ask for formal second opinions. Any time you hear a provider asking for advice on options for treatment-resistant cases, encourage consultation.

Practicing and Improving Clinical Skills

Deliberate practice is essential for continuing to improve levels of performance in all fields (Ericsson 2004). It is critical to remain current with our scientific literature and any changes in diagnostic categories. Clinical presentations (such as CME programs and grand rounds) at nearby treatment or educational facilities and state, regional, and national professional meetings offer excellent opportunities for clinical discussions with peers. Your knowledge can be self-assessed in many ways, including commercial board preparation tools, the American Psychiatric Association's Annual Meeting Self-Assessment in Psychiatry (American Psychiatric Association 2022), and the Psychiatrists In-Practice Examination (PIPE) of the American College of Psychiatrists (2021). Additionally, practicing important skills such as communication with patients and the way we keep and review records (see section "Record and Review" in Chapter 8, "Reducing Treatment Failure") can enhance treatment outcomes.

Patient noncompliance is estimated at between 25%–50% (DiMatteo 2004; Vermeire et al. 2001) and has been described as the key mediator between medical practice and patient outcomes (Kravitz and Melnikow 2004). It is also significantly associated with the communication skills of physicians. Better communication by a provider is linked to the retrieval of important clinical information; patient involvement in decision-making;

and discussion of barriers to compliance, trust, and rapport (Zolnierek and Dimatteo 2009). With accurate diagnoses and treatment plans, patients of physicians who communicate effectively are 19% more compliant; adherence to treatment plans has been shown to increase 12% after a provider receives communication skills training (Zolnierek and Dimatteo 2009). In fact, the very concept of patient compliance or adherence may be flawed: patients have their own circumstances and beliefs about illness and treatments (see section "Countertherapeutic Factors" in Chapter 4, "The Myth of Treatment Resistance?", and "Perceiving and Respecting Your Patient" in Chapter 5, "Essential Assessment and Reevaluation"). Clinically successful providers learn how to contribute to the decisions patients are making about treatments rather than merely dictating them (Donovan 1995; Kravitz and Melnikow 2004; Vermeire et al. 2001).

Improving your communication skills, then, is one clear way to reduce treatment failures. Training programs may include communication skills in their curricula. For practicing clinicians, print tools (see Coll et al. 2012; Silverman et al. 2017) and online tools, such as the Calgary-Cambridge Guide (Kurtz et al. 1998; Silverman et al. 1998; available for free download through GP-Training.net at www.gp-training.net/wp-content/uploads/2020/08/calgary-5.pdf), can be used to improve these essential skills (Iversen et al. 2021; Kuehl 2011; Kurtz and Silverman 1996).

Vague expressions of feelings by patients during interviews are more common than overt mention of negative emotions. Clinicians often do not respond to these feelings, particularly late in an interview. Providers may also suppress random expression of feelings because they prefer investigating feelings from direct questions they feel are linked to diagnoses. These spontaneous, but subtle, cues that clinicians are likely to suppress may relate directly to physiological or cognitive symptoms and help clarify a correct diagnosis, as well as strengthen the therapeutic alliance. If the provider hears the cue, is empathetic, repeats the cue, and provides and encourages space for open discussion, both diagnosis and treatment may be improved (Del Piccolo et al. 2012, 2014). Deliberate effort and practice to recognize and provide space for exploration of these expressions is warranted.

Additionally, the order and structure with which physicians proceed with a patient interview appear to bear little resemblance to what we were taught in training (Noble et al. 2022). Combining a thorough, semistructured interview (see section "Conduct Semistructured Clinical Interviews" in Chapter 8) (Putman 2020; Aboraya et al. 2006) with review of a patient's previous medical records leads to more accurate primary diagnoses, plus the identification of more secondary diagnoses than does relying on interview alone (Ramirez Basco et al. 2000). Obtaining outside information, such as from family, friends, and staff, also improves diagnosis (Hetmański 2020).

Because of our biased memory for symptoms once a diagnosis has been made (see section "Implications for Medical Practice"), it is important to record not only your diagnosis but all symptoms actually observed and reported at each patient encounter. This will prevent memory distortion that can grow over time because diagnoses are remembered better than the data on which they are based (Lingle and Ostrom 1979). Recording symptoms for subsequent review at any stage of treatment allows for revision of erroneous diagnoses and treatment plans rather than remaining at an impasse—that is, treatment failure (see section "Record and Review" in Chapter 8).

Summary

The conception of a problem implies a solution through discovering pathways to deliver desired situations. In medicine, we employ a range of decision-making and problem-solving skills but most usefully apply abductive reasoning: forming a hypothesis (e.g., a diagnosis or treatment plan), testing it, reformulating the hypothesis on the basis of new data, and then repeating the process. The actual value we offer to our patients is our problem-solving skill. Treatment failure resulting in the relabeling of a diagnosis as treatment resistance actually represents a failure of problem-solving.

Expertise in medical problem-solving develops as case material is reformulated into larger macro concepts as we generalize across increasingly complex cases, with expected and unexpected outcomes. These illness scripts, or diagnoses, may also be described as the templates discussed in Chapter 1 (see section "Chunking Theory and Expertise"). When new cases appear similar to past cases, recognition is rapid, but quick diagnosis may also cause the practitioner to ignore atypical or incompatible symptoms that might lead to the correct solution. We develop and maintain a long-term mental set that favors the most common answers, stifles creative thinking, and directs us away from alternative answers.

Our expertise can be maintained and improved only by recognizing that we overestimate the accuracy of our problem-solving efforts and by incorporating formal and informal feedback during the process. We enhance our skills by seeing a large number of patients with similar problems who require different treatment solutions. When a diagnostic or therapeutic impasse becomes evident, we must consciously deconstruct our encapsulated illness prototypes and recombine them, reconsidering previously ignored or rejected information. After the initial hypothesis is altered to fit the data from testing, it is then ready for retesting—a necessarily conscious process. Ask and listen for feedback and use it reflectively to improve your practice. Eschew informal second opinions in favor of complete reevaluations by respected colleagues; be prepared to offer only the same to them.

We tend to remember diagnoses, not symptoms, so it is important to keep a clear record of every symptom at each patient contact for subsequent review and reformulation. Perform standard semistructured interviews, review previous medical records, and obtain outside information. Our communication style with patients may suppress, or leave unexplored, information essential to achieving treatment success. How effective we are in using communication skills also has a significant impact on how we influence patients to consider valid therapeutic strategies. Practicing communication and record-keeping skills, in addition to incorporating feedback, will reduce your incidence of treatment failures.

Key Points

- Combine semistructured interviews with review of medical records.
- Obtain outside information.
- Be methodical, thorough, and consistent in all patient contacts.
- Do not ignore data that do not fit with your initial diagnoses.
- Access your biomedical knowledge when problems are difficult.
- Choosing a diagnosis causes us to miss important symptoms or cues, which are poorly remembered later. Keep a clear record of all symptoms for later review.
- Expect, don't underestimate, your errors.
- Seek active feedback on your problem-solving.
- Deliberately practice your skills.
- See many patients with similar problems and use feedback to develop methods for distinguishing among diagnoses requiring different treatments.

Self-Assessment Questions

1. Which of the following statements is *not* true?

    A. Expert practitioners automatically maintain and enhance their performance through routine practice.
    B. Years of medical practice may reinforce conceptual error.
    C. Without feedback, expertise narrows over time.
    D. Long-term mental sets constrain creative thinking and problem-solving.

    Correct answer: A. Expert practitioners automatically maintain and enhance their performance through routine practice.

    The quality of practitioner performance depends not only on the amount of time spent practicing relevant skills but also the quality of that practice. As the skills of experts narrow, it becomes increasingly difficult to consider alternatives. The most effective providers are alert for errors, seek feedback, and consciously recombine data to find creative solutions.

2. Which of the following statements is true about the diagnoses we make?

    A. They are often made too quickly.
    B. They often ignore atypical or inconsistent symptoms.
    C. They cause us to "remember" symptoms that were not present.
    D. All of the above.

    Correct answer: D. All of the above.

    The most common error among practitioners is making quick assessments on the basis of their experience, then searching for data to confirm the diagnosis. This results in ignoring symptoms that do not fit and imagining others to be present that are not. When inconsistent symptoms appear in an initial presentation, clinicians delaying diagnosis outperform those who make rapid conclusions.

3. All of the following are essential for effective clinical practice except which one?

   A. Recording every symptom at every patient contact.
   B. Informal consultation.
   C. Informal feedback.
   D. Communication skills.

   Correct answer: B. Informal consultation.

   Second opinions must be formal full evaluations by competent, respected peers who have the opportunity to review the complete record and interview the patient. Off-the-cuff chats only recapitulate the original formulation and may further misdirect treatment because they rely on partial information. However, informal feedback gleaned from patients, peers, and team members is reflectively considered by the most effective practitioners. Because we recall diagnoses rather than symptoms, each symptom must be available in the record for later reevaluation. Our communication skills directly impact diagnosis, the therapeutic alliance, and outcomes.

4. Best practices in problem-solving include which of the following?

   A. Continuous interaction between the solver and the environment.
   B. Breaking problems into subproblems and solving each.
   C. Breaking familiar patterns into components, then regrouping into new configurations.
   D. A and C.

   Correct answer: A and C.

   Ongoing, real-world feedback alerts the solver to errors and impending failure. When reaching an impasse, consciously reforming reinforced and progressively narrowed schema into creative new patterns is more effective than simply subdividing the problem.

5. More accurate primary and secondary diagnoses can best be obtained by which two of the following options?

    A. An interview honed by years of practice.
    B. Investigating feelings from direct questions.
    C. A semistructured interview and review of outside information.
    D. Review of previous medical records.

    Correct answer: C and D.

    Investigating feelings through direct questioning is inferior to providing space for exploration of their vague expression during a structured interview. Reviewing previous records and outside information improves the accuracy of the primary diagnosis and the number of secondary diagnoses.

Discussion Topics

1. A patient you have treated for 6 years with mixed success misses a routine appointment and does not respond to your calls. Three weeks later, you receive a request to transfer her records to another provider in your city. How can you use this informal feedback to assess your communication and problem-solving skills?
2. A relatively new patient has not experienced the treatment outcome you had hoped for but also evidences poor follow-through with your full recommendations. In addition to reconsidering your own problem-solving efforts, how would you explore your patient's circumstances and beliefs about illness and treatments and use this knowledge to contribute to his decisions about a treatment plan?

Additional Readings

Coll X, Papageorgiou A, Stanley A, Tarbuck A (eds): Communication Skills in Mental Health Care: An Introduction. Boca Raton, FL, CRC Press, 2012: *A collection of basic communication skills to be used in psychiatry, based on the Calgary-Cambridge model; useful for review*

Epstein D: Range: Why Generalists Triumph in a Specialized World. New York, Riverhead Books, 2019: *Offers evidence that super-specializing in a domain, rather than broadening one's knowledge once specialty expertise is achieved, limits problem-solving success*

Hardavella G, Aamli-Gaagnat A, Saad N, et al: How to give and receive feedback effectively. Breathe (Sheff) 13(4):327–333, 2017: *Describes various modes of feedback and best practices*

Silverman J, Kurtz S, Draper J: Skills for Communicating With Patients, 3rd Edition. New York, CRC Press, 2017: *A detailed guide for all practitioners to improve patient outcomes through improving their communication skills*

Waitzkin J: The Art of Learning: A Journey in the Pursuit of Excellence. New York, Free Press, 2007: *A chess and martial arts champion's process for learning, illustrating successful problem-solving skills; the introduction and Chapters 3–13 are particularly relevant*

References

Aboraya A, Rankin E, France C, et al: The reliability of psychiatric diagnosis revisited: the clinician's guide to improve the reliability of psychiatric diagnosis. Psychiatry (Edgmont) 3(1):41–50, 2006 21103149

Agre GP: The concept of problem. Educ Stud 13:121–142, 1982

Allen M: Post mortem: without autopsies, hospitals bury their mistakes. ProPublica, December 15, 2011. Available at: www.propublica.org/article/without-autopsies-hospitals-bury-their-mistakes. Accessed July 6, 2022.

American College of Psychiatrists: Psychiatrists In-Practice Examination® (PIPE®). St. Louis, MO, American College of Psychiatrists, 2021. Available at: https://www.acpsych.org/pipe. Accessed July 15, 2022.

American Psychiatric Association: 2022 APA Annual Meeting Self-Assessment in Psychiatry. Available at: https://education.psychiatry.org/diweb/catalog/item/eid/C2200101. Accessed July 15, 2022.

Archer J, Cameron N, Laugharn K, et al: UMbRELLA: Shaping the Future of Medical Revalidation, Interim Report. London, General Medical Council, January 2016. Available at: www.gmc-uk.org/UMbRELLA_interim_report_FINAL.pdf_65723741.pdf. Accessed July 18, 2022.

Arkes HR, Harkness AR: Effect of making a diagnosis on subsequent recognition of symptoms. J Exp Psychol Hum Learn 6(5):568–575, 1980 6448908

Baines R, Zahra D, Bryce M, et al: Is collecting patient feedback "a futile exercise" in the context of recertification? Acad Psychiatry 43(6):570–576, 2019 31309453

Barbieri JS, Fuchs BD, Fishman N, et al: The Mortality Review Committee: a novel and scalable approach to reducing inpatient mortality. Jt Comm J Qual Patient Saf 39(9):387–395, 2013 24147350

Barrows HS, Tamblyn RM: Problem-Based Learning: An Approach to Medical Education. New York, Springer, 1980

Bilalić M, McLeod P, Gobet F: Inflexibility of experts—reality or myth? Quantifying the Einstellung effect in chess masters. Cognit Psychol 56(2):73–102, 2008 17418112

Borasi R: On the nature of problems. Educ Stud Math 17:125–141, 1986

Boshuizen HPA, Gruber H, Strasser J: Knowledge restructuring through case processing: the key to generalise expertise development theory across domains? Educ Res Rev 29:100310, 2020

Campitelli G, Speelman C: Expertise and the illusion of expertise in gambling, in Problem Gambling: Cognition, Prevention and Treatment. Edited by Gobet F, Schiller M. London, Palgrave Macmillan, 2014 pp 41–60

Carlier IVE, Meuldijk D, Van Vliet IM, et al: Routine outcome monitoring and feedback on physical or mental health status: evidence and theory. J Eval Clin Pract 18(1):104–110, 2012 20846319

Coll X, Papageorgiou A, Stanley A, et al. (eds): Communication Skills in Mental Health Care: An Introduction. Boca Raton, FL, CRC Press, 2012

Connelly DP, Johnson PE: The medical problem solving process. Hum Pathol 11(5):412–419, 1980 7429488

David D, McAfee SG, Eth S: The impact of patient feedback on psychotherapy and supervision outcomes in psychiatry residency. Acad Psychiatry Apr 26, 2022 35474182Online ahead of print

Del Piccolo L, Mazzi MA, Goss C, et al: How emotions emerge and are dealt with in first diagnostic consultations in psychiatry. Patient Educ Couns 88(1):29–35, 2012 22326453

Del Piccolo L, Danzi O, Fattori N, et al: How psychiatrist's communication skills and patient's diagnosis affect emotions disclosure during first diagnostic consultations. Patient Educ Couns 96(2):151–158, 2014 24976629

DiMatteo MR: Variations in patients' adherence to medical recommendations: a quantitative review of 50 years of research. Med Care 42(3):200–209, 2004 15076819

Donovan JL: Patient decision making: the missing ingredient in compliance research. Int J Technol Assess Health Care 11(3):443–455, 1995 7591546

Egidi M: Decomposition patterns in problem solving, in Cognitive Economics: New Trends (Contributions to Economic Analysis, Vol. 280). Edited by Topol R, Walliser B. Bingley, UK, Emerald Group, 2006 pp 15–46

Einhorn HJ: Expert judgment: some necessary conditions and an example. J Appl Psychol 59(5):562–571, 1974

Einhorn HJ, Hogarth RM: Confidence in judgment: persistence of the illusion of validity. Psychol Rev 85(5):395–416, 1978

Ellis JJ, Reingold EM: The Einstellung effect in anagram problem solving: evidence from eye movements. Front Psychol 5:679, 2014 25071650

Ericsson KA: Deliberate practice and the acquisition and maintenance of expert performance in medicine and related domains. Acad Med 79(10)(suppl):S70–S81, 2004 15383395

Fann KT: Pierce's Theory of Abduction. The Hague, Netherlands, Martinus Nijhoff, 1970

Frensch PA, Sternberg RJ: Expertise and intelligent thinking: when is it worse to know better? in Advances in the Psychology of Human Intelligence, Vol 5. Edited by Sternberg RJ. Mahwah, NJ, Lawrence Erlbaum, 1989, pp 157–188

Frensch PA, Sternberg RJ (eds): Complex Problem Solving: Principles and Mechanisms. New York, Psychology Press, 2014

Gabriel A, Violato C: Problem-solving strategies in psychiatry: differences between experts and novices in diagnostic accuracy and reasoning. Adv Med Educ Pract 4:11–16, 2013 23745095

Gagnon R, Charlin B, Roy L, et al: The cognitive validity of the Script Concordance Test: a processing time study. Teach Learn Med 18(1):22–27, 2006 16354136

Gondek D, Edbrooke-Childs J, Fink E, et al: Feedback from outcome measures and treatment effectiveness, treatment efficiency, and collaborative practice: a systematic review. Adm Policy Ment Health 2016 43(3):325–343, 2016

Guest CB, Regehr G, Tiberius RG: The life long challenge of expertise. Med Educ 35(1):78–81, 2001 11123600

Hansen L, Vincent S, Harris S, et al: A patient satisfaction rating scale for psychiatric service users. Psychiatrist 34(11):485–488, 2010

Hardavella G, Aamli-Gaagnat A, Saad N, et al: How to give and receive feedback effectively. Breathe (Sheff) 13(4):327–333, 2017 29209427

Hawkins EJ, Lambert MJ, Vermeersch DA, et al: The therapeutic effects of providing patient progress information to therapists and patients. Psychother Res 14:308–327, 2004

Hetmański M: Expertise and expert knowledge in social and procedural entanglement. Eidos 4(2):6–22, 2020

Hoffman RR: How can expertise be defined? Implications of research from cognitive psychology, in Exploring Expertise: Issues and Perspectives. Edited by Williams R, Faulkner W, Fleck J. New York, MacMillan, 1998 pp 81–100

Hoyert DL: The changing profile of autopsied deaths in the United States, 1972–2007. NCHS Data Brief 67(67):1–8, 2011 22142988

Huang F, Tang S, Hu Z: Unconditional perseveration of the short-term mental set in chunk decomposition. Front Psychol 9:2568, 2018 30618985

Iversen ED, Wolderslund M, Kofoed PE, et al: Communication skills training: a means to promote time-efficient patient-centered communication in clinical practice. J Patient Cent Res Rev 8(4):307–314, 2021 34722798

Janis IL: Victims of Group Think: A Psychological Study of Foreign-Policy Decisions and Fiascoes. Boston, MA, Houghton Mifflin, 1972

Knaup C, Koesters M, Schoefer D, et al: Effect of feedback of treatment outcome in specialist mental healthcare: meta-analysis. Br J Psychiatry 195(1):15–22, 2009 19567889

Knoblich G, Ohlsson S, Haider H, Rhenius D: Constraint relaxation and chunk decomposition in insight problem solving. J Exp Psychol Learn Mem Cogn 25(6):1534–1555, 1999

Knoblich G, Ohlsson S, Raney GE: An eye movement study of insight problem solving. Mem Cognit 29(7):1000–1009, 2001 11820744

Kravitz RL, Melnikow J: Medical adherence research: time for a change in direction? Med Care 42(3):197–199, 2004 15076818

Kuehl SP: Communication tools for the modern doctor bag: physician patient communication part 1: beginning of a medical interview. J Community Hosp Intern Med Perspect 1(3): 8428, 2011 23882333

Kurtz SM, Silverman JD: The Calgary-Cambridge Referenced Observation Guides: an aid to defining the curriculum and organizing the teaching in communication training programmes. Med Educ 30(2):83–89, 1996 8736242

Kurtz SM, Silverman JD, Draper J: Teaching and Learning Communication Skills in Medicine. London, CRC Press, 1998

Lambert MJ, Whipple JL, Smart DW, et al: The effects of providing therapists with feedback on patient progress during psychotherapy: are outcomes enhanced? Psychother Res 11(1):49–68, 2001 25849877

Lambert M, Whipple J, Hawkins E, et al: Is it time for clinicians to routinely track patient outcome? A meta-analysis. Clin Psychol Sci Pract 10(3):288–301, 2003

Lingle JH, Ostrom TM: Retrieval and selectivity in memory-based impression judgement. J Pers Soc Psychol 37(2):180–194, 1979

Lockyer J, Armson H, Chesluk B, et al: Feedback data sources that inform physician self-assessment. Med Teach 33(2):e113–e120, 2011 21275533

Lovett MC, Anderson JR: History of success and current context in problem solving: combined influences on operator selection. Cogn Psychol 31(2):168–217, 1996

Neroni MA, Vasconcelos LA, Crilly N: Computer-based 'mental set' tasks: an alternative approach to studying design fixation. J Mech Des 139(7):071102, 2017

Noble LM, Manalastas G, Viney R, et al.: Does the structure of the medical consultation align with an educational model of clinical communication? A study of physicians' consultations from a postgraduate examination. Patient Educ Couns 105(6):1449–1456, 2022 34649752

Ohlsson S: Information-processing explanations of insight and related phenomena, in Advances in the Psychology of Thinking. London, Harvester Wheatsheaf, 1992, pp 1–44

Öllinger M, Jones G, Knoblich G: Investigating the effect of mental set on insight problem solving. Exp Psychol 55(4):269–282, 2008 18683624

Öllinger M, Jones G, Knoblich G: The dynamics of search, impasse, and representational change provide a coherent explanation of difficulty in the nine-dot problem. Psychol Res 78(2):266–275, 2014 23708954

Öllinger M, Fedor A, Brodt S, Szathmáry E: Insight into the ten-penny problem: guiding search by constraints and maximization. Psychol Res 81(5):925–938, 2017 27592343

Patel VL, Arocha JF, Zhang J: Thinking and reasoning in medicine, in Cambridge Handbook of Thinking and Reasoning. Edited by Holyoak K, Morrison R. Cambridge, UK, Cambridge University Press, 2005 pp 727–750

Putman HP: Rational Psychopharmacology: A Book of Clinical Skills. Washington, DC, American Psychiatric Association Publishing, 2020

Ramirez Basco M, Bostic JQ, Davies D, et al: Methods to improve diagnostic accuracy in community mental health. Am J Psychiatry 157(10):1599–1605, 2000 11007713

Reese RJ, Slone NC, Miserocchi KM: Using client feedback in psychotherapy from an interpersonal process perspective. Psychotherapy (Chic) 50(3):288–291, 2013 24000837

Ricks TR, Turley-Ames KJ, Wiley J: Effects of working memory capacity on mental set due to domain knowledge. Mem Cognit 35(6):1456–1462, 2007 18035641

Romanowicz M, Oesterle TS, Croarkin PE, et al: Measuring patient satisfaction in an outpatient psychiatric clinic: what factors play a role? Ann Gen Psychiatry 21(1):2, 2022 35042513

Royal College of Psychiatrists: Patient and Colleague Feedback. London, Royal College of Psychiatrists, 2022. Available at: https://www.rcpsych.ac.uk/members/supporting-your-professional-development/revalidation/revalidation-mythbusters/patient-and-colleague-feedback. Accessed July 19, 2022.

Ryback D: Confidence and accuracy as a function of experience in judgment-making in the absence of systematic feedback. Percept Mot Skills 24(1):331–334, 1967

Salvi C, Bowden EM: Looking for creativity: where do we look when we look for new ideas? Front Psychol 7:161, 2016 26913018

Sarathy V: Real world problem-solving. Front Hum Neurosci 12:261, 2018 29997490

Sargeant JM, Mann KV, van der Vleuten CP, et al: Reflection: a link between receiving and using assessment feedback. Adv Health Sci Educ Theory Pract 14(3):399–410, 2009 18528777

Schmidt HG, Boshuizen HPA: Encapsulation of biomedical knowledge, in Advanced Models of Cognition for Medical Training and Practice. Edited by Evans DA, Patel VL. New York, Springer, 1992 pp 265–282

Schultz PW, Searleman A: Rigidity of thought and behavior: 100 years of research. Genet Soc Gen Psychol Monogr 128(2):165–207, 2002 12194421

Scordo KA: Differential diagnosis: correctly putting the pieces of the puzzle together. AACN Adv Crit Care 25(3):230–236, 2014 25054528

Shanteau J, Phelps RH: Judgment and swine: approaches in applied judgment analysis, in Human Judgment and Decision Processes in Applied Settings. Edited by Kaplan MF, Schwartz S. New York, Academic Press, 1977 pp 255–271

Shipley K, Hilborn B, Hansell A, et al: Patient satisfaction: a valid index of quality of care in a psychiatric service. Acta Psychiatr Scand 101(4):330–333, 2000 10782555

Silverman JD, Kurtz SM, Draper J: Skills for Communicating With Patients. Oxford, UK, Radcliffe Medical Press, 1998

Silverman JD, Kurtz SM, Draper J: Skills for Communicating With Patients, 3rd Edition. New York, CRC Press, 2017

Spiro RJ: Remembering information from text: the "state of schema" approach, in Schooling and the Acquisition of Knowledge. Edited by Anderson RC, Spiro RJ, Montague WE, et al. New York, Lawrence Erlbaum Associates, 1977, pp 131–160

Solstad SM, Castonguay LG, Moltu C: Patients' experiences with routine outcome monitoring and clinical feedback systems: a systematic review and synthesis of qualitative empirical literature. Psychother Res 29(2):157–170, 2019 28523962

Sowden PT, Pringle A, Gabora L: The shifting sands of creative thinking: connections to dual-process theory. Think Reason 21(1):40–60, 2015

Sulin RE, Dooling DJ: Intrusion of a thematic idea in retention of prose. J Exp Psychol 103(2):255–262, 1974

Tang X, Pang J, Nie Q-Y, et al: Probing the cognitive mechanism of mental representational change during chunk decomposition: a parametric fMRI study. Cereb Cortex 26(7):2991–2999, 2016 26045566

Tay SW, Ryan P, Ryan CA: Systems 1 and 2 thinking processes and cognitive reflection testing in medical students. Can Med Educ J 7(2):e97–e103, 2016 28344696

't Hart P: Irving L. Janis' victims of groupthink. Polit Psychol 12(2):247–278, 1991

Upmeier zu Belzen A, Engelschalt P, Krüger D: Modeling as scientific reasoning—the role of abductive reasoning for modeling competence. Educ Sci (Basel) 11(9):495, 2021

Vargas-Rosendo R, Alemán-Velázquez P, Jasso-Gutiérrez L: El Comité de Mortalidad: una necesidad hospitalaria (The Mortality Committee: a hospital need). Bol Méd Hosp Infant México 49(10):683–688, 1992

Vermeire E, Hearnshaw H, Van Royen P, et al: Patient adherence to treatment: three decades of research. A comprehensive review. J Clin Pharm Ther 26(5):331–342, 2001 11679023

Violato C, Lockyer JM, Fidler H: Assessment of psychiatrists in practice through multisource feedback. Can J Psychiatry 53(8):525–533, 2008 18801214

Wiley J: Expertise as mental set: the effects of domain knowledge in creative problem solving. Mem Cognit 26(4):716–730, 1998 9701964

Yoruk S, Runco MA: The neuroscience of divergent thinking. Act Nerv Super 56:1–16, 2014

Zabelina D, Saporta A, Beeman M: Flexible or leaky attention in creative people? Distinct patterns of attention for different types of creative thinking. Mem Cognit 44(3):488–498, 2016 26527210

Zolnierek KB, Dimatteo MR: Physician communication and patient adherence to treatment: a meta-analysis. Med Care 47(8):826–834, 2009 19584762

Zoudji B, Thon B, Debû B: Efficiency of the mnemonic system of expert soccer players under overload of the working memory in a simulated decision-making task. Psychol Sport Exerc 11(1):18–26, 2010

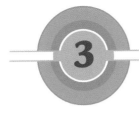

The Goal of Evidence-Based Practice

We practice psychiatry with the goal of providing satisfactory clinical outcomes for patients, so we choose treatments we believe will avoid treatment resistance (i.e., treatment failure). We have always presumed that the interventions we employ will work, and we have always based that expectation on some category of data: our experience, hearsay, theory, tradition, even availability, in addition to randomized clinical trials (RCTs). We independently consider each of these sources of information to be "evidence" if we base recommendations on them.

The practice of evidence-based medicine (EBM), however, refers to the conscious, overt, and consistent selection of the best current evidence of treatment efficacy to apply to treatment planning. This evidence must be demonstrable to a wide body of clinicians and not just based on individual experience or unexamined, shared opinions. We must understand this effort, discover data generally accepted as worthy of the title *evidence*, and routinely adhere to this method to offer our patients their soundest chance of avoiding treatment failure.

Evolution of Evidence-Based Medicine

There are ancient examples of EBM, and the efficacy of treatments was noted as far back as the eleventh century by Avicenna in *The Canon of Medicine* (Brater and Daly 2000; Nasir 2010). The practice reappeared in the 1700s as the effectiveness of bloodletting was challenged and a solution for scurvy was discovered. The next era of EBM stretched from the late nineteenth century to 1970, particularly involving surgical interventions.

Registries were initiated; controlled RCTs were developed and increasingly used as the double blind was eventually added to randomization (Claridge and Fabian 2005).

The modern era of EBM began with the publication of *Effectiveness and Efficiency: Random Reflections on Health Services* by Archibald Cochrane in 1972 as an attempt to improve the United Kingdom's National Health Service by evaluating clinical treatments and procedures through the results of RCTs (Claridge and Fabian 2005; Cochrane 1999; Cochrane Community 2022; Winkelstein 2009). David Eddy, M.D., Ph.D., first used the term *evidence based* when referring to practice guidelines based on the analysis of outcomes (Eddy 1990). A "systemic approach to analyze published research as the basis for clinical decision making" was aggressively pursued by David Sackett and Gordon Guyatt at Canada's McMaster University during the 1980s–1990s (Claridge and Fabian 2005, p. 547; Nasir 2010; Zimerman 2013). The term evidence-based medicine first appeared in the medical literature in 1992 (Guyatt et al. 1992). The idea and goals of EBM have also been propelled by medicine's response to questions about its relationship to society and issues of medical authority (Zimerman 2013).

The Cochrane Centre (now Cochrane) was founded in 1992 "to facilitate the preparation of systematic reviews of randomised controlled trials of health care" (Cochrane Community 2022) and was named to honor the important efforts of epidemiologist Archie Cochrane. It has since grown into a not-for-profit global network that synthesizes evidence of medical outcomes for use in medical decision-making. It currently offers more than 7,500 systematic reviews at the online Cochrane Library, making it an excellent resource for clinicians practicing EBM (Claridge and Fabian 2005; Cochrane 1999; Cochrane Community 2022; Winkelstein 2009).

Although some people distinguish between EBM and evidence-based practice (EBP), defining the former as research evidence and the latter as the actual practice of medicine, the term EBM is generally reserved for medical practice, and EBP is reserved for nonphysician providers (e.g., psychologists, physician extenders) or nonphysical treatments (e.g., psychotherapy) (Lilienfeld and Basterfield 2020; Nasir 2010). Both terms imply the same principles and, for the remainder of this chapter, will be used interchangeably.

Resistance to Evidence-Based Medicine

Some practitioners react to this new clinical ideology with the thought that this is what they have already been doing. They read journals and think that their years of clinical practice and experience also count as evidence, sometimes more than data from research that is not always relevant to a specific case. By the turn of the previous century, in fact, most psychiatrists indicated that they thought their practice was already consistent with the model (Carey and Hall 1999). Sackett and colleagues not only formalized but redefined EBM in 1996, attempting to return credence to subjective experience and the role of expertise in order that clinical practice not be "tyrannized" by good data that are not applicable or appropriate for a given patient. They also added patient preferences as the third pillar of this widely accepted definition of EBM: "clinical evidence from systematic research...[added to] the proficiency of judgement of individual physicians...[and] individual patients' predicaments, rights, and preferences" (Claridge and Fabian 2005; Eddy 2011; Sackett et al. 1996, p. 71).

During the past two decades, many authors have tenaciously held to the value of individual expert judgment based on clinical experience, stating that EBM is "idealism" and that clinical decision-making cannot be based solely on the evidence we have available (Fernandez et al. 2015; Hampton 2002; Nasir 2010). As demonstrated in Chapter 2, "Keys to Problem-Solving" (section "Obstacles to Problem-Solving"), however, expertise is hardly foolproof and is open to problem-solving error through many mechanisms, including narrowed consideration of data and the tendency to apply standard solutions to all problems.

Practitioners operating in isolation, as sole decision-makers, are unlikely to follow the practice guidelines that have proliferated in the past few decades and are usually thought of as evidence-based (Timmermans and Mauck 2005). However, these standards may have been established through expert consensus rather than RCTs and may not fully express the uncertainty of some data (Croft et al. 2011; Mandell 2021). Even guidelines based on systematic reviews quickly become obsolete as new evidence is found. Studies show that 20% of these recommendations become outdated within 3 years of publication and about half within 5 years (Clark et al. 2006; Martínez García et al. 2014; Shekelle et al. 2001).

Other providers are concerned, appropriately, about the significant holes in the evidence. These often result from gaps in research and research policies, particularly due to decisions made by commercial stakeholders. Too often in contemporary research, new pharmaceuticals are compared only with placebo and not with existing treatments. Vulnerable population groups are excluded, and long-term and rare effects are not explored (Mintzes 2013). Not all research is published, because of either lack of initiative when results are disappointing or the traditional bias of scientific publications to publish only new and positive results. Proprietary information may not be released for commercial reasons. Research into psychotherapy outcomes has often been quantitative and skewed toward short-term therapies, such as cognitive-behavioral therapy and interpersonal psychotherapy (Hoffman 2009). Additionally, psychotherapy studies are typically of small sample size, and efforts to draw broad conclusions from them through meta-analysis are hampered by strong heterogeneity (Eppel 2018).

EBM in medical school curricula is found most commonly during the first 2 years of training and is less evident during clinical rotations (Blanco et al. 2014). A bias toward the value of mechanistic explanations of treatments over even clear outcome data persists among providers, reminiscent of the historical delay in implementing diets shown to prevent scurvy because the pathophysiology was not understood or agreed on (Claridge and Fabian 2005).

Defining Evidence

An important distinction comes down to what we consider evidence: Which data are valid, which are not, and where is the authority for making these decisions? Do we consider our individual evaluations of data satisfactory, or should we believe our own impressions must be externally validated by others through a preponderance of outside data? To avoid treatment failure and ensure the best outcomes for our patients, we must base our clinical decisions on the best, not just *any*, evidence.

The scientific method must be the primary basis for obtaining data. In order to use it effectively and employ EBM, we must clarify the form of scientific reasoning we value as capable of providing us evidence. Traditionally, medicine, like the social and behavioral sciences, has been thought of as using hypothetico-deductive reasoning: using a theory to form a hypothesis, then following with tests to see whether the null hypothesis is defeated according to arbitrary definitions of significance (Mason et al. 2018). Recall that the null hypothesis asserts that there is no statistically significant difference between two experimental groups. Statistical significance is usually estimated with P values: low ones support the significance of a difference and high ones less so. Because there is no absolute value for P that dictates significance, researchers and practitioners must make their own judgments (Sterne and Davey Smith 2001).

The further limitations of this reductive method include its narrow, mechanistic, and deterministic view of natural phenomena. This does not allow the description of a context within the complex, dynamic, contextual environment in which we humans live (Bechtel 2009). For example, the complexity and heterogeneity of substance abuse prevention and treatment programs reduce the relevance of RCTs in evaluating narrowly defined interventions (Mason et al. 2018). Theories evaluated in isolation, rather than relative to alternative hypotheses, may result in the premature rejection of partially correct theories (Capaldi and Proctor 2008).

The use of abductive reasoning in clinical medicine (see Chapter 2, section "General Nature of Problems"), however, offers a better strategy for rigorous data collection and analysis, as well as the creation of a differential diagnosis (Stanley and Campos 2013). In the abductive theory of mind (ATOM), data are considered to be evidence only of phenomena that are observed. An observation is followed by the construction of a theory to describe the causal mechanism that produces that phenomenon. This theory is then tested and compared with competing theories (Capaldi and Proctor 2008). Confounding is controlled for either by randomization or by closely matching nonrandomized groups (Mason et al. 2018). ATOM seeks generalizability of relationships rather than just statistical significance.

Experiential and observational studies, considered individually, offer less quality information than do RCTs (Barton 2000). When randomized studies are not feasible for studying a given hypothesis, however, these naturalistic studies may be compared across multiple data sets that vary in sampling and setting, as with meta-analysis (Frieden 2017; Haig 2005). We may also find evidence beyond RCTs by employing multivariate longitudinal design (Tucker and Roth 2006), network modeling (Gilbert 2008; Heath 2000), and disease registries (Frieden 2017). ATOM abandons *certainty* (arbitrarily defined with *P*-test significance) for successive testing and competitive hypothesis revision, choosing the best hypothesis to fit the data at each step (Capaldi and Proctor 2008; Mason et al. 2018).

Gathering Evidence

The best research designs and methods of analysis offer researchers and clinicians the soundest guidance for treating patients. It is essential that the design of a study match the type of statistical analysis to be applied and that the research methods employed are able to provide the data sought for examination. All studies should be evaluated by the nature of their design *and* by how well they conform to that original design.

Randomness emerges as the key design element in good clinical research: volunteers must be randomly assigned to treatment or nontreatment groups. Researchers, as well as the participants, must be blind to the group assignment (i.e., a double-blind). Randomized, placebo-controlled, double-blind prospective studies have been the gold standard for clinical research. Although expensive and time-consuming, this design best avoids *confounding* (missing or confusing real causes), *cognitive bias*, and *sampling error*, all of which make it less likely a given patient will respond to treatment in the same way the study participants appeared to. When RCT data are available, they should be ranked as the highest evidence (Barton 2000), even, in most cases, over meta-analysis (LeLorier et al. 1997; Sivakumar and Peyton 2016). This is, of course, provided that the RCT was designed without flaws and was powered appropriately (i.e., enough participants were included in each study cell). As stated earlier, however, when RCTs are unavailable, infeasible, underpowered, or flawed, naturalistic observational studies and registries may help fill the knowledge gap (Croft et al. 2011; Frieden 2017).

Sample error is very difficult to avoid; randomization and prospective studies, as controlled experiments, observational studies, or registries, help. True randomness is difficult to achieve with retrospective studies. Further, sample size can skew significance: larger sizes are likelier to report a statistically significant response, whereas small ones carry an increased chance of missing a true effect (Levine et al. 2008). Also important is the definition of an end point to be measured. We need to be certain that measured treatment outcomes are patient-centered (e.g., symptoms, function, quality of life) rather than surrogate (e.g., biomarkers, intermediate findings) outcomes (Yu et al. 2015). In addition, because arbitrary statistical significance cannot fully describe the magnitude or likelihood of clinical effect we seek in our patients, we may better forecast them by considering number needed to treat (NNT) and number needed to harm (NNH), determined in settings more resembling clinical practice (Roose et al. 2016).

Often missing from our literature are studies that repeat the work of others or fail to show statistically significant outcomes (Turner et al. 2008). In addition to recent mandates from the World Health Organization, the United States, and Europe, the AllTrials petition attempts to resolve these omissions by requiring that individuals, companies, and organizations agree to register all past and current trials with their full methods and that all summary results be reported (All Trials 2014). The registration number of a trial, such as with ClinicalTrials.gov (National Institutes of Health 2021), should be included with both abstracts and full-text articles on publication.

Thorough familiarity with clinical research design *and* analysis is essential for us as practitioners as we evaluate studies for inclusion in our EBM database. Readers must ensure that they understand Phase I–IV studies, prospective and retrospective analyses, meta-analysis, intention to treat (ITT), risk ratio or relative risk (RR), odds ratio (OR), confidence interval (CI), *P* value, absolute risk reduction (ARR), NNT, and NNH (see Putman 2020).

We must also appreciate the level of proof that has been targeted by a publication. We do not hold open case reports to the same scientific rigor as RCTs or meta-analyses, yet may practitioners find them helpful as alerts to new insights or potential problems that can be studied by others more carefully. Similarly, small open-label studies commonly follow these reports as quicker and lower-cost evaluations of whether more expansive, difficult, and expensive studies may be justified. All have a place in the scientific canon, but it is imperative that practitioners never blur the level of evidence each of these efforts implies. Case reports and open-label studies may be suggestions for further study but are never evidence.

A "Crisis" of Reproducibility

Medical school graduation speeches commonly opine that half of what the graduates have been taught is wrong—the faculty just doesn't know which half. Although we expect that old knowledge will gradually be replaced by new, we still might not imagine that we cannot trust the conclusions published in our most revered journals. It is axiomatic in basic and clinical research that the validity of data is demonstrated by reproducibility (or replicability) of the data, an expectation we hold for the evidence of EBM. Many studies and surveys over the past two decades have suggested, however, that as many as half of the findings published in peer-reviewed journals throughout most of science, including psychology and medicine, are not replicated by further study (Baker 2016; Flier 2022; Hebert et al. 2002; Ioannidis 2005; Nieuwenhuis et al. 2011; Strasak et al. 2007a).

The role of unethical submission of plagiarized or falsified data must be considered (Krokoscz 2021). However, such data are currently estimated at an incidence of 2%–8%, so this is not the main reason for irreproducible data (Flier 2022; Gopalakrishna et al. 2022a, 2022b; Singh Chawla 2021). Given the difficulties in obtaining valid evidence reviewed here, the most common culprits of this "crisis" (Baker 2016) should not be surprising: inadequate understanding of research design and statistical methods; inability to accurately recreate methods or materials; and misaligned research and publishing incentives by usually well-intentioned researchers, granters, peer reviewers, and publishers. All of these easily lead to erroneous conclusions that are not supported by better design or even replicated with other random cohorts (Flier 2022).

A majority of the statistical analyses published in peer-reviewed medical science journals have been found to be invalid (Ercan et al. 2015). This results mostly from the evolution of complex study designs that require analytical sophistication beyond the elementary skills learned by both researchers and peer reviewers early in their scientific educations (Strasak et al. 2007b). Some journals provide guidelines or templates and hire statisticians to assist in peer review, although the participating percentage does not appear to have improved since 1998 (Goodman et al. 1998; Hardwicke and Goodman 2020). From the outset, in order to provide valid conclusions, a research design must be chosen that will fit with the method of statistical analysis selected. Observing that this intention has been registered through ClinicalTrials.gov (https://clinicaltrials.gov) or similar efforts in advance of patient enrollment can help clinicians avoid being misled by the publication of spurious significances eventually obtained from data dredging (Erasmus et al. 2022).

Publications are rarely withdrawn, even when the data are not supportable. However, the rate of withdrawal has increased steadily over the past few decades to 1 per 10,000 published articles (Azoulay et al. 2017). The time between publication and retraction is decreasing: since 2002, the average is just under 24 months (Singh et al. 2014; Steen et al. 2013). Unfortunately, a survey found that 40% of retracted papers in the mental health literature had not been flagged as such by library platforms, and 26.3% of available PDFs also did not indicate the retraction (Bakker and Riegelman 2018). Not only can clinicians locate these papers and inadvertently consider them useful data, but, unaware of the retractions, authors may cite or include them in a meta-analysis in other publications that may be correspondingly compromised. This degrades our EBM database and our patients' outcomes. Tainted articles often continue to be cited for years, even following withdrawal (Hagberg 2020). Additionally, articles identified for retraction often receive both critical and uncritical attention in social and news media and other platforms, elevating their visibility with the general public, as well as the professional community. As such, many readers may not be aware of the erroneous data of concern (Peng et al. 2022).

How can we be informed or made aware that evidence no longer thought valid is still available for us to base our treatments on? Development of a standardized process for highlighting articles that have been retracted has not yet occurred (De Cassai et al. 2022; Marcus et al. 2022; Rong et al. 2022). An article's retraction may be noted by a publisher but not by directories, such as PubMed or Google Scholar (Pfeil and Goldhammer 2022). Information in notices of retraction, including the details at issue and reasons for retraction, are also not standardized: some are detailed, and others offer no explanation (Azoulay et al. 2017).

Practitioners need to develop their own retraction strategy to search for and avoid discredited publications. It is prudent to routinely view articles on the publisher's website and not rely on abstracts from directories (just as we would never accept an abstract as evidence at face value without reviewing the structure and analysis of the data ourselves). Tools available to practitioners to help avoid considering retracted data as evidence include Retraction Watch of the Center for Scientific Integrity, which includes a detailed user guide (Retraction Watch Database 2018). Some bibliographic software (e.g., Crossmark, www.crossref.org/services/crossmark; Open Retractions, https://github.com/open-retractions/open-retractions; ReTracker, Dinh et al. 2019) can assist providers in culling retracted papers. Searching for retracted articles on databases such as PubMed, Google Scholar, BIOSIS, and PLoS One is complicated by the lack of a standard method (Table 3–1), but each platform has some discoverable technique to accomplish this (University of Massachusetts Amherst 2022). No single database is likely to discover every retracted article, however (Pastor-Ramón et al. 2022), so all clinicians must make sufficient efforts to protect the integrity and quality of the evidence to reduce the number of treatment failures and the perception of treatment resistance.

Effective Use of Evidence

Practicing EBM does not promise our patients and us the perfect solutions, just the best we can determine for the present. The correct answers will be fluid, so keeping up with the literature is essential for effective practitioners. Our sources must be valid, but we must also be able to correctly interpret any data we are going to apply as evidence (Horwitz 1996). As a busy practitioner, you have many new tools to rely on, includ-

Table 3–1. Retraction notices of popular databases

Database	Notice	References and web pages
PubMed	Citation for retraction notices: "Retraction of: [article title]"; citation for retracted articles: "Retraction in: [article title]" PDFs carry watermark	PubMed 2018
Google Scholar	Visual warning through Chrome extension RetractOmatic	Pastor-Ramón et al. 2022 Available at: https://chrome.google.com/webstore/detail/retractomatic/afopanbkaaojicelmcniljbdphjagpie/related?hl=en
BIOSIS	Retraction cited, text of statement becomes abstract, indexing copied to retraction citation	Atlas 2004
PLoS One	Notice posted at top of web page and linked to publication record	PLoS One 2023
Springer Link	Article watermarked "retracted"; explanation provided in a note linked to the watermarked article	Springer 2023
Web of Science	"RETRACTED" placed before title, with "Retracted article" and link to retraction following it	Tay 2020[a]
	Visual warning available through Chrome extension RetractOmatic	Pastor-Ramón et al. 2022 Available at: https://chrome.google.com/webstore/detail/retractomatic/afopanbkaaojicelmcniljbdphjagpie/related?hl=en

Note. Retraction notices for articles are not standardized among commonly used directories. Users must confirm the policy for each source.
[a]https://creativecommons.org/licenses/by/4.0/legalcode.

ing high-level resources such as the Cochrane Library that help you review and compare the complete literature (Cochrane Community 2022; Siwek 2018).

Contemporary EBP encompasses three elements: the best research, practitioner expertise, and patient preference (Sackett et al. 1996). Erroneous guidance may come from errors produced in any one or more of these areas. Gaps in research data may have negative impacts on practice because they leave us with inadequate information on which to base decisions (Mintzes 2013). Experts may routinely commit errors in their assessments (see Chapter 2, section "Obstacles to Problem-Solving"); as a result, the databases, goals, and perspectives of patients and family members may not be adequately understood or considered during treatment planning (Siminoff 2013).

Remember that we too often make quick diagnoses and then search for and cherry-pick data to support them rather than considering data that are inconsistent and contradictory. The same can be true in our evaluation of the medical literature (Carvour 2013). We are more likely to acknowledge data when they support our initial or long-term mindset (see section "Obstacles to Problem-Solving" in Chapter 2).

We should not just wait for new and better treatments but instead struggle to determine that we are proposing the right treatment for the right problem among the options currently available. We should also not delay in considering and suggesting newer treatments once they are validated as effective and safe. Collaborative treatments should be layered as indicated, such as psychotherapy with medication. Although genomics cannot yet tell us which treatments are most likely to work, they can help us predict which ones might not be well tolerated, and this can be quite useful in treatment planning (Greden 2022).

At any given time, clinicians may be called on to make treatment recommendations based on insufficient data. The Achilles heel of EBM, is, after all, that there so often appears to be insufficient evidence. Practitioners must then weigh what evidence is available and make their best choice as they endeavor to "do no harm" and avoid treatment failure or apparent resistance. Scholarship is an essential foundation for practitioners intending to achieve treatment success. The prepared mind will be able to sift through evidence, rank it according to the methods through which it was obtained, look at how others evaluate it, and, in the face of necessity, use it on the basis of quality.

Impact of Evidence-Based Medicine on Clinical Practice

Becoming the most effective practitioner demands releasing the role of sole, or even primary, authority when it comes to validating evidence. This is what we mean when we say to avoid anecdotal evidence—not only is it statistically invalid, but its use anoints the practitioner to become their own judge and jury, operating independently of shared, well-founded knowledge. As Scott Aaronson, M.D., director of Clinical Research at Sheppard Pratt, observed, "The plural of anecdote is not evidence" (S. Aaronson, personal communication, August 18, 2022). Just because you have experienced or heard about something more than once does not qualify it as the best data.

We talk often about countertransference in psychotherapy, but we mention it less in acute care and seldom in pharmacological practice (Jagarlamudi et al. 2012; Rubin 2001). How deeply do we examine ourselves, our motivations and perceptions, when choosing pharmacological treatments or treating an urgent case? How alert are we to the pressure of time and the narrowing of expertise through repeated evaluations and treatments of patients without adequate feedback (Tay et al. 2016; 't Hart 1991) (see section "Obstacles to Problem-Solving" in Chapter 2)?

EBP is not only about the data themselves but even more about a practitioner's self-appraisal and attitude. It is this long-term mental set that determines what type of authoritative data the practitioner will look for: subjective or objective, validated or experiential. In addition, we are stronger together: one mind alone is unlikely to routinely identify the best treatment decisions. Just like supercomputers, when we work in parallel with other professionals and researchers, we stand a better chance of finding the best solutions and avoiding treatment failure. We must always choose to cede authority in treatment options and decisions to collaboration and external validation, through RCTs, meta-analyses, competitive hypothesis revision, consensus, and new tools as they emerge—what we must define as the evidence in EBM (see Smalheiser 2017; Timmermans and Mauck 2005).

Summary

EBM, effectively synonymous with EBP, is the conscious and consistent application of the best and most current treatment outcome data to treatment planning and monitoring. It is the practice method most likely to avoid treatment failure. Honed in the last half-century to include clinical evidence from systematic research, clinical judgment, and patient preference, the practice is presumed, but often it is relegated to early didactics, its adoption limited by incomplete data sets, a lingering belief in anecdotal experience, and a bias toward mechanistic explanations of treatments over outcome data.

Abductive reasoning offers the most suitable scientific method for pursuing EBM, favoring successive testing and competitive hypothesis revision over arbitrary definitions of certainty. Outcome studies, such as RCTs and systematic reviews, when available, and prospective observational studies and registries when not, must be evaluated by the quality of their design and how well they conform to it. Practitioners must become completely familiar with the methods of clinical research design and analysis and aware of the risks of invalid and retracted research to propose the best evidence during treatment planning.

Employing forced metacognition—thinking about how we think—allows us to enhance opportunities for EBP and outcome success for our patients. Evidence must include data about our process, as well as outcomes, as we search for not only psychodynamic barriers to success but also limitations in our own processing of data (often dulled by repetition, time constraints, and acuity) that lead us to overvalue our individual clinical experience. Treatment planning must be a collaboration, not only with our patients but with colleagues through utilization of the best objective evidence.

Key Points

- Evidence-based medicine (EBM) is the deliberate use of the best outcome data for treatment planning.
- Overvaluation of clinical experience may threaten the objectivity of EBM.
- Evidence may be limited when relying solely on arbitrary significance, such as *P* values.
- Evidence may be expanded by successive theory testing and competitive hypothesis revision.
- We must possess the knowledge to correctly interpret any data we consider for evidence.
- Frequently cited articles may have been retracted.

- We are most likely to acknowledge data that fit our long-term mindset.
- We must defer authority over the validation of evidence to the best tools of our profession.

Self-Assessment Questions

1. The abductive theory of mind (ATOM) includes which of the following?

   A. Generalizability of relationships.
   B. A firm level of $P < 0.05$ for detecting statistical significance.
   C. Theories based on observation that are tested and compared with other theories.
   D. A and C.

   Correct answer: D. A and C.

   ATOM seeks generalizability of relationships rather than just statistical significance. An observation is followed by the construction of a theory to describe the causal mechanism that produces that phenomenon. This is then tested and compared with competing theories, choosing the best hypothesis to fit the data at each step. With hypothetico-deductive reasoning, when P values are used to estimate significance, there is never an absolute value for rejecting or accepting the null hypothesis. Low values support rejecting the null, indicating there is likely to be a true and important difference between experimental groups, but this judgment is up to the reader.

2. Evidence-based medicine and evidence-based practice encompass which of the following?

   A. Clinical outcome evidence from systematic research.
   B. The proficiency of the judgment of individual physicians.
   C. Individual patients' predicaments, rights, and preferences.
   D. All of the above.

   Correct answer: D. All of the above.

This is the revised and most cited definition from Sackett et al. (1996). However, clinicians should be wary of overvaluing individual judgment when strong outcome evidence is available.

3.   Which two of the following statements are true?

A. Retrospective studies help avoid sample error through true randomization.
B. Small sample sizes are more likely to miss a true effect.
C. Naturalistic observation studies are the gold standard for evidence.
D. About half of practice guidelines are outdated within 5 years.

Correct answer: B and D.

It is difficult to detect true effects with small sample sizes in randomized controlled trials (RCTs)—this is when systematic reviews using meta-analysis may be helpful. About 20% of practice guidelines are obsolete within 3 years of publication, and 50% are obsolete within 5 years. Prospective studies are more likely to approach true randomization and reduce sample error. RCTs that are well designed, executed, and analyzed are the traditional gold standard for clinical research, even over meta-analysis. When such studies are not available, observational studies may be compared across multiple data sets that vary in sampling and setting, as with meta-analysis.

4.   Number needed to treat (NNT) and number needed to harm (NNH) offer estimates of which of the following?

A. The magnitude of a clinical effect for a patient.
B. The likelihood of a clinical effect for a patient.
C. The nature of a clinical effect for a patient.
D. A and B.

Correct answer: D. A and B.

Arbitrary clinical significance from *P* values speaks to whether a particular clinical effect is possible from a given treatment. NNT and NNH estimate the likelihood that any one patient will experience benefit or harm, respectively.

5.   Which of the following offers no information beyond that obtainable from RCTs?

   A. Multivariate longitudinal design.
   B. Network modeling.
   C. Prospective registries.
   D. None of the above.

   Correct answer: D. None of the above.

   Every one of these methods may offer valid and useful data that RCT may not be designed to capture. After a thorough examination, the physician may confirm a diagnosis that an RCT may not be designed to capture.

Discussion Topics

1.   You are consulted by a patient who has undergone two unsuccessful trials of antidepressant treatment for severe major depression and learn that both treatments involved adequate doses and time allowed for response. You find no contributing health factors that might interfere with treatment, and she and her family assure you of her commitment to the treatment plans and of her compliance. Both medication trials used selective serotonin reuptake inhibitors. The family, now leery of medication, asks you to consider transcranial magnetic stimulation or cognitive-behavioral therapy for her next treatment. How will you consider the evidence for these treatments versus a third trial of medication for this patient, and how will you address the family's concerns about medication?

2.   A senior colleague mentions that a certain new treatment is being used for PTSD. What questions do you need to ask about this treatment, what sources will you search, and what criteria will allow you to consider it a valid treatment option for your patients?

Additional Readings

Flier JS: The problem of irreproducible bioscience research. Perspect Biol Med 65(3):373–395, 2022 36093772: *A thoughtful and useful exploration of irreproducibility in biomedical science, easily translatable to our field*

Mintz D: Psychodynamic Psychopharmacology: Caring for the Treatment-Resistant Patient. Washington, DC, American Psychiatric Association Publishing,

2022: *Explores psychodynamic contributions that may be leading or adding to treatment resistance*

Putman HP: Rational Psychopharmacology: A Book of Clinical Skills. Washington, DC, American Psychiatric Association Publishing, 2020: *Chapter 2, "Evidence-Based Medicine in an Era of Sparse Evidence," is a concise but comprehensive review of current clinical research design and analysis for practitioners*

Smalheiser NR: Rediscovering Don Swanson: the past, present and future of literature-based discovery. J Data Inf Sci 2(4):43–64, 2017 29355246: *An intriguing review of literature-based discovery and how it contributes evidence by linking research outcomes that would otherwise go unrecognized*

References

AllTrials: All Trials Registered, All Results Reported. London, Sense About Science, 2014. Available at www.alltrials.net/petition. Accessed August 24, 2022.

Atlas MC: Retraction policies of high-impact biomedical journals. J Med Libr Assoc 92(2):242–250, 2004 15098054

Azoulay P, Bonatti A, Krieger JL: The career effects of scandal: evidence from scientific retractions. Res Policy 46(9):1552–1569, 2017

Baker M: 1,500 scientists lift the lid on reproducibility. Nature 533(7604):452–454, 2016 27225100

Bakker C, Riegelman A: Retracted publications in mental health literature: discovery across bibliographic platforms. J Libr Sch Commun 6(1):eP2199, 2018

Barton S: Which clinical studies provide the best evidence? The best RCT still trumps the best observational study. BMJ 321(7256):255–256, 2000 10915111

Bechtel W: Looking down, around and up: mechanistic explanation in psychology. Philos Psychol 22(5):543–564, 2009

Blanco MA, Capello CF, Dorsch JL, et al: A survey study of evidence-based medicine training in US and Canadian medical schools. J Med Libr Assoc 102(3):160–168, 2014 25031556

Brater DC, Daly WJ: Clinical pharmacology in the Middle Ages: principles that presage the 21st century. Clin Pharmacol Ther 67(5):447–450, 2000 10824622

Capaldi EJ, Proctor RW: Are theories to be evaluated in isolation or relative to alternatives? An abductive view. Am J Psychol 121(4):617–641, 2008 19105581

Carey S, Hall D: Psychiatrists' views of evidence-based psychiatric practice. Psychiatr Bull 23(3):159–161, 1999

Carvour M: Teaching critical appraisal of medical evidence. Virtual Mentor 15(1):23–27, 2013 23356802

Claridge JA, Fabian TC: History and development of evidence-based medicine. World J Surg 29(5):547–553, 2005 15827845

Clark E, Donovan EF, Schoettker P: From outdated to updated, keeping clinical guidelines valid. Int J Qual Health Care 18(3):165–166, 2006 16613986

Cochrane AL: Effectiveness and Efficiency: Random Reflections on Health Services. Cambridge, UK, Royal Society of Medicine Press, 1999

Cochrane Community: Chronology of significant events and milestones in Cochrane's history. London, Cochrane, 2022. Available at https://community.cochrane.org/history. Accessed August 11, 2022.

Croft P, Malmivaara A, van Tulder M: The pros and cons of evidence-based medicine. Spine 36(17):E1121–E1125, 2011 21629165

De Cassai A, Geraldini F, De Pinto S, et al: Inappropriate citation of retracted articles in anesthesiology and intensive care medicine publications. Anesthesiology 137(3):341–350, 2022 35789367

Dinh L, Cheng Y-Y, Parulian N: ReTracker: An Open-Source Plugin for Automated and Standardized Tracking of Retracted Scholarly Publications. 2019 ACM/IEEE Joint Conference on Digital Libraries (JCDL), 2019, pp 406–407

Eddy DM: Practice policies: where do they come from? JAMA 263(9):1265–1272, 1990 2304243

Eddy DM: The origins of evidence-based medicine—a personal perspective. Virtual Mentor 13(1):55–60, 2011 23134763

Eppel A: A critical review of psychotherapy research, in Short-Term Psychodynamic Psychotherapy. Cham, Switzerland, Springer, 2018 pp 71–93

Erasmus A, Holman B, Ioannidis JPA: Data-dredging bias. BMJ Evid Based Med 27(4):209–211, 2022 34930812

Ercan I, Karadeniz PG, Cangur S, et al: Examining of published articles with respect to statistical errors in medical sciences. UHOD Uluslar Hematol Onkol Derg 25(2):130–138, 2015

Fernandez A, Sturmberg J, Lukersmith S, et al: Evidence-based medicine: is it a bridge too far? Health Res Policy Syst 13:66, 2015 26546273

Flier JS: The problem of irreproducible bioscience research. Perspect Biol Med 65(3):373–395, 2022 36093772

Frieden TR: Evidence for health decision making—beyond randomized, controlled trials. N Engl J Med 377(5):465–475, 2017 28767357

Gilbert GN: Agent-Based Models. London, Sage, 2008

Goodman SN, Altman DG, George SL: Statistical reviewing policies of medical journals: caveat lector? J Gen Intern Med 13(11):753–756, 1998 9824521

Gopalakrishna G, Ter Riet G, Vink G, et al: Prevalence of questionable research practices, research misconduct and their potential explanatory factors: a survey among academic researchers in The Netherlands. PLoS One 17(2):e0263023, 2022a 35171921

Gopalakrishna G, Wicherts JM, Vink G, et al: Prevalence of responsible research practices among academics in the Netherlands. F1000Res 11:471, 2022b 36128558

Greden JF: New interventional psychiatry treatments improve remission and/or prevention of difficult-to-treat depressions (TRD). 2021 Mood Disorders

Award Lecture presented at the American College of Psychiatrists 2022 Annual Meeting, Bonita Springs, FL, August 20, 2022

Guyatt G, Cairns J, Churchill D, et al: Evidence-based medicine: a new approach to teaching the practice of medicine. JAMA 268(17):2420–2425, 1992 1404801

Hagberg JM: The unfortunately long life of some retracted biomedical research publications. J Appl Physiol (1985) 128(5):1381–1391, 2020

Haig BD: An abductive theory of scientific method. Psychol Methods 10(4):371–388, 2005 16392993

Hampton JR: Evidence-based medicine, opinion-based medicine, and real-world medicine. Perspect Biol Med 45(4):549–568, 2002 12388887

Hardwicke TE, Goodman SN: How often do leading biomedical journals use statistical experts to evaluate statistical methods? The results of a survey. PLoS One 15(10):e0239598, 2020 33002031

Heath RA: Nonlinear Dynamics: Techniques and Applications in Psychology. Hillsdale, NJ, Lawrence Erlbaum Associates, 2000

Hebert RS, Wright SM, Dittus RS, Elasy TA: Prominent medical journals often provide insufficient information to assess the validity of studies with negative results. J Negat Results Biomed 1(1):1, 2002 12437785

Hoffman L: A brief history of psychotherapy outcome research: how history informs the current debate. Existential Psychology (blog), December 7, 2009. Available at: https://existentialpsychology.typepad.com/my_weblog/2009/12/a-brief-history-of-psychotherapy-outcome-research.html#:~:text=In%20the%201970s%20and%201980s%2C%20the%20field%20of,payer%20systems%20by%20counselors%2C%20therapists%2C%20psychologists%2C%20and%20psychiatrists. Accessed April 20, 2023.

Horwitz R: The dark side of evidence-based medicine. Cleve Clin J Med 63(6):320–323, 1996

Ioannidis JPA: Why most published research findings are false. PLoS Med 2(8):e124, 2005 16060722

Jagarlamudi K, Portillo G, Dubin W: Countertransference effects in acutely disturbed inpatients. J Psychiatr Intensive Care 8(2):105–112, 2012

Krokoscz M: Plagiarism in articles published in journals indexed in the Scientific Periodicals Electronic Library (SPELL): a comparative analysis between 2013 and 2018. Int J Educ Integr 17(1):1–22, 2021

LeLorier J, Grégoire G, Benhaddad A, et al: Discrepancies between meta-analyses and subsequent large randomized, controlled trials. N Engl J Med 337(8):536–542, 1997 9262498

Levine TR, Weber R, Hullett CR, et al: A critical assessment of null hypothesis significance testing in quantitative communication research. Hum Commun Res 34(2):171–187, 2008

Lilienfeld SO, Basterfield C: History of evidence-based practice. Oxford, UK, Oxford Research Encyclopedias, February 28, 2020. Available at: https://oxfordre.com/

psychology/display/10.1093/acrefore/9780190236557.001.0001/acrefore-9780190236557-e-633?rskey=LE40S2&result=1. Accessed August 9, 2022.

Mandell BF: Evidence-based medicine and clinical guidelines. Merck Manual Professional Version. Rahway, NJ, Merck Sharp and Dohme, 2021. Available at: www.merckmanuals.com/professional/special-subjects/clinical-decision-making/evidence-based-medicine-and-clinical-guidelines. Accessed August 11, 2022.

Marcus A, Abritis AJ, Oransky I: How to stop the unknowing citation of retracted papers. Anesthesiology 137(3):280–282, 2022 35984926

Martínez García L, Sanabria AJ, García Alvarez E, et al; Updating Guidelines Working Group: The validity of recommendations from clinical guidelines: a survival analysis. CMAJ 186(16):1211–1219, 2014 25200758

Mason WA, Cogua-Lopez J, Fleming CB, Scheier LM: Challenges facing evidence-based prevention: incorporating an abductive theory of method. Eval Health Prof 41(2):155–182, 2018 29719989

Mintzes B: Evidence-based medicine: strengths and limitations. Australian Prescriber, September 1, 2013. Available at www.nps.org.au/australian-prescriber/articles/evidence-based-medicine-strengths-and-limitations. Accessed August 9, 2022.

Nasir A: From evidence-based medicine to evidence-based practice: is there enough evidence? Middle East Fertil Soc J 15(4):294–295, 2010

National Institutes of Health: History, policies, and laws. ClinicalTrials.gov, last updated May 2021. Available at: https://clinicaltrials.gov/ct2/about-site/history#EmaExpands. Accessed September 1, 2022.

Nieuwenhuis S, Forstmann BU, Wagenmakers E-J: Erroneous analyses of interactions in neuroscience: a problem of significance. Nat Neurosci 14(9):1105–1107, 2011 21878926

Pastor-Ramón E, Herrera-Peco I, Agirre O, et al: Improving the reliability of literature reviews: detection of retracted articles through academic search engines. Eur J Investig Health Psychol Educ 12(5):458–464, 2022 35621514

Peng H, Romero DM, Horvát EÁ: Dynamics of cross-platform attention to retracted papers. Proc Natl Acad Sci USA 119(25):e2119086119, 2022 35700358

Pfeil DS, Goldhammer JE: Fake news in science: maybe they have a point? J Cardiothorac Vasc Anesth 36(2):412–413, 2022 34895965

PLoS One: Retractions, in Corrections, Expressions of Concern, and Retractions. San Francisco, CA, PLOS, 2023. Available at: https://journals.plos.org/plosone/s/corrections-and-retractions#:~:text=When%20retracting%20an%20article%2C%20PLOS,or%20by%20the%20journal%E2%80%99s%20editors. Accessed December 15, 2023.

PubMed: Retractions and retraction notices, in Errata, Retractions, and Other Linked Citations in PubMed. Bethesda, MD, National Library of Medicine, 2018. Available at: www.nlm.nih.gov/bsd/policy/errata.html#:~:text=The%

20Publication%20Type%20Retracted%20Publication,%3A%20%5Barticle% 20title%5D.%E2%80%9D. Accessed December 15, 2023.

Putman HP: Rational Psychopharmacology: A Book of Clinical Skills. Washington, DC, American Psychiatric Association Publishing, 2020

Retraction Watch Database. The Center for Scientific Integrity, New York, 2018. Available at http://retractiondatabase.org. Accessed April 7, 2023.

Rong LQ, Audisio K, Rahouma M, et al: A systematic review of retractions in the field of cardiothoracic and vascular anesthesia. J Cardiothorac Vasc Anesth 36(2):403–411, 2022 34600831

Roose SP, Rutherford BR, Wall MM, et al.: Practising evidence-based medicine in an era of high placebo response: number needed to treat reconsidered. Br J Psychiatry 208(5):416–420, 2016 27143006

Rubin J: Countertransference factors in the psychology of psychopharmacology. J Am Acad Psychoanal 29(4):565–573, 2001 11901553

Sackett DL, Rosenberg WM, Gray JA, et al: Evidence based medicine: what it is and what it isn't. BMJ 312(7023):71–72, 1996 8555924

Shekelle PG, Ortiz E, Rhodes S, et al: Validity of the Agency for Healthcare Research and Quality clinical practice guidelines: how quickly do guidelines become outdated? JAMA 286(12):1461–1467, 2001 11572738

Siminoff LA: Incorporating patient and family preferences into evidence-based medicine. BMC Med Inform Decis Mak 13(suppl 3):S6, 2013 24565268

Singh HP, Mahendra A, Yadav B, et al: A comprehensive analysis of articles retracted between 2004 and 2013 from biomedical literature—a call for reforms. J Tradit Complement Med 4(3):136–139, 2014 25161916

Singh Chawla D: 8% of researchers in Dutch survey have falsified or fabricated data. Nature: Jul 22, 2021 34294932Epub ahead of print

Sivakumar H, Peyton PJ: Poor agreement in significant findings between meta-analyses and subsequent large randomized trials in perioperative medicine. Br J Anaesth 117(4):431–441, 2016 28077529

Siwek J: Evidence-based medicine: common misconceptions, barriers, and practical solutions. Am Fam Physician 98(6):343–344, 2018 30215913

Smalheiser NR: Rediscovering Don Swanson: the past, present and future of literature-based discovery. J Data Inf Sci 2(4):43–64, 2017

Springer: Corrections and Retractions. New York, Springer, 2023. Available at: www.springer.com/gp/editorial-policies/corrections-and-retractions. Accessed December 15, 2023.

Stanley DE, Campos DG: The logic of medical diagnosis. Perspect Biol Med 56(2):300–315, 2013 23974509

Steen RG, Casadevall A, Fang FC: Why has the number of scientific retractions increased? PLoS One 8(7):e68397, 2013 23861902

Sterne JAC, Davey Smith G: Sifting the evidence—what's wrong with significance tests? BMJ 322(7280):226–231, 2001 11159626

Strasak AM, Zaman Q, Marinell G, et al: The use of statistics in medical research: a comparison of the New England Journal of Medicine and Nature Medicine. Am Stat 61(1):47–55, 2007a

Strasak AM, Zaman Q, Pfeiffer KP, et al: Statistical errors in medical research—a review of common pitfalls. Swiss Med Wkly 137(3–4):44–49, 2007b 17299669

Tay A: Understanding the current state of retractions and what you can do about it as an author to avoid citing them in papers (blog). Medium, November 17, 2020. Available at: https://medium.com/a-academic-librarians-thoughts-on-open-access/understanding-the-current-state-of-retractions-what-you-can-do-about-it-as-an-author-to-avoid-eb63a6632f1e. Accessed April 15, 2023.

Tay SW, Ryan P, Ryan CA: Systems 1 and 2 thinking processes and cognitive reflection testing in medical students. Can Med Educ J 7(2):e97–e103, 2016 28344696

't Hart P: Irving L. Janis' victims of groupthink. Polit Psychol 12(2):247–278, 1991

Timmermans S, Mauck A: The promises and pitfalls of evidence-based medicine. Health Aff (Millwood) 24(1):18–28, 2005 15647212

Tucker JA, Roth DL: Extending the evidence hierarchy to enhance evidence-based practice for substance use disorders. Addiction 101(7):918–932, 2006 16771885

Turner EH, Matthews AM, Linardatos E, et al: Selective publication of antidepressant trials and its influence on apparent efficacy. N Engl J Med 358(3):252–260, 2008 18199864

University of Massachusetts Amherst: Scientific publications: retracted publications and related topics, in Libraries. Amherst, University of Massachusetts, Amherst, 2022. Available at: https://guides.library.umass.edu/c.php?g=672689andp=4736833. Accessed August 31, 2022.

Winkelstein W Jr: The remarkable Archie: origins of the Cochrane Collaboration. Epidemiology 20(5):779, 2009 19680039

Yu T, Hsu YJ, Fain KM, et al: Use of surrogate outcomes in US FDA drug approvals, 2003–2012: a survey. BMJ Open 5(11):e007960, 2015 26614616

Zimerman AL: Evidence-based medicine: a short history of a modern medical movement. Virtual Mentor 15(1):71–76, 2013 23356811

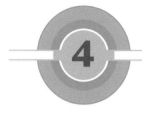

The Myth of Treatment Resistance?

In Chapter 1, "Conceptualization (and Failed Concepts)," we discussed the conceptual error of confusing the observation of a failed treatment effort with the concept of treatment resistance. Treatment resistance is a nonempirical, subjective concept that is not a standardized diagnosis, yet it is broadly applied. Does it exist? Are there data supporting the existence of any entity in psychiatry that is usually responsive, although occasionally immune, to treatment, or is it always a misconception based on limited data? To paraphrase Gertrude Stein, "Is there any there there?" (Stein 1971, p. 289).

References to patients not responding to trusted treatments have been logged since the initiation of psychotherapeutic, symptomatic, occupational, somatic, and pharmacological interventions (Ball and Kiloh 1959; Sargant 1961; Watts 1947; Young et al. 1979). Treatment-resistant schizophrenia (TRS), initially labeled *therapy resistant* or *treatment refractory*, has been discussed in the literature for more than 50 years (Itil et al. 1966). Treatment-resistant (or refractory) depression (TRD) as a specific term first appeared in the 1970s (Cowen 1988; Malhi and Byrow 2016), mostly referring to resistance to a particular treatment, such as tricyclic antidepressants (Extein 1989). Starting around 1990, TRD became both an entity and a consistent term in the literature (Gitlin 1991; Nierenberg and Amsterdam 1990; Nierenberg and White 1990). The percentage of articles addressing treatment resistance compared with total articles published in psychiatry has increased by about 75% during the past two decades (Howes et al. 2022).

Because early studies of treatment-refractory cases focused more on the inadequacy of a treatment's efficacy, there was essentially no effort to define a new diagnosis. In considering treatment resistance, we may be indicating our inability to predict response for a single patient more than we are saying that treatment never works (Anderson 2018). Some authors have explored the possibility that iatrogenic alterations from therapies may be contributing to treatment failure, and the question of in vivo tachyphylaxis remains unclear (Fornaro et al. 2019; Malhi et al. 2019; Targum 2014). Much work originally centered on finding the right treatments for the right patient, and this activity should continue to reflect our current efforts (Akiskal 1985; Pare and Mack 1971; Remick 1986).

Inconsistent Criteria

Although the term *treatment resistance* is now all too common, from the beginning there has been insufficient consensus on its definition and criteria. Issues of number, type, and quality of treatment attempts still elude the proper application of treatment resistance within most diagnoses, most notably depression, schizophrenia, OCD, and PTSD (Anderson 2018; Malhi and Byrow 2016; Malhi et al. 2019; McAllister-Williams et al. 2018; Sheitman and Lieberman 1998; Sippel et al. 2018; Voineskos et al. 2020). Most authors have found difficulty incorporating variables other than previous pharmacological treatments (Bennabi et al. 2015). The calculations of incidence and prevalence of treatment resistance, as well as meta-analysis of interventional strategies, are stymied by these inconsistent definitions (Howes et al. 2022; Zhdanava et al. 2021). However, although 100% of practitioners queried in one recent expert consensus survey still sought an operational definition, 92% of psychiatrists considered TRD a useful concept, and 85% reported they used the concept in clinical practice (Rybak et al. 2021).

Inherent in any discussion of the concept of treatment resistance is the necessity of restricting its application, withholding its use in conditions we do not currently expect to treat successfully. Cases of schizophrenia and OCD are particularly difficult to label as treatment resistant because we do not currently expect any treatment to result in a full remission (Sharma and Math 2019; Sheitman and Lieberman 1998). Positive symptoms of schizophrenia have responded well to many pharmacological treatments, whereas negative symptoms, although more amenable to treatment with atypical second-generation antipsychotic medications, still prevail for most patients (Correll and Schooler 2020; Erhart et al.

2006). Outcome expectations for OCD therapies were similarly low until clomipramine, first reported in 1966 (Lopez-Ibor 1966), was confirmed effective more than two decades later (Clomipramine Collaborative Study Group 1991; Insel et al. 1983). Currently, 40%–60% of OCD cases are likely to respond to treatment, although still without resolution, and perhaps with episodic remission. Researchers are now targeting cases refractory to this recent treatment progress (Abudy et al. 2011; Fallon et al. 1998; Sharma and Math 2019). It appears useful to restrict cases of distinct treatment failure (and any consideration of treatment resistance) to exclude irreversible medical conditions for which there is currently no effective treatment for any patient with the diagnosis.

Authors have often considered the issue of pseudo resistance, indicating that treatments attempted were flawed and inadequate in their execution rather than that competent application of state-of-the-art, previously proven procedures had failed. In fact, a review of the literature shows much more effort in ruling out true treatment resistance than providing evidence for it. Declining response rates with subsequent pharmaceutical trials may be more a factor of lower placebo response rates and less spontaneous improvement than treatment resistance to a specific therapy (Anderson 2018). Although there is support for the idea that psychiatric and medical comorbidities increase the likelihood of treatment failure, adequate testing of criteria for treatment resistance is lacking (Fava 2003). It has been proposed that the term treatment resistance be restricted to when the most promising treatments have been applied. For some authors, this includes the competent application of cognitive-behavioral therapy before affixing a label of treatment resistance or drug resistance (Fava et al. 1997, 2020; Hollinghurst et al. 2014; Wiles et al. 2013).

There are also important differences in the assessment of and reaction to 1) no response, 2) partial response, and 3) insufficient response (i.e., response compared with remission) (Malhi et al. 2019; Nierenberg and DeCecco 2001). Since the Sequenced Treatment Alternatives to Relieve Depression (STAR*D) study, it is more common to see TRD "diagnosed" following the failure of two attempts at pharmacological treatment. Occasionally, only one trial is still used, such as in the pivotal study and indication for transcranial magnetic stimulation (O'Reardon et al. 2007; Rush et al. 2006; Rybak et al. 2021). *Response* generally refers to a 50% decline in symptomatology measured by a peer-reviewed and published scale, such as the Hamilton Rating Scale for Depression (HAM-D; Hamilton 1960, 1976), the Montgomery-Åsberg Depression Rating Scale (MADRS; Montgomery and Asberg 1979), or the Clinical Global Impression (CGI;

Bobo et al. 2016; Demyttenaere and Jaspers 2020). Although *remission* is still difficult to define for schizophrenia and OCD (Andreasen et al. 2005; Davidson et al. 2008), many authors accept a HAM-D score ≤7 for major depression. The STAR*D 1-year naturalistic follow-up study showed better longer-term outcomes for patients reaching this level of response to one or more treatment attempts (Warden et al. 2007). *Recovery* is reserved for a symptom-free status (Nierenberg and DeCecco 2001). Some authors urge changing the definition of treatment resistance from nonresponse to nonremission, as used in the STAR*D study (Sinyor et al. 2010), seeking functional rather than syndromal change (National Institute of Mental Health 2022; Smith-Apeldoorn et al. 2019).

Staging

To help clarify the wide description of states that have come to be described as treatment resistant, many efforts have been made to stage degrees of treatment effort and response (Cosci and Fava 2013, 2022). The methods most commonly applied to TRD are the Thase and Rush model (Thase and Rush 1997), the Massachusetts General Hospital staging method (Fava 2003; Petersen et al. 2005), Maudsley criteria (Fekadu et al. 2009, 2018), and the Dutch Measure for Quantification of Treatment Resistance in Depression (DM-TRD; Peeters et al. 2016). Unfortunately, these staging criteria differ as widely as the original disparate definitions of TRD. It has been proposed that a categorical approach could be used to initially define treatment resistance, followed by continuous, rather than dichotomous, dimensional (functional) staging to evaluate progression and plan strategies (Rybak et al. 2021; Salloum and Papakostas 2019; van Dijk et al. 2019).

In practice, however, the value of staging TRD has not been adequately assessed for its predictive value, largely because of heterogeneity, and few methods include even limited options for psychotherapy, as do DM-TRD and a strategy proposed by Conway and associates (Anderson 2018; Conway et al. 2017; Markowitz et al. 2022; Ruhé et al. 2012). A recent meta-analysis (van Bronswijk et al. 2019) showed no superiority of psychotherapy over treatment as usual (TAU) in TRD but did show moderate effect size from combining TAU with psychotherapy (0.42 [95% CI 0.29–0.54]; Chu et al. 2020; Sullivan and Feinn 2012; van Bronswijk et al. 2019). Although following a consistent staging strategy may help a single clinician methodically work through various treatment options (Cosci and Fava 2022), it is not yet clear which method will lead to the best results.

Countertherapeutic Factors

Rather than seeking a new, unknown diagnostic category to attach to each existing classification, it seems valid to consider factors that may co-exist with our current categorical diagnoses and that fight against successful remission in a particular case (De Las Cuevas and de Leon 2017; Malhi et al. 2019). Many apparent risks factors are actually more descriptive than predictive or etiological. In addition, lifestyle decisions and behaviors commonly contribute to treatment success or failure and may masquerade as treatment resistance (Putman 2020, pp. 219–245); see also section "Lifestyle Factors" in Chapter 7, "Underappreciated Causes of Treatment Failure".

Illness behavior, which may be ameliorated or exacerbated by the doctor-patient relationship (see Chapter 9, "Managing a Sustained Therapeutic Relationship During Treatment Failure"), may contribute to treatment failure or inadequacy in three different ways: 1) what a patient perceives leads to their experience of the attempt at therapeutic alliance, 2) the patient's cognitive style and abilities affect their interpretation of these perceptions, and, thus 3) the patient's behavior and degree of collaboration interact with a proposed or prescribed treatment plan (Cosci and Fava 2016; Fava et al. 2020). At the very least, we must be aware that treatment outcomes are contingent on our therapeutic alliances; we must work to improve our understanding of patients' disease and treatment concepts and their treatment satisfaction (Fava et al. 2017; Murphy et al. 2013). See also section "Genetic and Epigenetic Factors" later in this chapter.

Cognitive impairment is a symptom in many psychiatric diagnoses and may affect executive functioning, processing speed, and working memory (particularly with unstructured and unguided tasks during depression). Dysfunctional cognitive schemata associated with depression include negative self-referential biases and trouble inhibiting or updating negative information in working memory. This is often linked to rumination, more common in females, which is likely to lead to and sustain depressive episodes (De Carlo et al. 2016; Grant et al. 2004; LeMoult and Gotlib 2019; Nolen-Hoeksema et al. 1999). Emotion regulation in depression is further impaired by a reduced ability to distract and reappraise. Altering these cognitive schemata is the basis for cognitive-behavioral therapy and similar interventions, such as emotion regulation therapy for generalized anxiety disorder and major depression and cognitive processing therapy for PTSD (LeMoult and Gotlib 2019; Renna et al. 2017; Resick et al. 2017, pp. 5–9, 25–27).

The STAR*D study was designed to be more pragmatic and informative to the average office psychiatrist than a strict randomized controlled
trial (RCT) by being open label and using patient reports and functional
(dimensional) assessments as secondary outcome measurements. It determined that although no differences were found among types of treatment
attempts at any level, patients with longer index episodes, more psychiatric
or general medical comorbidities, and/or lower measures of baseline function were less likely to achieve remission, the primary end point. Many patients reached remission if treatment continued up to 14 weeks, longer
than the standard 6- to 8-week trials of many RCTs (Sinyor et al. 2010;
Warden et al. 2007).

The literature does show that being widowed or separated is associated with lack of remission. Nonresponse to additional treatments is associated with longer duration of an episode, moderately high suicidal
risk ($P=0.001$, odds ratio [OR] 2.2), more hospitalizations, and use of
higher doses of antidepressants and antipsychotics; older age has a weak
correlation (De Carlo et al. 2016; Souery et al. 2007); for discussion of
odds ratio, see Szumilas (2010). The broader term treatment resistance
is associated with earlier onset in cases of major depression ($P=0.009$,
OR 2.0), bipolar disorder, schizophrenia, and anxiety as the number of
recurrent episodes and duration of episodes extend (Smith-Apeldoorn et
al. 2019; Souery et al. 2007). In other words, most authors agree that
greater severity is linked to treatment failure.

Coexisting conditions can also play a role in disappointing treatment
results. Anxiety symptoms alongside a diagnosis of depression reduce
the chances of remission ($P<0.001$, OR 2.6), and the concomitant presence of either panic disorder ($P<0.001$, OR 3.2) or social anxiety disorder
($P=0.008$, OR 2.1) reduces response (De Carlo et al. 2016; Souery et al.
2007). Comorbidity with other psychiatric disorders, in general, does indicate that each diagnosis may be more difficult to treat, with response
rates being 25%–30% lower (Smith-Apeldoorn et al. 2019). For this reason, some authors suggest beginning treatment for comorbidities concurrently.

There are some situations in which concurrent treatment may be ill-
advised and may contribute to treatment failure, however, such as when
ADHD is prematurely and incorrectly diagnosed and treated, simply on
the basis of the presence of poor concentration in mood disorders. Stimulants are unnecessary in the treatment of routine major depression and
may inadvertently worsen mood, anxiety, sleep, and appetite (Bahji and
Mesbah-Oskui 2021; Berman et al. 2009; Efron et al. 1997). A logical pro-

gression in diagnosis and careful planning to avoid iatrogenic outcomes are recommended (Spencer et al. 1999; Turgay and Ansari 2006).

There is no association with TRD and specific drugs or molecules, nor with augmentation or switching strategies. The number of previous treatment trials is predictive in some reviews but not prognostic in others. Data supporting associations with personality disorders are weak or nonconfirmatory ($P=0.049$, OR 1.7) (De Carlo et al. 2016; Papakostas et al. 2003; Petersen et al. 2002; Smith-Apeldoorn et al. 2019; Souery et al. 2007). Although there is inconsistent evidence for subtypes of depression (De Carlo et al. 2016; Gronemann et al. 2018), randomization erases important distinctions among subtypes of nonresponders and also obscures iatrogenic factors (or iatrogenic comorbidity). To avoid this, clinical studies might use homogeneous samples of symptoms or treatment history to provide new and useful information for practitioners (Malhi et al. 2019).

Genetic and Epigenetic Factors

There is some evidence that genetic factors play a role in TRD and psychosis (including TRS), as there is for a decreased volume of gray matter and enlarged lateral and third ventricles. Some genetic polymorphisms are linked to our broad definition of treatment resistance (Smith-Apeldoorn et al. 2019). Many antidepressant and antipsychotic medications cross the blood-brain barrier via the transporter protein P-glycoprotein (P-gp), coded for by the *ABCB1* gene. This transporter also limits toxins entering the brain. It has been theorized that as P-gp function is decreased during neuroinflammatory events, it may contribute to the development of depression and psychosis. Further, P-gp single-nucleotide polymorphisms (SNPs) rs2032583 and rs2235015 have been found to have a significant impact on the outcome of antidepressant therapy (Boiso Moreno et al. 2013; Breitenstein et al. 2015; Mossel et al. 2021, pp. 45–81).

The brain-derived neurotrophic factor gene (*BDNF*) and its top three SNPs are linked to symptomatology and resistance to clozapine treatment in schizophrenia, respectively (OR 2.57, 2.19, and 2.08) (Suchanek-Raif et al. 2020; Zhang et al. 2013). TRD is three times more likely in patients carrying both the 5-HT1A C1019G polymorphism GG genotype and the A allele of *BDNF* G196A (Val66Met) polymorphism (Anttila et al. 2007). The SNP *BDNF* rs6265 in the presence of *NTRK2* gene variants (rs1387923, rs2769605, and rs1565445) in Han Chinese patients likely contributes to TRD (OR 1.43, 95% CI 1.16–1.76, $P=0.0008$; OR 1.41, 95% CI 1.14–1.74, $P=0.0014$) (Li et al. 2013). A discrete functional polymorphism (rs1805502) of *GRIN2B*, which in humans codes for the 2B subunit of the *N*-methyl-D-aspartate receptor, has been linked to increased risk of TRD when there is an excess of the G allele (OR 1.55, 95% CI 1.18–2.05, corrected $P = 0.008$) (Bennabi et al. 2015; Zhang et al. 2014). *FKBP5* and *CACNA1C* SNPs may also have an impact on antidepressant response and TRD through reduced negative feedback of the hypothalamic-pituitary-adrenal axis and L-type calcium channel activity affecting neuroplasticity, respectively (Fabbri et al. 2018).

It is important to remember that gene expression is influenced by environmental exposure; causes and effects have cross-influences. We must also take into account, then, the social milieu in which our treatments take place, including economic situation, education, resource allocation, lifestyle, and personal understanding of disease. Stressors, which are potentially unrecognized, may contribute to observations of treatment resistance (Tripathi et al. 2019); see Chapter 3, "The Goal of Evidence-Based Practice," sections "Resistance to Evidence-Based Medicine" and "Effective Use of Evidence."

We have become increasingly conscious of ethnic and socioeconomic factors that likely add to the number of treatment failures, particularly in cases of TRS but of other disorders as well (Smith-Apeldoorn et al. 2019; Teo et al. 2013). Ethnicity linked to social factors has been associated with TRS through delay in initial treatment (Singh and Grange 2006) and access to newer, more effective, and better tolerated medications (de Freitas et al. 2022; Herbeck et al. 2004). In psychiatric research, African Americans have a higher noncompletion rate in RCTs, such as in the STAR*D study, largely due to lower levels of treatment satisfaction, despite higher objective estimates of depressed mood (Lesser et al. 2011; Murphy et al. 2013). Sample error in RCTs misses many racial and ethnic minority patients, potentially skewing outcomes and obscuring important physiological differences. This includes SNP-mediated differences in cytochrome P450 drug metabolism (McGraw and Waller 2012) but perhaps also the impact of issues such as experienced racism and economic disparity on gene expression (Price et al. 2022).

Metabolic Factors

In addition to the common medical conditions discussed in Chapter 6, "Successful Outcomes," and Chapter 7, evidence exists of rare metabolic disorders that infrequently preclude response to standard treatments. Metabolomics examines patterns of metabolic intermediates to characterize dysfunctional metabolic pathways that may relate to neuropsychiatric symptoms. Failure to address these inborn errors of metabolism will likely result in treatment failure or treatment resistance, even in the absence of systemic disease (Pan et al. 2017). In a case-control study of 33 cases of conservatively diagnosed TRD (at least three failed maximum-dose, adequate-duration medication treatment attempts), Pan et al. (2017) detected 21 patients with metabolite abnormalities. Cerebral folate deficiency was the most common (12/33), and all of these patients showed clinical improvement when treated with folinic acid. One patient also had low levels of tetrahydrobiopterin metabolites in the cerebrospinal fluid and responded to treatment with sapropterin. Five patients had an acylcarnitine profile abnormality. One case of each of the following conditions was also found in this group of patients: a low guanidinoacetate level (and a creatine/creatinine ratio consistent with a creatine synthesis deficit), Fabry's disease, a 20p12.1 microdeletion, and a 15q13.3 microduplication on microarray analysis.

In a larger study, 32 of 124 patients with TRD were found to have one of three metabolic deficiencies for which they were screened (McClain et al. 2020). In an investigation of recurrent major depression, metabolomics was able to explain up to 43% of the phenotypic variance (Mocking et al. 2021). There is a rare inherited error of metabolism that leads to lower levels of folate and vitamin B_{12}, cofactors in the synthesis of *S*-adenosyl methionine (SAMe; see section "Lifestyle Factors" in Chapter 7, "Underappreciated Causes of Treatment Failure"). This interferes with myelination and the biosynthesis of monoamine neurotransmitters, resulting in dementia and depression. Given the poor quality of studies to this point, there is only low-quality evidence of the effectiveness of oral administration of SAMe in reversing depression, compared with placebo or other single or combined treatments (Galizia et al. 2016; Sharma et al. 2017). Although use of metabolomics to examine treatment-resistant conditions in psychiatry is just beginning, metabolomics does inform us that a wide range of inborn errors of metabolism may be an unidentified factor in some rare cases that resist treatment.

Insufficient Evidence

The lack of consensus on definition, due to myriad subdivisions of possible outcomes, argues against any useful conception of treatment resistance. Heterogeneous biotypes respond to different mechanisms of action (Nasrallah 2021) or other necessary interventions. The prepon-

derance of evidence tells us that treatment resistance is not a discrete entity but instead is the result of many different origins—an individual
situation that must be determined for each treatment failure, with specific causes that are unlikely to be identical to many other cases. Adopting treatment resistance as an explanation, rather than treatment failure
as a stage, misdirects the clinician from discovering critical solutions to
improve the sometimes desperate, and always initially undesirable, conditions of the patient. It also threatens to worsen prognosis by unneces-
sarily extending the length of an index or recurrent episode (Drake et al.
2020; Kraus et al. 2019; Severe et al. 2020; Sharma and Math 2019) and
increases the risk of death and burden of disease by prolonging categorical and functional impairments (Carney and Freedland 2009; Demyttenaere and Van Duppen 2019; Greden 2001; Jaffe et al. 2019; Kennedy et
al. 2014). It has been wisely suggested that the term *difficult to treat* may
be more useful (Demyttenaere 2019).

Pharmaceutical companies (joining manufacturers of transcranial
magnetic stimulation machines) have begun to seek indications for marketing products targeting treatment resistance (Cristea and Naudet
2019; Moncrieff 2003; Singh et al. 2020; Turner 2019, 2020). However,
because there is no official definition of treatment resistance, there can
be no specific treatment for it, and the effort begins to resemble a snipe
hunt. If a condition is treatable, it is not, logically, treatment resistant.

The application of the term treatment resistance is unnecessary, tau-
tological, and misconceptualized from misdiagnosis and treatment error, a reification that too many people have come to believe exists apart
from the conditions that lead to this mirage (Anderson 2018; Malhi et al.
2019). Rather than persisting in a search for the proverbial needle in the
haystack that has defied identification over more than four decades, examination and organization of the hay appears to be more productive because it appears there is only biomass. At the very least, this awareness
should constantly redirect us to consider and explore the individual
characteristics of cases and the circumstances around treatment failures
rather than adopting an assault on a poorly characterized and operation-
ally nonexistent entity.

Case Example

Colin (not his real name) experienced his first episode of psychosis in
2012 at age 19 while attending college. According to his family, he was
treated with antipsychotic medication for some period of time, with resolution of positive symptoms, including hyperreligiosity and strong sex-

ual thoughts. It is not known how well he continued his treatment, and he experienced a second episode a year later that led to treatment with second-generation antipsychotics. He was considered functional for a brief period while he was taking medication, which he then discontinued. He was hospitalized for a third time in 2014, was diagnosed with schizophrenia, and was treated once more with antipsychotic medications. His history between that hospitalization and his fourth known hospitalization in 2021 in another state is murky. At the time of that admission, his medications were aripiprazole 300 mg IM monthly, with olanzapine 10 mg and escitalopram 10 mg daily. On discharge 2 months later, he was prescribed aripiprazole 400 mg IM monthly, with daily oral aripiprazole 20 mg, olanzapine 10 mg, and escitalopram 30 mg.

Nine months later, Colin was admitted to an academic medical center for his fifth psychiatric hospitalization. By this time, he had acquired a diagnosis of TRS. He was mute and unable to participate in an interview; ultimately, a diagnosis of catatonia was made, and he was transferred to the psychiatric intensive care unit, where he was initially given oral aripiprazole 15 mg/day and lorazepam 2 mg q 8 hours. The aripiprazole was then tapered and discontinued, olanzapine was restarted and titrated to 20 mg/day, and his dose of lorazepam was increased to 3 mg qid. He became more verbal and responsive, and his behavior was not as repetitive, but he still showed severe speech latency, as well as strong sexual thoughts and hyperreligiosity, as reported with previous episodes.

Right unilateral electroconvulsive therapy (ECT) was begun, but Colin experienced hypotension following the second treatment. He was evaluated in the emergency department (ED), where a chest X-ray was normal. After several additional ECT treatments, he developed hypoxia with pink, frothy sputum and returned to the ED, where, after finding consolidation of the lower lobe of his right lung, staff transferred him to the medical ICU. During Colin's stay there, the psychiatric consultation team continued his olanzapine at 20 mg qhs, changed his lorazepam to 5 mg bid, and suspended ECT until he was medically stable. Diagnosed with aspiration pneumonia, acute hypoxemic respiratory failure, and severe sepsis, he was treated with antibiotics for 7 days. He improved and was returned to the psychiatric floor.

On arrival, Colin stated that he felt hopeful and wanted to get better during the hospital stay; he allowed the treatment team to contact his family, who provided additional history. His consistent goal was ultimately to stop all medications, but he was amenable to restarting ECT. He continued to be somewhat hyperreligious and persisted with his plan to go to a monastery out of state after leaving the hospital. When ECT was restarted, glycopyrrolate 0.4 mg was added to reduce oral secretions, and the subsequent seven ECT treatments proceeded without complication.

Attempts were made to decrease Colin's lorazepam from 5 mg bid to 4 mg qam and 5 mg qhs and to increase his olanzapine from 20 mg qhs to 30 mg qhs, but on discharge his dosages were 5 mg bid and 20 mg qhs, respectively. Maintenance ECT was also continued by the academic center, and his treatment was managed by a local community health center. The treatment team wished to reintroduce a selective serotonin reuptake inhibitor (SSRI), particularly paroxetine, for his obsessive thoughts, but Colin declined: he thought moving to a monastery would be the best solution for his persistently strong sexual thoughts. Overall, this fifth in-patient treatment was able to reverse his symptoms of catatonia and moderate his positive symptoms of psychosis.

Melvin J. Thomas, M.D., assistant professor in the Department of Psychiatry at the University of Texas at Austin Dell Medical School, the attending psychiatrist who generously provided this case example, shared the feelings of inadequacy he and the treatment team felt in attempting to help this patient previously classified with TRS. He acknowledged how discouraging applying a label of treatment resistance is for providers, as well as patients and family (Demyttenaere and Van Duppen 2019).

We must always remember the alternative categories under which such a case may be listed. In this example, a diagnosis of bipolar disorder was considered, but the clinicians could not identify symptoms they thought were consistent with mania, and they considered the patient's negative symptoms to not be indicative of depression. They also linked his hypersexuality to his obsessive thoughts. However, affective disorders, particularly bipolar disorder, are frequently the cause of catatonia (Abrams and Taylor 1976; Jaimes-Albornoz et al. 2022; Morrison 1973; Rasmussen et al. 2016) and might also explain the patient's hypersexuality and response to ongoing ECT once the catatonia had resolved. Additionally, although most authors consider one or two failed trials of antipsychotic medications to indicate treatment resistance in schizophrenia, it is not at all clear from the history that this patient showed enough sustained compliance with medication to meet criteria for failed trials; we do know that he persistently expressed a preference for any treatment other than medication, choosing continuation ECT over clozapine and repeatedly telling providers he planned to not be taking medication long term. Further, remembering how schizophrenia is never likely to respond fully to any antipsychotic treatment (see section "Inconsistent Criteria"), the response of the patient's positive symptoms, from either ECT or antipsychotic medication, more than once appears standard, not treatment resistant. This case could also be labeled response, not remission, noncompliant, or, possibly, alternative diagnosis and illustrates how the label of treatment resistant adds no value to treatment planning.

Summary

The occasional lack of response to all types of otherwise validated interventions has been documented in the literature since modern treatment began early in the twentieth century. Whereas early reports centered on the lack of consistent therapeutic effect of a specific treatment, the last three decades have seen an explosion in the concept of treatment resistance, now often referred to as an entity, rather than a treatment phase category (i.e., treatment failure). The focus has shifted from evaluation of a treatment to description of a patient's condition.

Broad literature review, however, shows more success in identifying individual explanations for treatment failure than actually identifying a "diagnosis" of treatment resistance. Some patients require treatment plans that differ from the needs of others with the same diagnosis. Efforts to confirm or reject the hypothesis of treatment resistance as a valid concept are stymied by a lack of consensus on criteria for every diagnostic category: the number, type, length, assessment methods, and quality of treatment efforts examined are not standardized for definition. Proposed staging criteria are just as variable and currently appear most useful for organizing methodical treatment planning.

The presence of psychiatric and other medical comorbidities lowers treatment response rates by 25%–30%; whether the simultaneous treatment of all conditions present is optimal depends on logical, accurate diagnosing and thoughtful treatment planning in order to avoid iatrogenic complications. The weight of evidence shows that treatment failure is linked most specifically to the severity and length of symptoms but also sometimes to illness behavior; cognitive impairment (especially rumination); and genetic, epigenetic, and rare metabolic factors. Understanding how a patient perceives illness and treatment recommendations can help mitigate treatment failure. Clinicians must approach every case of treatment failure individually, applying labels carefully and searching for one or more unique causes, rather than conceptualizing a global origin that evades reproducibility, explanation, and validity.

Key Points

- Failed treatment efforts have been reported throughout the modern era of treatment.

- *Treatment resistance* originally referred to the efficacy of treatments.
- There is insufficient consensus on treatment resistance criteria for every diagnosis.
- Comorbidities and severity increase the possibility of treatment failure.
- Outcomes are often based on the quality of the therapeutic alliance.
- A wide variety of medical, social, and cognitive factors lead to treatment failure.
- Treatment resistance is not a discrete entity but results from many unique causes.
- Having a standard treatment for treatment resistance is illogical and incorrect.

Self-Assessment Questions

1. Declining response rates to subsequent treatment attempts may be related to which of the following?

   A. Lower placebo response rates.
   B. Treatment resistance.
   C. Less spontaneous improvement.
   D. A and C.

   Correct answer: D. A and C.

   Placebo response, in particular, is more likely to appear earlier in treatment. In the STAR*D study, many patients achieved remission if treatment continued up to 14 weeks, longer than the standard 6–8 weeks used in many RCTs. Treatment resistance is not a valid entity and should be considered to be treatment failure.

2. Dysfunctional cognitive schemata linked to depression include which of the following?

   A. Negative self-referential biases.
   B. Reduced ability to distract and reappraise.

C. Rumination.

D. All of the above.

Correct answer: D. All of the above.

Trouble inhibiting or updating negative information in working memory is one reason standard treatments may fail. Altering these cognitive schemata is the focus of cognitive-behavioral therapy and emotion regulation therapy.

3. A 50% decline in symptomatology measured by peer-reviewed and published scales is a common criteria for which of the following?

A. Remission.

B. Response.

C. Recovery.

D. None of the above.

Correct answer: B. Response.

Remission criteria vary according to diagnosis, and recovery refers to symptom-free status. Commonly used validated scales include the HAM-D, MADRS, and CGI.

4. Which of the following statements is false?

A. There is no association between TRD and specific switching strategies.

B. There is inconsistent evidence for subtypes of depression.

C. Randomization highlights distinctions among subtypes of TRD.

D. Randomization obscures iatrogenic comorbidity.

Correct answer: C. Randomization highlights distinctions among subtypes of TRD.

Randomization erases important distinctions among subtypes. Studying homogeneous samples of symptoms or treatment history may help avoid this artifact.

5.   There is evidence in TRD and TRS for which of the following?

   A. Genetic factors.
   B. An increased volume of gray matter.
   C. Smaller lateral and third ventricles.
   D. No influence of SNPs.

   Correct answer: A. Genetic factors.

   Multiple SNPs have been linked to TRD and TRS, along with a decreased volume of gray matter and larger lateral and third ventricles.

Discussion Topics

1. A patient previously diagnosed as having TRS is brought to you by her sister and brother-in-law. Her previous provider wanted to treat her with clozapine, given that it is the only medication to have an indication from the FDA for TRS. They are concerned about side effects. How would you discuss the "diagnosis" of TRS, the FDA indication, and treatment options with them?
2. A patient seeks a second opinion from you about beginning transcranial magnetic stimulation after a failure of one trial of an SSRI from his primary care physician; he is concerned about the cost. Given the FDA indication for transcranial magnetic stimulation use in those who have not achieved satisfactory improvement from prior antidepressant medication, how would you approach your assessment and discussion of options with him?

Additional Readings

Howes OD, Thase ME, Pillinger T: Treatment resistance in psychiatry: state of the art and new directions. Mol Psychiatry (27):58–72, 2022: *A concise review of current competing theories of treatment resistance, problems with definition, neurobiological possibilities, and direction of future efforts*

Nemeroff CB (ed): Management of Treatment-Resistant Major Psychiatric Disorders. New York, Oxford University Press, 2012: *Discussion by leaders in the field of how treatment resistance may be considered and approached in each subspecialty; although published a decade ago, the frameworks and conceptualizations remain valid and informative today*

References

Abrams R, Taylor MA: Catatonia: a prospective clinical study. Arch Gen Psychiatry 33(5):579–581, 1976 1267574

Abudy A, Juven-Wetzler A, Zohar J: Pharmacological management of treatment-resistant obsessive-compulsive disorder. CNS Drugs 25(7):585–596, 2011 21699270

Akiskal HS: A proposed clinical approach to chronic and "resistant" depressions: evaluation and treatment. J Clin Psychiatry 46(10 Pt 2):32–37, 1985 3930475

Anderson IM: We all know what we mean by treatment-resistant depression—don't we? Br J Psychiatry 212(5):259–261, 2018 29693539

Andreasen NC, Carpenter WT Jr, Kane JM, et al: Remission in schizophrenia: proposed criteria and rationale for consensus. Am J Psychiatry 162(3):441–449, 2005 15741458

Anttila S, Huuhka K, Huuhka M, et al: Interaction between 5-HT1A and BDNF genotypes increases the risk of treatment-resistant depression. J Neural Transm (Vienna) 114(8):1065–1068, 2007 17401528

Bahji A, Mesbah-Oskui L: Comparative efficacy and safety of stimulant-type medications for depression: s systematic review and network meta-analysis. J Affect Disord 292:416–423, 2021 34144366

Ball JR, Kiloh LG: A controlled trial of imipramine in treatment of depressive states. BMJ 2(5159):1052–1055, 1959 13796229

Bennabi D, Aouizerate B, El-Hage W, et al: Risk factors for treatment resistance in unipolar depression: a systematic review. J Affect Disord 171:137–141, 2015 25305428

Berman SM, Kuczenski R, McCracken JT, et al: Potential adverse effects of amphetamine treatment on brain and behavior: a review. Mol Psychiatry 14(2):123–142, 2009 18698321 (Correction Mol Psychiatry 15(11):1121, 2010)

Bobo WV, Angleró GC, Jenkins G, et al: Validation of the 17-item Hamilton Depression Rating Scale definition of response for adults with major depressive disorder using equipercentile linking to Clinical Global Impression scale ratings: analysis of Pharmacogenomic Research Network Antidepressant Medication Pharmacogenomic Study (PGRN-AMPS) data. Hum Psychopharmacol 31(3):185–192, 2016 26999588

Boiso Moreno S, Zackrisson AL, Jakobsen Falk I, et al: ABCB1 gene polymorphisms are associated with suicide in forensic autopsies. Pharmacogenet Genomics 23(9):463–469, 2013 23820292

Breitenstein B, Brückl TM, Ising M, et al: ABCB1 gene variants and antidepressant treatment outcome: a meta-analysis. Am J Med Genet B Neuropsychiatr Genet 168B(4):274–283, 2015 25847751

Carney RM, Freedland KE: Treatment-resistant depression and mortality after acute coronary syndrome. Am J Psychiatry 166(4):410–417, 2009 19289455

Chu B, Liu M, Leas EC, et al: Effect size reporting among prominent health journals: a case study of odds ratios. BMJ Evid Based Med 26(4):184, 2020 33303479

Clomipramine Collaborative Study Group: Clomipramine in the treatment of patients with obsessive-compulsive disorder. Arch Gen Psychiatry 48(8):730–738, 1991 1883256

Conway CR, George MS, Sackeim HA: Toward an evidence-based, operational definition of treatment-resistant depression: when enough is enough. JAMA Psychiatry 74(1):9–10, 2017 27784055

Correll CU, Schooler NR: Negative symptoms in schizophrenia: a review and clinical guide for recognition, assessment, and treatment. Neuropsychiatr Dis Treat 16:519–534, 2020 32110026

Cosci F, Fava GA: Staging of mental disorders: systematic review. Psychother Psychosom 82(1):20–34, 2013 23147126

Cosci F, Fava GA: The clinical inadequacy of the DSM-5 classification of somatic symptom and related disorders: an alternative trans-diagnostic model. CNS Spectr 21(4):310–317, 2016 26707822

Cosci F, Fava GA: Staging of unipolar depression: systematic review and discussion of clinical implications. Psychol Med 52(9):1621–1628, 2022 35655409

Cowen PJ: Depression resistant to tricyclic antidepressants. BMJ 297(6646):435–436, 1988 3139133

Cristea IA, Naudet F: US Food and Drug Administration approval of esketamine and brexanolone. Lancet Psychiatry 6(12):975–977, 2019 31680013

Davidson L, Schmutte T, Dinzeo T, Andres-Hyman R: Remission and recovery in schizophrenia: practitioner and patient perspectives. Schizophr Bull 34(1):5–8, 2008 17984297

De Carlo V, Calati R, Serretti A: Socio-demographic and clinical predictors of non-response/non-remission in treatment resistant depressed patients: a systematic review. Psychiatry Res 240:421–430, 2016 27155594

de Freitas DF, Patel I, Kadra-Scalzo G, et al: Ethnic inequalities in clozapine use among people with treatment-resistant schizophrenia: a retrospective cohort study using data from electronic clinical records. Soc Psychiatry Psychiatr Epidemiol 57(7):1341–1355, 2022 35246709

De Las Cuevas C, de Leon J: Reviving research on medication attitudes for improving pharmacotherapy: focusing on adherence. Psychother Psychosom 86(2):73–79, 2017 28183085

Demyttenaere K: What is treatment resistance in psychiatry? A "difficult to treat" concept. World Psychiatry 18(3):354–355, 2019 31496099

Demyttenaere K, Jaspers L: Trends in (not) using scales in major depression: a categorization and clinical orientation. Eur Psychiatry 63(1):e91, 2020 32962793

Demyttenaere K, Van Duppen Z: The impact of (the concept of) treatment-resistant depression: an opinion review. Int J Neuropsychopharmacol 22(2):85–92, 2019 29961822

Drake RJ, Husain N, Marshall M, et al: Effect of delaying treatment of first-episode psychosis on symptoms and social outcomes: a longitudinal analysis and modelling study. Lancet Psychiatry 7(7):602–610, 2020 32563307

Efron D, Jarman F, Barker M: Side effects of methylphenidate and dexamphetamine in children with attention deficit hyperactivity disorder: a double-blind, crossover trial. Pediatrics 100(4):662–666, 1997 9310521

Erhart SM, Marder SR, Carpenter WT: Treatment of schizophrenia negative symptoms: future prospects. Schizophr Bull 32(2):234–237, 2006 16492797

Extein IL (ed): Treatment of Tricyclic-Resistant Depression. Washington, DC, American Psychiatric Press, 1989

Fabbri C, Corponi F, Albani D, et al: Pleiotropic genes in psychiatry: calcium channels and the stress-related FKBP5 gene in antidepressant resistance. Prog Neuropsychopharmacol Biol Psychiatry 81:203–210, 2018 28989100

Fallon BA, Liebowitz MR, Campeas R, et al: Intravenous clomipramine for obsessive-compulsive disorder refractory to oral clomipramine: a placebo-controlled study. Arch Gen Psychiatry 55(10):918–924, 1998 9783563

Fava GA, Savron G, Grandi S, et al: Cognitive-behavioral management of drug-resistant major depressive disorder. J Clin Psychiatry 58(6):278–284, 1997 9228899

Fava GA, Tomba E, Bech P: Clinical pharmacopsychology: conceptual foundations and emerging tasks. Psychother Psychosom 86(3):134–140, 2017 28490035

Fava GA, Cosci F, Guidi J, et al: The deceptive manifestations of treatment resistance in depression: a new look at the problem. Psychother Psychosom 89(5):265–273, 2020 32325457

Fava M: Diagnosis and definition of treatment-resistant depression. Biol Psychiatry 53(8):649–659, 2003 12706951

Fekadu A, Wooderson S, Donaldson C, et al: A multidimensional tool to quantify treatment resistance in depression: the Maudsley staging method. J Clin Psychiatry 70(2):177–184, 2009 19192471

Fekadu A, Donocik JG, Cleare AJ: Standardisation framework for the Maudsley staging method for treatment resistance in depression. BMC Psychiatry 18(1):100, 2018 29642877

Fornaro M, Anastasia A, Novello S, et al: The emergence of loss of efficacy during antidepressant drug treatment for major depressive disorder: an integrative review of evidence, mechanisms, and clinical implications. Pharmacol Res 139:494–502, 2019 30385364

Galizia I, Oldani L, Macritchie K, et al: S-adenosyl methionine (SAMe) for depression in adults. Cochrane Database Syst Rev 10(10):CD011286, 2016 27727432

Gitlin MJ: Treatment-resistant depression. West J Med 155(5):521, 1991 1815398

Grant KE, Lyons AL, Finkelstein JA, et al: Gender differences in rates of depressive symptoms among low-income, urban, African American youth: a test of two mediational hypotheses. J Youth Adolesc 33(6):523–533, 2004

Greden JF: The burden of disease for treatment-resistant depression. J Clin Psychiatry 62(Suppl 16):26–31, 2001 11480881

Gronemann FH, Jorgensen MB, Nordentoft M, et al: Incidence of, risk factors for, and changes over time in treatment-resistant depression in Denmark: a register-based cohort study. J Clin Psychiatry 79(4):17m11845, 2018

Hamilton M: A rating scale for depression. J Neurol Neurosurg Psychiatry 23(1):56–62, 1960 14399272

Hamilton M: The role of rating scales in psychiatry. Psychol Med 6(3):347–349, 1976 996197

Herbeck DM, West JC, Ruditis I, et al: Variations in use of second-generation antipsychotic medication by race among adult psychiatric patients. Psychiatr Serv 55(6):677–684, 2004 15175466

Hollinghurst S, Carroll FE, Abel A, et al: Cost-effectiveness of cognitive-behavioural therapy as an adjunct to pharmacotherapy for treatment-resistant depression in primary care: economic evaluation of the CoBalT trial. Br J Psychiatry 204(1):69–76, 2014 24262818

Howes OD, Thase ME, Pillinger T: Treatment resistance in psychiatry: state of the art and new directions. Mol Psychiatry 27(1):58–72, 2022 34257409

Insel TR, Murphy DL, Cohen RM, et al: Obsessive-compulsive disorder: a double-blind trial of clomipramine and clorgyline. Arch Gen Psychiatry 40(6):605–612, 1983 6342562

Itil TM, Keskiner A, Fink M: Therapeutic studies in "therapy resistant" schizophrenic patients. Compr Psychiatry 7(6):488–493, 1966 4382831

Jaffe DH, Rive B, Denee TR: The humanistic and economic burden of treatment-resistant depression in Europe: a cross-sectional study. BMC Psychiatry 19(1):247, 2019 31391065

Jaimes-Albornoz W, Ruiz de Pellon-Santamaria A, Nizama-Vía A, et al: Catatonia in older adults: a systematic review. World J Psychiatry 12(2):348–367, 2022 35317341

Kennedy JL, Altar CA, Taylor DL, et al: The social and economic burden of treatment-resistant schizophrenia: a systematic literature review. Int Clin Psychopharmacol 29(2):63–76, 2014 23995856

Kraus C, Kadriu B, Lanzenberger R, et al: Prognosis and improved outcomes in major depression: a review. Transl Psychiatry 9(1):127, 2019 30944309

LeMoult J, Gotlib IH: Depression: a cognitive perspective. Clin Psychol Rev 69:51–66, 2019 29961601

Lesser IM, Zisook S, Gaynes BN, et al: Effects of race and ethnicity on depression treatment outcomes: the CO-MED trial. Psychiatr Serv 62(10):1167–1179, 2011 21969643

Li Z, Zhang Y, Wang Z, et al: The role of BDNF, NTRK2 gene and their interaction in development of treatment-resistant depression: data from multicenter, prospective, longitudinal clinic practice. J Psychiatr Res 47(1):8–14, 2013 23137999

Lopez-Ibor JJ: Monochlorimipramine clinical trial, paper presented at the Fourth World Congress of Psychiatry, World Psychiatric Association, Madrid, 1966

Malhi GS, Byrow Y: Is treatment-resistant depression a useful concept? Evid Based Ment Health 19(1):1–3, 2016 26767390

Malhi GS, Das P, Mannie Z, et al: Treatment-resistant depression: problematic illness or a problem in our approach? Br J Psychiatry 214(1):1–3, 2019 30565539

Markowitz JC, Wright JH, Peeters F, et al: The neglected role of psychotherapy for treatment-resistant depression. Am J Psychiatry 179(2):90–93, 2022 35105164

McAllister-Williams RH, Christmas DMB, Cleare AJ, et al: Multiple-therapy-resistant major depressive disorder: a clinically important concept. Br J Psychiatry 212(5):274–278, 2018 30517072

McClain LL, Shaw P, Sabol R, et al: Rare variants and biological pathways identified in treatment-refractory depression. J Neurosci Res 98(7):1322–1334, 2020 32128872

McGraw J, Waller D: Cytochrome P450 variations in different ethnic populations. Expert Opin Drug Metab Toxicol 8(3):371–382, 2012 22288606

Mocking RJT, Naviaux JC, Li K, et al: Correction to: Metabolic features of recurrent major depressive disorder in remission, and the risk of future recurrence. Transl Psychiatry 11(1):115, 2021 33558468

Moncrieff J: Clozapine v. conventional antipsychotic drugs for treatment-resistant schizophrenia: a re-examination. Br J Psychiatry 183:161–166, 2003 12893670

Montgomery SA, Asberg M: A new depression scale designed to be sensitive to change. Br J Psychiatry 134(4):382–389, 1979 444788

Morrison JR: Catatonia. Retarded and excited types. Arch Gen Psychiatry 28(1):39–41, 1973 4683142

Mossel P, Bartels AL, de Deyn PP, et al: The role of P-glycoprotein at the blood-brain barrier in neurological and psychiatric disease, in PET and SPECT in Psychiatry. Edited by Dierckx RA, Otte A, de Vries EFJ, et al. Cham, Switzerland, Springer, 2021, pp 45–81

Murphy EJ, Kassem L, Chemerinski A, et al: Retention and attrition among African Americans in the STAR*D study: what causes research volunteers to stay or stray? Depress Anxiety 30(11):1137–1144, 2013 23723044

Nasrallah H: From the editor: treatment resistance is a myth! Current Psychiatry 20(3):14–16, 2021

National Institute of Mental Health: Research Domain Criteria (RDoC). Bethesda, MD, National Institute of Mental Health, 2022. Available at www.nimh.nih.gov/research/research-funded-by-nimh/rdoc. Accessed September 23, 2022.

Nierenberg AA, Amsterdam JD: Treatment-resistant depression: definition and treatment approaches. J Clin Psychiatry 51(suppl):39–50, 1990 2112132

Nierenberg AA, DeCecco LM: Definitions of antidepressant treatment response, remission, nonresponse, partial response, and other relevant outcomes: a focus on treatment-resistant depression. J Clin Psychiatry 62(Suppl 16):5–9, 2001 11480882

Nierenberg AA, White K: What next? A review of pharmacologic strategies for treatment resistant depression. Psychopharmacol Bull 26(4):429–460, 1990 2087539

Nolen-Hoeksema S, Larson J, Grayson C: Explaining the gender difference in depressive symptoms. J Pers Soc Psychol 77(5):1061–1072, 1999 10573880

O'Reardon JP, Solvason HB, Janicak PG, et al: Efficacy and safety of transcranial magnetic stimulation in the acute treatment of major depression: a multisite randomized controlled trial. Biol Psychiatry 62(11):1208–1216, 2007 17573044

Pan LA, Martin P, Zimmer T, et al: Neurometabolic disorders: potentially treatable abnormalities in patients with treatment-refractory depression and suicidal behavior. Am J Psychiatry 174(1):42–50, 2017 27523499

Papakostas GI, Petersen TJ, Farabaugh AH, et al: Psychiatric comorbidity as a predictor of clinical response to nortriptyline in treatment-resistant major depressive disorder. J Clin Psychiatry 64(11):1357–1361, 2003 14658951

Pare CM, Mack JW: Differentiation of two genetically specific types of depression by the response to antidepressant drugs. J Med Genet 8(3):306–309, 1971 5097136

Peeters FPML, Ruhe HG, Wichers M, et al: The Dutch Measure for Quantification of Treatment Resistance in Depression (DM-TRD): an extension of the Maudsley staging method. J Affect Disord 205(Suppl C):365–371, 2016 27568174

Petersen T, Hughes M, Papakostas GI, et al: Treatment-resistant depression and Axis II comorbidity. Psychother Psychosom 71(5):269–274, 2002 12207107

Petersen T, Papakostas GI, Posternak MA, et al: Empirical testing of two models for staging antidepressant treatment resistance. J Clin Psychopharmacol 25(4):336–341, 2005 16012276

Price JL, Bruce MA, Adinoff B: Addressing structural racism in psychiatry with steps to improve psychophysiologic research. JAMA Psychiatry 79(1):70–74, 2022 34613345

Putman HP: Critical lifestyle supports to successful clinical psychopharmacology, in Rational Psychopharmacology: A Book of Clinical Skills. Washington, DC, American Psychiatric Association Publishing, 2020, pp 219–246

Rasmussen SA, Mazurek MF, Rosebush PI: Catatonia: our current understanding of its diagnosis, treatment and pathophysiology. World J Psychiatry 6(4):391–398, 2016 28078203

Remick RA: Antidepressants: which one? Can Fam Physician 32:587–592, 1986 21267155

Renna ME, Quintero JM, Fresco DM, et al: Emotion regulation therapy: a mechanism-targeted treatment for disorders of distress. Front Psychol 8:98, 2017 28220089

Resick PA, Monson CM, Chard KM: Cognitive Processing Theory for PTSD: A Comprehensive Manual. New York, Guilford, 2017

Ruhé HG, van Rooijen G, Spijker J, et al: Staging methods for treatment resistant depression: a systematic review. J Affect Disord 137(1–3):35–45, 2012 21435727

Rush AJ, Trivedi MH, Wisniewski SR, et al: Acute and longer-term outcomes in depressed outpatients requiring one or several treatment steps: a STAR*D report. Am J Psychiatry 163(11):1905–1917, 2006 17074942

Rybak YE, Lai KSP, Ramasubbu R, et al: Treatment-resistant major depressive disorder: Canadian expert consensus on definition and assessment. Depress Anxiety 38(4):456–467, 2021 33528865

Salloum NC, Papakostas GI: Staging treatment intensity and defining resistant depression: historical overview and future directions. J Clin Psychiatry 80(4):18r12250, 2019

Sargant W: Drugs in the treatment of depression. BMJ 1(5221):225–227, 1961 20789042

Severe J, Greden JF, Reddy P: Consequences of recurrence of major depressive disorder: is stopping effective antidepressant medications ever safe? Focus Am Psychiatr Publ 18(2):120–128, 2020 33162849

Sharma A, Gerbarg P, Bottiglieri T, et al: S-adenosylmethionine (SAMe) for neuropsychiatric disorders: a clinician-oriented review of research. J Clin Psychiatry 78(6):e656–e667, 2017 28682528

Sharma E, Math SB: Course and outcome of obsessive-compulsive disorder. Indian J Psychiatry 61(Suppl 1):S43–S50, 2019 30745676

Sheitman BB, Lieberman JA: The natural history and pathophysiology of treatment resistant schizophrenia. J Psychiatr Res 32(3–4):143–150, 1998 9793867

Singh JB, Daly EJ, Mathews M, et al: Approval of esketamine for treatment-resistant depression. Lancet Psychiatry 7(3):232–235, 2020 32087801

Singh SP, Grange T: Measuring pathways to care in first-episode psychosis: a systematic review. Schizophr Res 81(1):75–82, 2006 16309892

Sinyor M, Schaffer A, Levitt A: The Sequenced Treatment Alternatives to Relieve Depression (STAR*D) trial: a review. Can J Psychiatry 55(3):126–135, 2010 20370962

Sippel LM, Holtzheimer PE, Friedman MJ, et al: Defining treatment-resistant posttraumatic stress disorder: a framework for future research. Biol Psychiatry 84(5):e37–e41, 2018 29752073

Smith-Apeldoorn SY, Veraart JKE, Schoevers RA: Definition and epidemiology of treatment resistance in psychiatry, in Treatment Resistance in Psychiatry. Edited by Kim YK. Singapore, Springer, 2019, pp 3–22

Souery D, Oswald P, Massat I, et al: Clinical factors associated with treatment resistance in major depressive disorder: results from a European multicenter study. J Clin Psychiatry 68(7):1062–1070, 2007 17685743

Spencer T, Biederman J, Wilens T: Attention-deficit/hyperactivity disorder and comorbidity. Pediatr Clin North Am 46(5):915–927, 1999 10570696

Stein G: Everybody's Autobiography. New York, Cooper Square, 1971

Suchanek-Raif R, Raif P, Kowalczyk M, et al: An analysis of five Trkb gene polymorphisms in schizophrenia and the interaction of its haplotype with rs6265 BDNF gene polymorphism. Dis Markers 2020:4789806, 2020

Sullivan GM, Feinn R: Using effect size—or why the p value is not enough. J Grad Med Educ 4(3):279–282, 2012 23997866

Szumilas M: Explaining odds ratios. J Can Acad Child Adolesc Psychiatry 19(3):227–229, 2010 20842279

Targum SD: Identification and treatment of antidepressant tachyphylaxis. Innov Clin Neurosci 11(3–4):24–28, 2014 24800130

Teo C, Borlido C, Kennedy JL, De Luca V: The role of ethnicity in treatment refractory schizophrenia. Compr Psychiatry 54(2):167–172, 2013 23017781

Thase ME, Rush AJ: When at first you don't succeed: sequential strategies for antidepressant nonresponders. J Clin Psychiatry 58(Suppl 13):23–29, 1997 9402916

Tripathi A, Das A, Kar SK: Biopsychosocial model in contemporary psychiatry: current validity and future prospects. Indian J Psychol Med 41(6):582–585, 2019 31772447

Turgay A, Ansari R: Major depression with ADHD: in children and adolescents. Psychiatry (Edgmont) 3(4):20–32, 2006 21103168

Turner EH: Esketamine for treatment-resistant depression: seven concerns about efficacy and FDA approval. Lancet Psychiatry 6(12):977–979, 2019 31680014

Turner EH: Approval of esketamine for treatment-resistant depression—author's reply. Lancet Psychiatry 7(3):236, 2020 32087803

van Bronswijk S, Moopen N, Beijers L, et al: Effectiveness of psychotherapy for treatment-resistant depression: a meta-analysis and meta-regression. Psychol Med 49(3):366–379, 2019 30139408

van Dijk DA, van den Boogaard TM, Deen ML, et al: Predicting clinical course in major depressive disorder: the association between DM-TRD score and symptom severity over time in 1115 outpatients. Depress Anxiety 36(4):345–352, 2019 30474901

Voineskos D, Daskalakis ZJ, Blumberger DM: Management of treatment-resistant depression: challenges and strategies. Neuropsychiatr Dis Treat 16:221–234, 2020 32021216

Warden D, Rush AJ, Trivedi MH, et al: The STAR*D project results: a comprehensive review of findings. Curr Psychiatry Rep 9(6):449–459, 2007 18221624

Watts CA: Endogenous depression in general practice. BMJ 1(4487):11–14, 1947 20278514

Wiles N, Thomas L, Abel A, et al: Cognitive behavioural therapy as an adjunct to pharmacotherapy for primary care based patients with treatment resistant depression: results of the CoBalT randomised controlled trial. Lancet 381(9864):375–384, 2013 23219570

Young JP, Lader MH, Hughes WC: Controlled trial of trimipramine, monoamine oxidase inhibitors, and combined treatment in depressed outpatients. BMJ 2(6201):1315–1317, 1979 391342

Zhang C, Li Z, Wu Z, et al: A study of N-methyl-D-aspartate receptor gene (GRIN2B) variants as predictors of treatment-resistant major depression. Psychopharmacology (Berl) 231(4):685–693, 2014 24114429

Zhang J-P, Lencz T, Geisler S, et al: Genetic variation in BDNF is associated with antipsychotic treatment resistance in patients with schizophrenia. Schizophr Res 146(1–3):285–288, 2013 23433505

Zhdanava M, Pilon D, Ghelerter I, et al: The prevalence and national burden of treatment-resistant depression and major depressive disorder in the United States. J Clin Psychiatry 82(2):20m13699, 2021

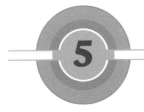

5

Essential Assessment and Reevaluation

The solution for treatment failure lies within the practitioner, not the patient or the diagnosis. How you approach the problem determines how well it will be solved. The questions that you ask of your patients, of the data, of yourself, and of your paradigms determine the treatment you provide and the chances of therapeutic success for your patients. Outcomes are determined largely by your mindset and its relation to that of your patients.

A large number of published articles conflate treatment failure and treatment resistance and lament our lack of full understanding of the processes that lead to this result. Many of these articles also remind readers of everything that could be interfering with successful treatment outcomes and encourage detailed methodical assessment to detect causes and find solutions. Shallow approaches to assessment at every step in the treatment process lead to treatment failure and treatment resistance situations. Inadequate initial assessment, in the absence of serendipity, almost certainly requires detailed reassessment later if a disappointing outcome is to be reversed. An ongoing insufficiency of information usually leads to sustained treatment failure. The best clinicians consistently *begin* with detailed, thorough, and methodical general medical and psychiatric examinations.

Return to the Biopsychosocial Model

Psychodynamics, particularly psychoanalysis, had control over North American psychiatry in the middle of the twentieth century. As medicine then began to reassert the influence it had wielded at the beginning of that century (Kawa and Giordano 2012; Ruffalo 2018), departments of psychiatry researched, treated, and educated along clearly demarcated lines: biological or psychological. Even in the early 1980s, it was difficult to find a training program that would adequately teach residents both psychopharmacology and psychotherapy. Gradually, departments became *eclectic*, meaning that they contained faculty who could teach residents both treatment methods, but with scant guidance for integration in an individual patient. In fact, much effort was put into deciding which patients would be offered psychotherapy and which would be offered medication (Friedman 1975; Klerman et al. 1974; Sotsky et al. 1991). Pluralistic, integrative approaches did not find much traction until later in the decade.

George Engel coined the term *biopsychosocial model* in 1977 to remind psychiatrists and other physicians that illness and disease take place not in an isolated organ but also in psychological and cultural milieus that influence symptom course and treatment response (Engel 1977; Fassino 2010; Papadimitriou 2017). Although the model is sometimes criticized for failure to provide detailed explanations of how the three realms are functionally connected, routine adoption of this tripartite paradigm cues us to remember and investigate broad contributions to pathogenesis, exacerbation, chronicity, and treatment failure, as well as paths to amelioration. The template invites contribution from genetic susceptibility and expression, personality, stress, and environmental conditions, both biological and socioeconomic. Rather than tell us how to connect the dots, it reminds us that the puzzle is larger and more multifaceted than categorical diagnosis might indicate, prompting us to constantly address the complexity in assessment, treatment planning, and monitoring. Rather than a model, it really is a mentality of the more successful practitioner, a tool for ferreting out contributions to actual or potential treatment failures: a long-term mindset that hopefully broadens, rather than narrows, our powers of assessment and problem-solving (see section "Obstacles to Problem-Solving" in Chapter 2, "Keys to Problem-Solving"). We want to avoid the either/or of bio/psycho/social milieus and become pluralistic, truly addressing all three at every step with every single patient.

Given our current diagnostic criteria, three approaches to assessment and formulation can be imagined that might avoid treatment failure and the assumption of treatment resistance. The first solution is to approach diagnosis symptomatically (categorically), hoping for the best, considering treatment resistance only when something fails—a paradigm shift to alert that a deep dive is necessary. To adopt this model is to accept a 50%–60% chance of at least initial treatment failure.

The second solution is to approach formulation functionally (dimensionally) once the first solution has led to failure, looking for additional biopsychosocial factors that have led to it. Structural features, such as race, ethnicity, economic opportunity, and status, may all affect development, psychiatric symptoms, and treatment selection and no doubt will eventually be integrated into evolving diagnostic systems (Alarcón 2009). Of course, although we could also begin with the second solution, most practitioners find purely dimensional groupings novel compared with their usual clinical assessments, and they also find such groupings awkward, given the categorical language of DSM-5-TR (American Psychiatric Association 2022; Kotov et al. 2011; National Institute of Mental Health 2022); see section "Classification of Concepts" in Chapter 1, "Conceptualization (and Failed Concepts)." Nevertheless, the groupings do point to important features that are valid for assessment and consideration in treatment planning.

The third solution is to embrace both categorical and dimensional approaches with full biopsychosocial methodology, searching from the outset for early answers at each level, finding solutions, and avoiding treatment failure from the beginning. After all, this is what many patients expect from us as medical therapists.

General Medical Assessment

Although it may sound like heresy, thorough general medical history and examination are not only essential in every case but are equal in importance to the mental status examination (MSE). A missed nonpsychiatric medical diagnosis can derail your assessment and treatment planning from the start. Rather than retracing steps to uncover the problem once treatment failure develops, begin with a strong effort to identify every problem initially (see section "Psychiatrists as Generalists" in Chapter 7, "Underappreciated Causes of Treatment Failure").

Many practitioners assume that a referring medical provider has already completed a thorough history and examination, but this is not always the case. Some patients do not want to tell the primary care provider (PCP) with whom they have a decades-long relationship that they are using cannabis or not taking the prescribed medication correctly; however, they might tell you, a relative stranger (see section "A

Case of Impaired Therapeutic Alliance" in Chapter 6, "Successful Outcomes"). Plus, unfortunately, not all busy and rushed PCPs are as complete and holistic as we must be, and not all specialists look outside their field. Start every evaluation from scratch, as though you are the first provider the patient has seen, even when you are not. If medical records from any provider are available, review them following your initial assessment. This will limit any bias these documents may lead to and also encourage you to perform a complete history yourself.

If you do not perform your own physical examinations, develop a working relationship with a physician who understands the needs of a proper psychiatric medical examination, including, but certainly not limited to, developmental, endocrine, and neurological findings. Table 5–1 lists important areas to cover in the general medical history and review of systems and to investigate in the physical examination. A detailed description of a complete initial general assessment can be found in my previous book, *Rational Psychopharmacology: A Book of Clinical Skills* (Putman 2020, pp. 61–74). Content and methods for monitoring during follow-up sessions (Tables 5–2 and 5–3) are covered in the same text (Putman 2020, pp. 281–285). Always remember that there may be more than one cause for each instance of treatment failure, and each cause, such as hypothyroidism, may come and go during treatment of a chronic psychiatric condition.

Psychiatric Assessment

Initial psychiatric assessments attempt to accomplish at least three tasks: building rapport that will hopefully develop into a healthy and functional therapeutic alliance, gathering the information needed to begin treatment planning, and motivating the patient to proceed for their own benefit; there will be some teaching, as well as inquiry. Part of that education is demonstrating to patients how specific and detailed our assessment must become. Although psychotherapy may become part of our treatment interaction, the initial assessment requires detailed, unambiguous answers to precise questions. Providers may have to ask the same questions several times, perhaps in different ways, until enough data are accumulated. If patients are unable to provide information, we certainly need to know that as well. For this reason, it is often best to initially examine patients alone so that well-meaning significant others do not prompt or answer for them.

The detailed elements of initial psychiatric evaluations—chief complaint and current, past, and family psychiatric history (Table 5–4) and

Table 5–1.   General medical history and review of symptoms

	Symptoms and conditions
Appearance	Weight
Birth and development	Perinatal complications, delays, learning disorders
Past medical problems	Injuries (especially to head), surgeries, cancers, infections
Allergies	Allergies to medication and food
Current medications	Prescription and over the counter, including as-needed medications
Substance use	Alcohol, nicotine, caffeine, legal and illegal drugs
Neurological history	LOC; CVA; seizures; headaches; memory, motor and sensory problems: balance, gait, tremor, vision, hearing, olfaction
Endocrine history	DM; hypoglycemia; thyroid and PTH levels
Sexual history	Desire, arousal, tumescence, ejaculation, orgasm, activity, STDs
Pregnancy	Menarche, G/P/A, LMP, contraception, plans
Cardiovascular history	Heart block, arrhythmias, DVT; blood pressure
Respiratory history	Asthma, COPD, cough
Gastrointestinal history	Issues with swallowing, nausea, diarrhea, constipation; hepatic issues
Orthopedic history	Fractures, mineralization
Hematological history	Anemia, bleeding

Note.   COPD = chronic obstructive pulmonary disease; CVA = cerebrovascular accident; DM = diabetes mellitus; DVT = deep vein thrombosis; G/P/A = gravidity, parity, abortus; LMP = last menstrual period; LOC = loss of consciousness; PTH = parathyroid hormone.

MSE (Table 5–5)—and techniques for interviewing are comprehensively covered in *Rational Psychopharmacology: A Book of Clinical Skills* (Putman 2020, pp. 43–61). Ongoing monitoring (Table 5–6) is discussed in the same text (Putman 2020, pp. 277–281). Developing an effective therapeutic alliance includes helping your patient understand how important accurate and detailed information is to their outcome. This not only provides you with the best data to guide treatment recommendations but also focuses the patient's self-observations and reinforces many of your lifestyle recommendations.

Table 5–2.   Follow-up visit review of systems and laboratory checklist

	Symptoms and conditions
Appearance	Weight
Allergies	Update allergies
New medical problems	Injuries, infections, exacerbations or return of old problems, new diagnoses
Neurological system	New head injuries (even mild); seizures; syncope; headaches; motor and sensory problems: tremor, weakness, involuntary movements, rigidity, gait, balance, vision (diplopia, blurred vision), olfaction
Gastrointestinal system	Swallowing, nausea, vomiting, diarrhea, constipation, pain, bleeding
Cardiovascular system	Abnormal rhythm (including tachycardia); chest pain; blood pressure, especially with stimulant and some antidepressant treatment (may include postural hypotension)
Respiratory system	Dyspnea (a check on allergy), cough, shortness of breath, snoring, sleep apnea
Sexual issues	Desire, arousal, tumescence, ejaculation, orgasm, infection, changes in menstruation
Orthopedic system	Mineralization changes, joint problems (a check on allergy), injury (good check on head injury)
Endocrine system	Changes in blood sugar, nocturia, kidney stones, thyroid status
Dermatological system	Rash, swelling, pain, pruritus
Relevant serum levels of medications	May include prescription of new medication by another provider; essential when brand or dose is changed or drug interaction is possible
Liver profile	As indicated
Electrolytes and serum creatinine	As indicated
Complete blood count	As indicated
Vitamin D level (as 25[OH]D)	When replacing, otherwise annually
Thyroid-stimulating hormone	Initial screen and as indicated; during replacement every 6–12 months
Thyroid antibodies	Initial screen and as indicated

Note.   25[OH]D = 25-hydroxy vitamin D.

Table 5–3.   Follow-up medications and adverse event checklist

	Information to obtain
Medications taken	Nonpsychiatric, over the counter, and as needed
Supplements taken	Including new ones
New medications	List of new medications
Stopped medications	Reason
Brand changes	To and from (and to alternative) generics with dates
Dosage changes	Timing and reasons
Side effects	Degree, timing
Adverse events	Degree, timing, treatment
Menstrual cycle	Date of last menstrual period
Birth control	Including compliance
Pregnancy	Method of testing, stage, complications
Nursing	Including schedule
Alcohol	Amount
Nicotine	Form, amount
Caffeine	All sources, including chocolate, plus amounts
Psychoactive drugs	Legal and illegal, recreational and self-treatment

Accounting for Every Symptom or Dysfunction

Jesse L. Hite, M.D., who practiced anesthesiology as well as becoming a board-certified psychiatrist, frequently encountered patients during his 45 years of psychiatric practice who had endured multiple failed attempts at treatment for major depression. He contributes the case of a 16-year-old Black girl brought to him by her mother following treatment failures with several standard antidepressants; the young woman had made six suicide attempts and had been hospitalized four times in a psychiatric facility during the 2 years prior to his initial consultation with her.

During Dr. Hite's evaluation, the patient confirmed experiencing up to 5 or 6 hours of initial insomnia nightly and sustained rapid thinking. She also endorsed depressed mood and denied any symptoms of increased energy or inappropriate social behavior. In fact, she was an honor student. On the basis of these previously uncovered or underappreciated symptoms, Dr. Hite changed her diagnosis to bipolar disorder, mixed state. He prescribed risperidone 0.5 mg in the morning and 1.5 mg

Table 5–4. Psychiatric history

	Information needed
Chief complaint	Detailed information on current and neurovegetative symptoms: what, when, length, antecedents, context, onset, change
Current psychiatric history	Current professional treatments and self-treatments, contributions or alterations by other providers, follow-through, results; suicidality, violent ideation
Developmental history	Perinatal diagnoses or complications, developmental milestones and delays, learning problems or disorders, social behavior and connections, education, employment and military service
Past psychiatric history	Past psychiatric symptoms and diagnoses, with dates of onset and any remissions; details of all past treatments and responses—pharmacological, somatic, psychotherapeutic (including type); abuse or other trauma; head injury
Family psychiatric history	Pertinent medical conditions (e.g., neurological, endocrine); psychiatric symptoms and diagnoses, with details of any treatment attempts; suicidality or violence

in the evening, tapered her antidepressants, and started titration of valproate, eventually achieving a therapeutic and effective serum level. The patient achieved a remission of her symptoms and continued this treatment under the care of her PCP. Eighteen months later, Dr. Hite learned that the PCP had discontinued the valproate for unknown reasons, but the risperidone was still being used effectively for sleep and mood; the patient had had no serious episodes of depressed mood during the interval.

Thorough symptom evaluations are always essential. When we meet patients who have undergone multiple unsuccessful treatments for the same diagnosis with several previous providers, we must strive to appreciate present symptoms or dimensions that were not included in the previous diagnosis and account for them. As we saw in Chapter 2, an early or previous diagnosis blunts a clinician's awareness of and sensitivity to symptoms that do not fit with that diagnosis, increasing the risk of treatment failure (see sections "Obstacles to Problem-Solving" and "Implications for Medical Practice" in Chapter 2). Dr. Hite's experience with similar patients broadened his mindset, allowing him to consider an underdiagnosed problem (Ghaemi et al. 1999; Hu et al. 2014; McElroy 2008; Nusslock and Frank 2011) and proceed with successful treatment for it

Table 5–5. Mental status examination

	What to look for
Appearance	Eye contact, clothing, grooming, motor activity
Speech	Volume, speed, prosody, delay
Orientation	Orientation to person, place, time, situation
Memory	Immediate, short-term, long-term
Concentration	Length
Anxiety	Subjective
Mood	Subjective
Affect	Objective appearance of mood/anxiety and congruity
Thought process	Association, speed
Thought content	Hallucinations, illusions, delusions
Self-harm and violence	Suicidality, homicidal ideation, plan and intent; lesser degrees of both
Insight	Awareness of the situation
Judgment	Subjective assessment from historical details
Reliability	Cooperation; impacts on therapeutic alliance

rather than accepting the case as treatment resistant, which would have offered no new therapeutic direction.

Perceiving and Respecting Your Patient

Highly educated segments of a population may use very different conceptualizations to predict outcomes than the general populace does (see Christian 2022, Chapter 5), making it essential that we communicate bidirectionally and appreciate how each of our patients will be sharing information and responding to our suggestions. Whether cultural or educational differences, a dysfunctional cognitive schema, or illness behavior is at work (see section "Countertherapeutic Factors" in Chapter 4, "The Myth of Treatment Resistance?"), we must more deeply understand our patients rather than blaming them for a failure. This is, after all, the third pillar of evidence-based medicine (see sections "Resistance to Evidence-Based Medicine" and "Effective Use of Evidence" in Chapter 3, "The Goal of Evidence-Based Practice"). Thinking about psychosocial aspects is much more than being polite, being considerate, and considering the patient to be a person. It is also more than listening to what a

Table 5–6.　Follow-up visit checklist

	What to look for
Appearance	Grooming, clothing, eye contact, motor activity
Orientation	Orientation to person, place, time, situation
Speech	Prosody, speed, volume, pitch
Sleep	Degree and quality, daytime drowsiness
Appetite	Changes in appetite
Weight	Gain or loss
Memory	Immediate, short-term, long-term
Concentration	Length
Anxiety	Example: avoidance
Interest in pleasurable activities	Examples: socialization, sex
Motivation for activities of daily living	Examples: work, school, cleaning, purchases
Physical energy	Distinguished from sleepiness
Mood	Subjective
Affect	Objective appearance of mood/anxiety with congruence
Irritability	Presence of irritability
Thought processing	Associations, speed of thoughts
Thought content	Hallucinations, illusions, delusions
Self-harm	Suicidal ideation, plan, or intent
Violence	Examples: aggression, aggressive ideation; homicidal ideation, plan, intent
Insight	Awareness of situation
Judgment	Subjective
Reliability	Including cooperation
Compliance	Acceptance of treatment; follow-through

patient wants before telling them what to do. Correctly approached, it offers keys to greater treatment success by reducing barriers to understanding by both patient and provider, as well as barriers to compliance.

Data show that we clinicians often misperceive how patients view us, our communication, the illness, and their own role in the therapeutic alliance (Hall et al. 1999; Rohrbaugh and Rogers 1994). We also underestimate how much of a partnership they desire with us. Providers primarily view increased patient education as the principal tool for enhancing compliance. Patients are likely to value the education we can provide, but they also indicate that compliance is based more on shared understanding, which creates trust in us. This does not mean simply that they understand the medical information we are delivering, but rather that we understand their experience and viewpoints just as well (Kennedy et al. 2017).

The more successful providers, then, will work to understand not only the preferences but also the beliefs and values of their patients. When patients are able to more fully share their perspective, the therapeutic alliance is enhanced, and clinical decision-making leads to better outcomes. Bidirectional communication is essential to reducing error from providers' decision-making and patient decisions about compliance. Patients notice when we take time, speak *with* rather than *at* them, and listen without cutting them off (even in psychiatry). They also indicate that such behaviors directly determine how well they receive our opinions and advice, even more than their understanding of their disease, which is often better than we suspect (Haidet and Paterniti 2003; Kennedy et al. 2017).

Cultural Influences

The task of assessing and advising patients is even more difficult when provider and patient do not share the same race, ethnicity, or culture. According to the United Nations, 3.6% of the world population migrated in 2020 (International Organization for Migration 2021). The greatest relocation was from developing economies to larger ones, such as the United States, United Arab Emirates, Saudi Arabia, and Germany; the second highest was from the Syria to Turkey. Since then, Europe has experienced more than 7.8 million additional relocations due to geopolitical conflict in Ukraine (U.N. Refugee Agency 2022). Further, the United Nations expects international migration to increase because of environmental and technological changes (International Organization for Migration 2021; U.N. Refugee Agency 2022). Patients who are refugees require a particularly sensitive, careful, and time-generous approach because trust is major challenge for many in this population (Byrow et al. 2020; Shannon et al. 2016).

The United States is becoming more racially and ethnically diverse. Changes since 2010 are due to demographic shifts, as well as improvements in the way race and ethnicity data are collected and processed (U.S. Census Bureau 2021). The United States considered five races and six ethnic groups in its 2020 census (Hispanic being an ethnicity spread across races): White (61.2%), Hispanic (18.8%), Black (12.1%), Asian (5.8%), American Indian and Alaska Native (1.0%), and Native Hawaiian and other Pacific Islander (0.2%) (U.S. Census Bureau 2021). The Census Bureau also calculates a diversity index (DI), indicating how likely it is that one person will encounter another from a different ethnicity. In 2020, the DI (converted to a percentage) indicates that there is a 61.1% chance that any two people in the United States, chosen at random, will be from different ethnic groups (up from 54.9% in 2010). Hawaii currently holds the highest DI (76%), followed by states in the west (California and Nevada), south (Maryland and Texas), and northeast (New York and New Jersey) (Jensen et al. 2021; U.S. Census Bureau 2021). The top 10 states are shown in Table 5–7.

A diffusion score (DS) has additionally been calculated that measures the percentage of a population that is not in the three largest racial and ethnic groups combined; DS correlates directly with diversity (U.S. Census Bureau 2021). These data show us that although a single, or several, ethnicities may predominate in an area, it is important to remember that additional ethnicities are also prominent and are less clustered into specific regions. Oklahoma, for example, is ranked 17th in DI but 3rd in DS. Alaska, Washington, and Massachusetts rank 2nd, 8th, and 9th, respectively, in DS but 12th, 20th, and 26th in DI (Table 5–8). This illustrates just how diverse our societies are. Practitioners should expect to routinely encounter patients with ethnicities and cultural and health beliefs different from their own.

Ben Raimer, M.D., a pediatrician and former president of the University of Texas Medical Branch, often shared with students how, when the antibiotics he prescribed did not work, a member of his own medical office staff rubbed an egg over her son's body, then cracked the egg into a glass of water and placed it under his bed. She reported that he recovered from this application of *curanderismo* (a folk healing method from Mexican Indian culture, popular in Hispanic society), which was intended to absorb bad energy and protect him from *mal de ojo* (the evil eye) (Padilla et al. 2001; Ramirez 2018; Tafur et al. 2009).

The Gullah culture along the coastal southeast United States is particularly noted for how strongly it has retained its African linguistic and belief traditions (Pollitzer 1999). Practitioners in the low country must learn not only much of Gullah vocabulary and syntax but also the beliefs about how spirits and hexes influence health for better or worse (Pellegrini and Putman 1984). Significant efforts to work collaboratively with this society to improve health outcomes has demonstrated how academic

Table 5–7. **Ten U.S. states with highest diversity index in 2020 (U.S. score 61.1%)**

State	Diversity index 2010, %	Diversity index 2020, %	Increase, %
Hawaii	75.1	76.0	0.9
California	67.7	69.7	2.0
Nevada	62.5	68.8	6.3
Maryland	60.7	67.3	6.6
District of Columbia	61.9	67.2	5.3
Texas	63.8	67.0	3.2
New Jersey	59.4	65.8	6.4
New York	59.4	65.8	5.5
Georgia	58.8	64.1	5.3
Florida	59.1	64.1	5.1

Note. The diversity index represents the likelihood that one person will encounter another from a different ethnicity.

Source. U.S. Census Bureau, 2010 Redistricting Data (Public Law 94-171) Summary File; 2020 Census Redistricting Data (Public Law 94-171). Information on analysis and definitions is available at www2.census.gov/programs-surveys/decennial/2020/technical-documentation/complete-tech-docs/summary-file.

practitioners must acknowledge the strength, value, and culture of their community; consider community members equal partners; and seek the community's collective wisdom and knowledge (Spruill et al. 2013).

We need to reach out to patients in a manner that will encourage them not only to try treatment plans we agree on but to return to us if results are initially unsuccessful. In order to do this, we must learn about other cultures, especially those with whom we have frequent contact, and how our behavior is interpreted from those contexts. Even differing expectations about handshaking during initial contact may determine whether or not there will be a cooperative relationship (Maduro 1983). Clinicians working to develop cultural competence, an appreciation of the complexity of a culture beyond stereotypes, will further enhance clinical outcomes through shared understanding and mutuality, offering the opportunity to reduce both treatment failure and health disparities (Betancourt and Green 2010; Teal and Street 2009).

Whether you are a new member of a society or treating a member of a different one in your home community, cultural sensitivities, humility,

Table 5–8.   Ten U.S. states with highest diffusion scores and their corresponding diversity index in 2020

Area	2020 diffusion score, %	2020 diversity index, %	2020 rank
U.S. total	11.4	61.1	
Hawaii	21.8	76.0	1st
Alaska	17.9	62.8	12th
Oklahoma	17.8	59.5	17th
Nevada	16.0	68.8	3rd
New York	14.3	65.8	8th
New Jersey	14.2	65.8	7th
Washington	13.0	55.9	20th
Massachusetts	12.6	51.6	26th
Maryland	12.0	67.3	4th

Note.   Diffusion score measures the percentage of a population that is not in the three largest racial and ethnic groups combined. A higher score indicates a lower concentration of the population in its three largest races and ethnicities and thus greater diversity (U.S. Census Bureau 2021).

Source.   U.S. Census Bureau, 2010 Redistricting Data (Public Law 94-171) Summary File; 2020 Census Redistricting Data (Public Law 94-171). Information on analysis and definitions is available at www2.census.gov/programs-surveys/decennial/2020/technical-documentation/complete-tech-docs/summary-file.

and, hopefully, even competencies, in ourselves and our office staff are now more than a nice idea for the future or for rare, random encounters. They are essential in developing a successful therapeutic alliance and achieving good clinical outcomes with the majority of patients we encounter today (Roncoroni et al. 2014; Shim 2023; Tucker et al. 2014, 2015).

Essential Value of Bayesian Inference

As clinicians, we are essentially involved with the process of assessing the present in order to predict the future. The beauty and success of our efforts to help our patients through our knowledge and problem-solving skills lie in the fact that we do not cease appraisal even after thorough initial evaluations—we repeat assessment and self-assessment in some form at every patient contact. This gives us the opportunity—in fact, mandate—to question our initial assessments repeatedly. Did we understand what the patient was telling us? Did they understand our diagnosis and treatment plan? Does our diagnosis appear correct? Are conditions optimal for the treatment plan to work? Is the treatment leading to improvement?

As we focus on *change* at every contact, eliciting, describing, and measuring it, we have the opportunity to confirm or amend our initial conceptualizations and problem-solving strategies because we can obtain and use *new information*. This is the essence of abductive reasoning: assessing, hypothesizing, testing, then reassessing, improving our hypothesis, and retesting, repeating this pattern throughout our entire relationship with a patient. Complacency and overconfidence easily lead to treatment failure.

This process of continually refining our impression of what the problem(s) is (are) and how to solve it (them) is more formally described as *Bayesian inference*: initial modeling altered to fit new data as soon as they arrive. When a treatment fails, we must examine the nature of our assault on the clinical challenge, as well as the target. Are we using the best methods to treat accurate diagnoses? If not, it is likely that treatment failure will result.

Modeling a clinical problem well, then, is key to treatment success. Few models are correct on initial assessment, and almost all benefit from refinement. As the statisticians George E.P. Box and N.R. Draper helpfully observed, "Essentially, all models are wrong, but some are useful" (Box and Draper 1987, p. 424). They go on to point out that we must always recall the *approximate* nature of models and search for two types of errors: systematic (or bias) errors and random errors. They write that systematic errors, always to be expected, are nevertheless often ignored, leading to misleading predictions. A recent survey found that 46.9% of first psychiatric diagnoses are revised to alternative diagnoses within the next 10 years; cases involving psychosis, single episodes of major depression, and substance abuse have the greatest diagnostic variability (Høj Jørgensen et al. 2023). Further, expert clinicians are even less skillful at prognosis than they are at diagnosis, often due to optimistic bias and anchoring (see section "Implications for Medical Practice" in Chapter 2 and section "Errors in Conceptualization" in Chapter 1) (Bieganski 1990; Chiffi and Zanotti 2017; Christakis and Lamont 2000).

It is not necessary for clinicians to mathematically solve Bayes' theorem to avoid treatment failure—understanding the concept is sufficient. Thomas Bayes' work essentially legitimized the science of probability by providing a tool for estimating its degree of confidence, making our ignorance explicit and quantifying it (Osimani 2009). This is the foundation of the sequential estimations we must employ to become effective practitioners. In Bayesian terminology, we convert a *prior probability* into a *posterior probability*.

Practicing psychiatry is in many ways a task of layering probabilities: the chance that your diagnoses are correct; the likelihood that you understand your patient and that they will understand, agree with, and comply with your recommendations; the degree of risk of treatments or lack of treatment; and the probabilities that each intervention you employ will work for a particular patient (hopefully based on randomized clinical trials, valid meta-analyses, and tools such as number needed to treat and number needed to harm; see section "Gathering Evidence" in Chapter 3). As a clinician, you must manipulate these probabilities in your mind and begin with an initial estimation of success—what Bayesians call prior probability. Although certain fields calculate a mathematical score for this, in our practice this synthesis of multiple probabilities is largely subjective, but it must nevertheless be conscious.

After determining the prior probability, you can employ the Bayesian effect. Through thorough reevaluation of general medical and psychiatric conditions (as well as compliance) during each visit, new information is collected. This may include new symptoms, adverse events, and new contributing factors, in addition to responses to psychotherapy or medication. All of this additional information must be added to the original (subjective) equation, and a new probability of success should be calculated. This posterior probability is predicated on amendments we make to our model (possibly new diagnoses, possibly new treatment plans), so the importance of this process is not merely calculating a more precise probability but showing us more accurately how to achieve our original goal of remission: by generating alternative hypotheses and changing direction as soon as the data indicate (Johnson 2020). We update our conceptualizations of the treatment scenario (our model) so that our problem-solving will be more exact and successful.

A professional baseball player seeking to catch a fly ball in the outfield does not simply go to the spot he caught the last one and wait. He uses his senses in real time to gather increasing amounts of information so that he can predict the ball's path and arrive waiting at the new, correct location. Given his distance from the plate, the sound of the ball hitting the bat alerts him to contact. He scans the area in front of him to detect the direction the orb is heading. If it is coming toward him, he estimates the angle of ascent and speed. As it gets closer, he adjusts to his right or left, at the same time moving closer or farther away in order to find the right distance for its arrival. His skin may detect a sudden gust of wind, and he must use this information to recalculate the ball's predicted trajectory. At the same time, he is alert to other outfielders also tracking the ball who might collide with him, makes a judgment as to who is best able to make the catch, and signals to his teammates whether he or another player should make the grab. Will he have to dive or slide for it, or should he remain standing? He keeps his eye on the ball, making perhaps scores of final adjustments until it is safely in his glove. Certainly, we can be as assiduous with our treatments. Unquestionably, a professional player would not have stood in the same position for the previous play and declared the ball "uncatchable."

A Clinical Example of Bayesian Inference

Case Example
Grace (not her real name), a 28-year-old woman, comes to you complaining of moderately depressed mood. Following a thorough general medical and psychiatric assessment, you diagnose major depressive disorder, moderate, and together you and she agree to a trial of a serotonin-norepinephrine reuptake inhibitor (SNRI); she agrees to cease moderate alcohol use as well. At her next appointment 3 weeks later, she shows worsening in her neurovegetative symptoms: sleep is now excessive, 12–14 hours a day, and never restful. Her appetite is increasing and is accompanied by a 3- to 4-pound weight gain. Her anxiety and agitation have also increased. You discover that although she has reduced her alcohol intake, she still drinks about 3 ounces of alcohol a week. The SNRI you prescribed was given to her in generic form, and she confirms taking it as directed. At this point, you consider the effects ongoing alcohol use may be having on her mood and response, and you strongly encourage her to refrain from all use, as well as tapering off caffeine because of her anxiety. She agrees. You note the generic brand of her SNRI and ask her to monitor any change. Noting that improvement may take another 4–5 weeks or so, you reassess the probability that your diagnosis and treatment plan are correct and will benefit this patient (a posterior probability), eventually agreeing to continue treatment for this diagnosis with these changes.

Two weeks later, Grace calls the office to report further deterioration: her anxiety is now severe, and she is taking 2–3 hours to fall asleep before sleeping 14–16 hours; she can no longer go to work. Her appetite and weight have continued to increase, and she has now gained 6 pounds. The brand of her SNRI was changed last week when she refilled her prescription, and she has not used any alcohol in 2 weeks nor any caffeine in the past week. On reexamination the next day, her concentration and short-term memory are both worse, and she is now reporting paranoia. Her speech is slightly pressured, and she confirms increased irritability.

The dose of the SNRI is adequate, and she has been taking it 5 weeks with not only no improvement but also worsening of her condition.

You continue to reevaluate the prior probability that continuing this SNRI in its various generic forms, with variable bioavailability, will eventually be successful, while at the same time reestimating the probability that your initial diagnosis of major depression is neither correct nor complete. Is there an alternative or supplemental diagnosis that would better fit this patient's situation? You make efforts to confirm that you are understanding her symptoms and dysfunctions well and that she grasps, agrees with, and is making every effort to comply with your mutually agreed-on treatment. You also reevaluate how new treatments may be layered into the plan and conclude that given her new thought content, cognitive-behavioral therapy may increase her chances of remission.

Considering that the majority of patients show at least a partial response to an SNRI within the first 5 weeks of treatment, you decide that the chance of eventual recovery with this SNRI is lower than you originally estimated, even taking into account the generic bioavailability issue (see section "Polypharmacy and Bioavailability Complications" in Chapter 7). Because of increases in Grace's sleep and appetite, you have also changed your mind about the probability your diagnosis is correct. These features, along with paranoia, are atypical for major depression, and this leads you to reconsider many other diagnoses, including bipolar disorder, schizoaffective disorder, hyperthyroidism, and hyperparathyroidism. On deeper examination with the MSE, you learn that Grace's thoughts are also coming more quickly than her speech can keep up with, consistent with her pressured speech. Layering probabilities, you conclude that the most likely diagnosis is now bipolar II disorder, depressed episode, severe. Hyperparathyroidism might also be correct but is much less common. Having estimated a new posterior probability, you recommend treatment for bipolar disorder: tapering the SNRI; initiating a mood stabilizer; and checking her parathyroid hormone (PTH), calcium, and phosphate levels.

Within 3 weeks, Grace is significantly improved. Weekly cognitive-behavioral therapy is helping her reverse the ruminative paranoia that was beginning to develop. Her anxiety is now mild, her thoughts are no longer coming too fast, and her speech is not pressured. Her appetite is still strong, but the weight gain has stopped. She can now fall asleep more quickly, and the length of her sleep has begun to decrease toward 8 hours. Her PTH, calcium, and phosphate levels are normal. At this reevaluation, you conclude that your new diagnosis is reasonable and that the treatment plan based on it has a strong probability of becoming increasingly effective. Careful successive approximations have allowed you to change your prior probability to a posterior probability, with significant benefits for your patient.

Additional clinical examples are as easy to identify as an initial diagnosis of major depression that turns out to be bipolar disorder: avoidant personality disorder that responds to treatment for social anxiety disorder; treatment failure for panic disorder reversing when an additional diagnosis of substance use disorder is eventually made and treatment is started; and psychosis abated through cessation of steroid use. Hyperparathyroidism may underlie unstable mood; what seemed to be bipolar disorder can disappear after parathyroidectomy; symptoms of ADHD might disappear once daily cannabis use is stopped for several months; and dementia may resolve once statins are discontinued.

Summary

We practice in the domain of prediction, and the tools and processes we choose determine clinical outcomes for our patients. We must identify, learn, and employ the best practices for their benefit. Routine adoption of the biopsychosocial model broadens our clinical mindset and opportunities for problem-solving.

Many treatment failures result from inadequate gathering of information from the literature and from the patient during initial and ongoing assessment. A comprehensive general medical evaluation is as essential as an MSE for every patient; we cannot assume this has been accomplished by other professionals. Initial psychiatric evaluations attempt to glean as much data as possible while building a therapeutic alliance and instructing patients on the necessity of detailed answers to precise questions, as well as alertness to small features. Lifestyle behaviors strongly influence outcomes. In order to avoid treatment failures, these behaviors must be explored and encouraged at every patient contact.

A clinician and their patient may approach treatment efforts with very different cognitive schemata. It is incumbent on each provider to consistently seek a deeper understanding of how the patient views the treatment process in order to support the most effective therapeutic alliance and to practice truly evidence-based medicine. Patients must feel that we share their understanding and are not just attempting to impart our own. To accomplish this, we must learn the beliefs and values of all of our patients, particularly when race and culture differ, and especially with populations under stress. Identifying and adjusting for our cultural biases, in addition to paradigmatic biases, are essential.

Constant vigilance for and incorporation of new, broad data are the key to avoiding and reversing treatment failure. Bayesian inference instructs us how to test our initial hypotheses and revise them (and, therefore, our outcome probabilities) as new information becomes available—additional data that we must anticipate, seek, and integrate. Providers must achieve a balance between rigid adherence to models that clearly do not fit evolving data and impulsively abandoning models while data are still insufficient, such as when an effective dose and expected time to response have not yet been achieved. Collection and consideration of all available data, from the patient and from the literature, best inform when and what changes should be made. As each model for problem-solving evolves, informed by probability theory, our chances of encountering treatment failure (or treatment resistance) decrease.

Key Points

- Treatment success is determined by our entire approach.
- The biopsychosocial model encourages the most helpful mindset.
- Begin with thorough general medical and psychiatric assessments.
- Patients must know we hear their beliefs and values.
- Cultural and ethnic humility, sensitivity, and competency aid outcomes.
- Adjusting our assessments and plans to new information is critical.

Self-Assessment Questions

1.   Which of the following describes Bayesian inference?

     A. It quantifies uncertainty.
     B. It is an application of probability theory.
     C. It is a step in abductive reasoning.
     D. All of the above.

     Correct answer: D. All of the above.

     Revising or choosing an alternate hypothesis on the basis of new data results in a new and measurable probability of success.

2. Why are cultural humility and competencies important to outcomes?

    A. There is a high chance that your next patient will have a different ethnicity from you.
    B. Refugee patients are likely to be very trusting of caregivers.
    C. They help reduce treatment failure (treatment resistance) and health disparities.
    D. A and C.

Correct answer: D. A and C.

In 2020, the U.S. Census Bureau determined from its diversity index that there is a 61.1% chance that any two people in the United States, chosen at random, are from different ethnicities. Canada, Mexico, Switzerland, Belgium, India, South Africa, Micronesia, United Arab Emirates, Pakistan, Bolivia, Spain, and most of Africa are ranked even higher by a variety of researchers and methods (Fearon 2003; Gören 2013). Refugee patients, as a group, struggle strongly with trust in authorities such as caregivers. Improving treatment outcomes helps reduce health disparity among racial and ethnic groups.

3. Which of the following describes the biopsychosocial model?

    A. It is eclectic.
    B. It is pluralistic.
    C. It is reductive.
    D. It is a detailed explanation of how the three realms are functionally connected.

Correct answer: B. It is pluralistic.

Rather than choosing among approaches to treat an individual patient or detailing how the realms are connected, this model reminds us that illness and disease take place in psychological and cultural milieus that influence symptom course and treatment response. Consideration of all three realms with every patient strengthens the chances of satisfactory outcomes.

4.   Clinicians often misperceive how patients view which of the following?

     A. The provider.
     B. Their illnesses.
     C. Communication with them.
     D. All of the above.

     Correct answer: D. All of the above.

     As clinicians, we often misunderstand how patients view their own role in the partnership and how much they want to have an alliance with us. Compliance is based mostly on achieving shared understanding, not our ability to convey scientific information.

5.   Which of the following statements is true?

     A. Almost half of initial psychiatric diagnoses are altered within 10 years.
     B. Bidirectional communication often degrades treatment planning.
     C. Two random people in the United States are likely to be from the same ethnic group.
     D. Early diagnosis of an atypical presentation enhances outcomes.

     Correct answer: A. Almost half of initial diagnoses in psychiatry are altered within 10 years.

     Diagnoses involving psychosis, single episodes of major depression, and substance abuse are the most variable. Bidirectional communication facilitates understanding for both sides, improving diagnosis and treatment planning, as well as compliance and outcomes. There is a 61.1% chance that any two people chosen randomly in the United States are from *different* ethnic groups, so providers should expect to encounter different cultures in practice. Early diagnosis more frequently leads to error though the exclusion of atypical features that point to an alternative diagnosis or additional diagnoses.

Discussion Topics

1. A 55-year old man who emigrated from Croatia in 2000 comes to you for help with insomnia that his primary care physician could not treat effectively. He is friendly and fluent in your language, but he is guarded and largely silent about most of his history. Although acknowledging current nightmares, he will discuss neither the content of the dreams nor whether he was exposed to any trauma prior to leaving Croatia. He provides only cursory answers to questions about his physical and sexual health and generally denies any other psychiatric problems. He does acknowledge some moderate use of alcohol. How would you approach further assessment and treatment planning with him?

2. A 36-year-old woman seeks to transfer to your care from another local provider because she is unhappy with his treatment attempts for her mood problems. She reports many failed romantic, platonic, and business relationships and was recently pushed out of a high position at a large local company. She also reports several significant health problems, including hyperthyroidism, kidney stones, undiagnosed headaches, and petit mal epilepsy as a child. She admits that she probably changes providers too often to have benefited from psychotherapy and often does not complete medication trials that are prescribed. Nevertheless, she promises you that she is tired of feeling so bad and wishes to commit to a serious doctor-patient relationship with you. How can you use the biopsychosocial model to formulate initial working hypotheses about her diagnoses, further evaluation methods, and treatment planning?

Additional Readings

Christian D: Future Stories: What's Next? New York, Little, Brown Spark, 2022: *Exploration of the human process of prediction, including a useful discussion of causation, probability theory, and information technology*

Kinzie JD, Keepers GA (eds): The Psychiatric Evaluation and Treatment of Refugees. Washington, DC, American Psychiatric Association Publishing, 2020: *A valuable resource for practitioners seeking more effective alliances and better outcomes when working with displaced patients who have experienced intense trauma and stigmatization*

Putman HP: Rational Psychopharmacology: A Book of Clinical Skills. Washington, DC, American Psychiatric Association Publishing, 2020: *For detailed expansions of medical and psychiatric assessment and reassessment, see Chapter 3, "Thorough Assessment Techniques," and Chapter 12, "Rational and Methodical Treatment Monitoring"*

Trapp NT, Martyna MR, Siddiqi SH, Bajestan SN: The neuropsychiatric approach to the assessment of patients in neurology. Semin Neurol 42(2):88–106, 2022: *A guide to evaluation of conditions on the cusp of psychiatry and neurology*

References

Alarcón RD: Culture, cultural factors and psychiatric diagnosis: review and projections. World Psychiatry 8(3):131–139, 2009 19812742

American Psychiatric Association: Diagnostic and Statistical Manual of Mental Disorders, 5th Edition, Text Revision, Washington, DC, American Psychiatric Association, 2022

Betancourt JR, Green AR: Commentary: linking cultural competence training to improved health outcomes: perspectives from the field. Acad Med 85(4):583–585, 2010 20354370

Bieganski W: The logic of medicine or the critique of medical knowledge, in The Polish School of Philosophy of Medicine: From Tytus Chalubinski (1820–1889) to Ludwik Fleck (1896–1961) (Philosophy and Medicine, Vol 37). Compiled and translated by Löwy I. Edited by Engelhardt HT Jr., Spiker SF. Dordrecht, Kluwer Academic, 1990

Box GPE, Draper NR: Empirical Model-Building and Response Surfaces (Wiley Series in Probability and Statistics), 1st Edition. New York, Wiley, 1987

Byrow Y, Pajak R, Specker P, Nickerson A: Perceptions of mental health and perceived barriers to mental health help-seeking amongst refugees: a systematic review. Clin Psychol Rev 75:101812, 2020 31901882

Chiffi D, Zanotti R: Fear of knowledge: clinical hypotheses in diagnostic and prognostic reasoning. J Eval Clin Pract 23(5):928–934, 2017 27882636

Christakis NA, Lamont EB: Extent and determinants of error in doctors' prognoses in terminally ill patients: prospective cohort study. BMJ 320(7233):469–472, 2000 10678857

Christian D: Future Stories: What's Next? New York, Little, Brown Spark, 2022

Engel GL: The need for a new medical model: a challenge for biomedicine. Science 196(4286):129–136, 1977 847460

Fassino S: Psychosomatic approach is the new medicine tailored for patient personality with a focus on ethics, economy, and quality. Panminerva Med 52(3):249–264, 2010 21045782

Fearon JD: Ethnic and cultural diversity by country. J Econ Growth 8:195–222, 2003

Friedman AS: Interaction of drug therapy with marital therapy in depressive patients. Arch Gen Psychiatry 32(5):619–637, 1975 1092282

Ghaemi SN, Sachs GS, Chiou AM, et al: Is bipolar disorder still underdiagnosed? Are antidepressants overutilized? J Affect Disord 52(1–3):135–144, 1999 10357026

Gören E: Economic Effects of Domestic and Neighbouring Countries' Cultural Diversity. ZenTra Working Paper in Transnational Studies No 16/2013. Social Science Research Network, April 27, 2013. Available at: https://ssrn.com/abstract=2255492. Accessed November 30, 2022.

Haidet P, Paterniti DA: "Building" a history rather than "taking" one: a perspective on information sharing during the medical interview. Arch Intern Med 163(10):1134–1140, 2003 12767949

Hall JA, Stein TS, Roter DL, Rieser N: Inaccuracies in physicians' perceptions of their patients. Med Care 37(11):1164–1168, 1999 10549618

Høj Jørgensen TS, Osler M, Jorgensen MB, Jorgensen A: Mapping diagnostic trajectories from the first hospital diagnosis of a psychiatric disorder: a Danish nationwide cohort study using sequence analysis. Lancet Psychiatry 10(1):12–20, 2023 36450298

Hu J, Mansur R, McIntyre RS: Mixed specifier for bipolar mania and depression: highlights of DSM-5 changes and implications for diagnosis and treatment in primary care. Prim Care Companion CNS Disord 16(2):PCC.13r01599, 2014

International Organization for Migration: World Migration Report 2022. Geneva, Switzerland, International Organization for Migration, 2021. Available at: https://publications.iom.int/system/files/pdf/WMR-2022.pdf. Accessed November 15, 2022.

Jensen E, Jones N, Rabe M, et al: 2020 U.S. population more racially and ethnically diverse than measured in 2010: the chance that two people chosen at random are of different race or ethnicity groups has increased since 2010, in America Counts: Stories. Washington, DC, U.S. Census Bureau, August 12, 2021. Available at: www.census.gov/library/stories/2021/08/2020-united-states-population-more-racially-ethnically-diverse-than-2010.html. Accessed November 14, 2022.

Johnson DK: Inference to the best explanation and avoiding diagnostic error, in Ethics and Medical Error. Edited by Allhoff F, Borden S. New York, Routledge, 2020, pp 243–261

Kawa S, Giordano J: A brief historicity of the Diagnostic and Statistical Manual of Mental Disorders: issues and implications for the future of psychiatric canon and practice. Philos Ethics Humanit Med 7:2, 2012 22243976

Kennedy BM, Rehman M, Johnson WD, et al: Healthcare providers versus patients' understanding of health beliefs and values. Patient Exp J 4(3):29–37, 2017 29308429

Klerman GL, Dimascio A, Weissman M, et al: Treatment of depression by drugs and psychotherapy. Am J Psychiatry 131(2):186–191, 1974 4587807

Kotov R, Ruggero CJ, Krueger RF, et al: New dimensions in the quantitative classification of mental illness. Arch Gen Psychiatry 68(10):1003–1011, 2011 21969458

Maduro R: Curanderismo and Latino views of disease and curing. West J Med 139(6):868–874, 1983 6364577

McElroy SL: Understanding the complexity of bipolar mixed episodes. J Clin Psychiatry 69(2):e06, 2008 18363450

National Institute of Mental Health: RDoC (Research Domain Criteria). Bethesda, MD, National Institute of Mental Health, 2022. Available at: www.nimh.nih.gov/research/research-funded-by-nimh/rdoc. Accessed September 23, 2022.

Nusslock R, Frank E: Subthreshold bipolarity: diagnostic issues and challenges. Bipolar Disord 13(7–8):587–603, 2011 22085472

Osimani B: "Modus tollens" probabilized: deductive and inductive methods in medical diagnosis. MEDIC 17(1–3):43–59, 2009

Padilla R, Gomez V, Biggerstaff SL, Mehler PS: Use of curanderismo in a public health care system. Arch Intern Med 161(10):1336–1340, 2001 11371263

Papadimitriou G: The "Biopsychosocial Model": 40 years of application in psychiatry. Psychiatriki 28(2):107–110, 2017 28686557

Pellegrini AJ, Putman P III: The amytal interview in the diagnosis of late onset psychosis with cultural features presenting as catatonic stupor. J Nerv Ment Dis 172(8):502–504, 1984 6747622

Pollitzer W: The Gullah People and Their African Heritage. Athens, University of Georgia Press, 1999

Putman HP: Rational Psychopharmacology: A Book of Clinical Skills. Washington, DC, American Psychiatric Association Publishing, 2020

Ramirez D: Curandero belief runs strong on campus. The South Texan, October 4, 2018. Available at: https://thesouthtexan.com/index.php/2018/10/04/curandero-belief-runs-strong-on-campus. Accessed November 14, 2022.

Rohrbaugh M, Rogers JC: What did the doctor do? When physicians and patients disagree. Arch Fam Med 3(2):125–129, 1994 7994433

Roncoroni J, Tucker CM, Wall W, et al: Patient perceived cultural sensitivity of clinic environment and its association with patient satisfaction with care and treatment adherence. Am J Lifestyle Med 8(6):421–429, 2014

Ruffalo M: The psychoanalytic tradition in American psychiatry: the basics. Psychiatric Times, January 24, 2018. Available at: www.psychiatrictimes.com/view/psychoanalytic-tradition-american-psychiatry-basics. Accessed December 18, 2023.

Shannon PJ, Vinson GA, Cook TL, Lennon E: Characteristics of successful and unsuccessful mental health referrals of refugees. Adm Policy Ment Health 43(4):555–568, 2016 25735618

Shim R: Social (in)justice and mental health. Lecture, Department of Psychiatry and Behavioral Sciences grand rounds, Austin, University of Texas at Austin Dell Medical School, February 28, 2023

Sotsky SM, Glass DR, Shea MT, et al: Patient predictors of response to psychotherapy and pharmacotherapy: findings in the NIMH Treatment of Depression Collaborative Research Program. Am J Psychiatry 148(8):997–1008, 1991 1853989

Spruill IJ, Leite RS, Fernandes JK, et al: Successes, challenges and lessons learned: community-engaged research with South Carolina's Gullah population. Gateways 6: 2013 25364473

Tafur MM, Crowe TK, Torres E: A review of curanderismo and healing practices among Mexicans and Mexican Americans. Occup Ther Int 16(1):82–88, 2009 19222054

Teal CR, Street RL: Critical elements of culturally competent communication in the medical encounter: a review and model. Soc Sci Med 68(3):533–543, 2009 19019520

Tucker CM, Moradi B, Wall W, Nghiem K: Roles of perceived provider cultural sensitivity and health care justice in African American/Black patients' satisfaction with provider. J Clin Psychol Med Settings 21(3):282–290, 2014 24913783

Tucker CM, Arthur TM, Roncoroni J, et al: Patient-centered, culturally sensitive health care. Am J Lifestyle Med 9(1):63–77, 2015

U.N. Refugee Agency: Ukraine Refugee Situation. Operational Data Portal, 2022. Available at https://data.unhcr.org/en/situations/ukraine. Accessed November 1, 2022.

U.S. Census Bureau: Racial and Ethnic Diversity in the United States: 2010 Census and 2020 Census. Washington, DC, U.S. Census Bureau, August 12, 2021. Available at: www.census.gov/library/visualizations/interactive/racial-and-ethnic-diversity-in-the-united-states-2010-and-2020-census.html. Accessed April 16, 2023.

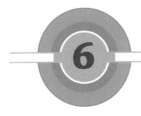

Successful Outcomes

Clinicians, as we have seen, have myriad opportunities for misconceptualization, errors in problem-solving, practicing non-evidence-based medicine, and performing inadequate initial and ongoing assessment. It is no wonder, then, that such a large number of treatment attempts result in treatment failure (Howes et al. 2022). Happily, though, knowledge of these potential pitfalls, conscientious efforts to avoid them, and abductive reasoning (see sections "General Nature of Problems" in Chapter 2, "Keys to Problem-Solving," and "Defining Evidence" in Chapter 3, "The Goal of Evidence-Based Practice") can either reverse treatment failure or avoid it altogether. In this chapter, I discuss eight actual case vignettes from clinical practices that illustrate how reexamination and additional data can lead to reconceptualization, then progression from treatment failure to satisfactory clinical results.

Note that when clinical progress is defined by the patient and based on their goals, it may include more functionality than categorical diagnosis measures; see sections "Return to the Biopsychosocial Model" in Chapter 5, "Essential Assessment and Reevaluation," and "Classification of Concepts" in Chapter 1, "Conceptualization (and Failed Concepts)," and the two case examples in Chapter 9, "Managing a Sustained Therapeutic Relationship During Treatment Failure." The cases reviewed in this chapter give equal weight to the more traditional view of symptom reduction traditionally favored by the practitioner. Also observe that in many of these cases, the treatment course was eventually reversed by the same practitioner who initially failed to help the patient.

A Case of Overspecialization and Inadequate Assessment

Frank (not his real name), a 57-year-old man, accompanied by his wife, consulted a psychiatrist in 2012 about memory problems. He had quit working because of poor executive function 9 months prior to the evaluation, having become less competent at managing grants over the years. He had been assessed by neurologists at a major academic medical center's Alzheimer's disease clinic (ADC), where he had two neuropsychiatric assessments. The clinicians diagnosed mild cognitive impairment (MCI) and prescribed donepezil 5 mg/day, which he was taking. He had also had symptoms of depressed mood for the previous 2 years, and his primary care physician (PCP) had treated him with antidepressants during the past year. The initial medication, escitalopram 20 mg/day, had made him foggy, but when the medication was changed to fluoxetine, the fogginess immediately lifted; he then became more active, with less social isolation. However, he was subsequently found to have concentration problems, with rapid thinking but not rapid speech: his attention capacity was reduced and he was unable to stay on topic or task. A previous psychiatric consultation had not led to further improvement, and the PCP had increased his dose of fluoxetine from 20 mg to 40 mg 5 days prior to the visit to this new psychiatrist.

Additional medical history revealed that Frank also had diabetes mellitus, and his blood glucose levels were not always ideal. Hypertension was under control, but he also had a cardiac arrhythmia of unknown cause. In addition to having osteoarthritis in both knees, he saw a nephrologist for "abnormal labs" but was not on dialysis. He was told by his endocrinologist 9 months previously that his thyroid function was normal, but she followed him quarterly for thyroid nodules: one had been biopsied and was found benign; he did not know if he had antibodies to his thyroid. He had had a kidney stone 2 years previously and did not know if his parathyroid hormone level (PTH) had also been assessed.

Frank had been overweight most of his life and had undergone lap band surgery two and a half years before, leading to a sustained decrease of 65 pounds; he did not know his current calorie intake, however. Fatty liver had been confirmed on biopsy. He had been taking medicine to lower his cholesterol levels for years, and he was also taking vitamin D replacement, without serum level monitoring. He had experienced erectile dysfunction for the previous 2 years that responded well to tadalafil. His sexual desire was currently low, and he had been told his testosterone levels were normal. Frank had also been diagnosed with obstructive sleep apnea, confirmed by polysomnogram, but he had not used continuous positive airway pressure in months. He had taken zolpidem 5 mg qhs for the past 5 years, but recently his PCP had begun to taper the medication, using trazodone.

Frank played football and baseball when he was young, no boxing or soccer, but could not recall any closed head injuries or loss of consciousness. His brain imaging at the ADC had been noncontributory, as had an electroencephalogram (EEG). He did not endorse a personal or family history of seizures, although his mother had had chronic depression and thyroid disease. He was also taking acetylsalicylic acid 81 mg/day, multiple vitamins, and Brain Sustain (a proprietary preparation containing *N*-acetylcysteine, phosphatidylserine, acetyl-L-carnitine, alpha lipoic acid, coenzyme Q10, and glucoraphanin). He also consumed five to six doses of caffeine a day, took occasional decongestants, and consumed three to four alcoholic drinks twice a week. His only use of recreational or illegal drugs was cannabis while in college, which produced a pleasant euphoria, and he denied ever using nicotine.

Frank's neurovegetative symptoms included middle or terminal insomnia, averaging 5.5 hours of deep sleep (according to monitoring) and 7.5 hours total. He had been rested in the morning prior to initiation of the trazodone, with good daytime energy that was never excessive. His moderate appetite was stable, as was his weight (BMI 29.0). He complained of impaired short-term memory and concentration and rapid thoughts. He denied diurnal mood variation and described pervasive anhedonia worsening over the past 2 years (although slightly improved recently) and mild social withdrawal. He had become progressively less agitated, and his irritability, prominent 5 years ago, was now infrequent and brief. Mental status examination (MSE) was significant only for impaired short-term memory and flat affect.

When Frank's wife joined the assessment, she added that his cognition and alertness had improved with the donepezil, but his short-term memory was still better on some days than others (e.g., he sometimes forgot to wash the dishes). She confirmed that the escitalopram had "put him in a fog" but also disclosed that nefazodone taken several years ago for depression and insomnia had definitely helped. She reported that beginning 13 years ago, Frank had sustained two long episodes of dysphoria with middle insomnia. She saw him now as "lackadaisical" but not depressed. She had not noticed problems with rosuvastatin, his current medication for high cholesterol; she thought his cognitive decline began when he did not take the prescribed nutritional supplements following his lap band placement.

The couple hoped that the psychiatrist would manage treatment for Frank's mood and help in any way he could with memory and concentration. The doctor diagnosed unspecified depressive disorder, executive dysfunction, and mild cognitive impairment. He proceeded to confirm thyroid function and levels of vitamins B_{12} and D. He requested a copy of the EEG, recommended a maximum daily intake of 1,500 calories with no alcohol or caffeine, and suggested reevaluation in 4 weeks once the new steady-state serum level of the fluoxetine was achieved.

Although he fell off a motorcycle and broke three ribs before his next appointment, Frank returned a month later reporting noticeable improvement in his mood, sleep, short-term memory, and concentration. His thyroid and vitamin levels were in acceptable ranges. He had not yet stopped his alcohol use, but he again agreed to do so and also to seek further improvement by changing to brand-name fluoxetine (Prozac) for the following 6 weeks. His mood did respond fully to this plan, but his short-term memory did not completely improve. Citing the current literature, and with the approval of Frank's cardiologist, the psychiatrist initiated a medication holiday with the rosuvastatin, although Frank's endocrinologist doubted this would be effective (Carlsson et al. 2009; Etgen et al. 2011; King et al. 2003; Rojas-Fernandez and Cameron 2012).

Within 3 months, Frank was fully euthymic, with no neurovegetative symptoms of a depressive disorder. He also had no cognitive impairment: short- and long-term memory and concentration were fully intact, with no rapid thoughts. Executive function was also now intact. In place of the rosuvastatin, he was now taking ezetimibe, a nonstatin, at 10 mg/day. He had stopped the donepezil on his own and returned to the ADC: they confirmed he no longer met criteria for MCI and, because repeat positron emission tomography (PET) and neuropsychological testing there confirmed no impairment, agreed he should not take the donepezil. Frank also said they would not admit that the statin, depression, or his myriad other medical problems may have led to the MCI diagnosis, but they also had no alternative explanation.

Frank continued to do well for the next 5 years. Minor perturbations in mood were occasionally produced by changes in bioavailability of his generic antidepressant and occasional problems with absorption due to his lap band. A consistent generic brand of sertraline was available and eventually was used long term at 200–250 mg/day; therapeutic serum levels were documented. Episodic alcohol and caffeine use also provoked minor symptoms that were easily corrected by a return to abstinence.

In late 2015, mild depression and cognitive impairment returned, and Frank noticed that he was not absorbing all of his oral medications because of his lap band placement (which had not been reevaluated in 2 years). Also, in early 2016, he used edible cannabis while vacationing in Colorado, and acute additional cognitive impairment followed: impaired short-term memory and concentration, evidenced by frequently forgetting and not staying on tasks, repeating trips to accomplish tasks, and limited ability to redirect if interrupted. At the same time, his thyroid function, which had been carefully monitored, began to show persistently elevated thyroid-stimulating hormone (TSH) levels. Further, he had resumed daily alcohol use, and he also now complained of irritability. During this multifactorial episode, the ADC asked to reevaluate Frank with neuropsychiatric testing and a PET scan; they had previously enrolled him in a study and wished him to continue it.

Frank stopped the alcohol and cannabis use, the lap band placement was reevaluated and adjusted, and subsequent therapeutic serum levels of sertraline were again confirmed. Treatment with brand-name levothyroxine (Synthroid) from a new endocrinologist was also initiated. Frank's mood symptoms again improved, as did his cognition. He continued to have no complaints about short- or long-term memory, which he and his wife both believed to be good: he readily recalled conversations, completed tasks, and denied misplacing things or getting lost. Additionally, his concentration remained intact: he stayed on tasks and completed them and was able to redirect his focus if interrupted. He denied racing thoughts. His only cognitive complaint was the intermittent return of an executive function problem: occasional difficulty initially organizing his thoughts to solve a problem. He also started a successful business that year.

Repeat testing at the ADC showed improvement, except for the executive function problem. Staff then diagnosed nonamnestic MCI and reenrolled Frank in their study, asking him to again resume donepezil. This was discussed with his psychiatrist, who considered the multiple possible contributions to his memory issues over the years, including statin side effects that resolved following discontinuation, possible nutritional deficiencies after bariatric surgery, his thyroid status, diabetes mellitus, depressive disorder status, alcohol and cannabis use, and untreated sleep apnea. Any cognitive impairment had been variable and appeared secondary to these obvious other factors. Frank had consistently refused treatment for his sleep apnea, although its persistence was documented. The psychiatrist, noting the assertion that his apnea was largely positional, suggested sleeping with a tennis ball attached to the back of his shirt (Eijsvogel et al. 2015; Kavey et al. 1982). He also suggested that they confirm thyroid status prior to resuming a cholinesterase inhibitor, wanting to be sure that any reversible causes of cognitive impairment could first be fully addressed (Quinlan et al. 2010; Ritchie and Yeap 2015).

By mid-2017, Frank was again euthyroid. His mood, memory, and concentration were again fully intact, except for occasional difficulty coming up with a plan to solve a problem, which was not endorsed as a symptom at every visit. Although the psychiatrist still considered Frank's poor compliance with the treatment for sleep apnea to be an ongoing factor in his mild and occasional executive function complaint, the neurologist running his study at the ADC had convinced Frank to resume donepezil "to prevent progression into dementia." The medication had been well tolerated previously, so they agreed to 5 mg/day, noting that eventual decline in cognition, if it occurred, would only be slowed by such a treatment and that confirmation of donepezil benefit would be impossible to achieve because of lack of a control. Frank's psychiatrist retired, and transfer of Frank's care to another psychiatrist was completed 3 months later.

Pseudodementia (cognitive impairment secondary to other medical and psychiatric conditions, such as major depressive disorder) has been described for decades and is generally considered reversible (Kang et al. 2014). Although some authors have demonstrated the persistence of MCI symptoms during and after treatment for mood disorders, the incidence reported is low: 14% for persistent nonamnestic MCI (Bhalla et al. 2009). The issue is further clouded by variations in criteria for mood symptoms and MCI among various studies (Panza et al. 2010). Multiple studies also show that reversion from MCI to normal cognition without intervention is at least as likely as progression to dementia, particularly in patients with high cognitive reserve (often estimated by degree of education) (Iraniparast et al. 2022).

This case is included to show how, when multiple factors appear to be contributing to symptoms that also respond to intervention against these causes, ignoring them, while adopting an additional, unrelated diagnosis that is nonreversible with proposed treatment, is a disservice compared with helping a patient discover and recover from each of the reversible causes. Abraham Maslow famously observed, "I suppose it is tempting, if the only tool you have is a hammer, to treat everything as if it were a nail" (Maslow 1966, pp. 15–16). The dangers of practitioners functioning as narrow but high-level specialists are described in Chapter 2, sections "Obstacles to Problem Solving" and "Implications for Medical Practice." Such providers are prone to diagnostic error from rapid conclusion and their failure to perceive data that do not fit with preferred diagnoses. It is not suggested that the neurologists in this case held on to a questionable diagnosis in order to fill slots in their studies. Their comfort, however, in asking the patient to accept a diagnosis with a limited to poor prognosis and a treatment not designed to lead to improvement led them to ignore how management of his mood disorder, hypothyroidism, and sleep apnea, in addition to avoiding side effects of certain medications and substance use, could restore him to higher levels of functionality. Blinders apparently led them to consistently deny the value of these other solutions, even in the face of their own evidence.

It is helpful for you as the practitioner to consistently view yourself as a generalist, perhaps with interest and additional strength in two or three areas. This has been proposed to foster creativity through paradigm shifts that specialists may not recognize because of cognitive biases (Epstein 2019). The path taken by the psychiatrist in this case gave the patient at least 5 years of symptom resolution and full functioning, including the ability to open a successful business and participate fully in activities with his friends and family. The alternative was to accept persistent cognitive impairment due to misdiagnosis.

A Case of Impaired Therapeutic Alliance

Tyler (not his real name), a 26-year-old man, was referred to a psychiatrist by his long-term PCP for treatment of ADHD. The PCP had attempted treatment with lisdexamfetamine dimesylate (Vyvanse) up to 40 mg qam and then methylphenidate osmotic release oral system (a generic form of

Concerta) up to 54 mg. Each trial produced only modest improvement in concentration for about 7 hours, leaving Tyler so impaired in the evening hours that he and the PCP both considered these trials failures.

The psychiatrist began with his own thorough evaluation. Tyler did not describe a history consistent with ADHD: onset of impaired concentration appears to have begun only around age 20, and there was no evidence of current or previous hyperactivity. He denied any problems with completing schoolwork as a child or adolescent, although he was now having significant problems staying on and completing tasks at work, the reason he sought help from his PCP. His medical history and review of systems appeared noncontributory: no developmental problems, head injuries, or neurological or endocrine illnesses. His MSE was significant only for impaired concentration, without rapid thoughts, and impaired immediate- and short-term memory. He was anxiety-free and appeared euthymic. No additional diagnoses were found that could explain Tyler's symptoms, except that on direct questioning he did admit that he was smoking cannabis daily for recreational reasons, and had been for more than 5 years. He did not see it as a problem. When asked whether the referring physician was aware of this cannabis use, the patient replied that he had not disclosed this information to his PCP, who had cared for him since he was young, because of embarrassment.

The psychiatrist nodded that he understood and explained to Tyler how cannabis use might be negatively affecting his concentration and, therefore, short-term memory (Gruber et al. 2003; Hall and Degenhardt 2014; Hartman and Huestis 2013; Harvey et al. 2007; Messinis et al. 2006; Petker et al. 2020; Solowij et al. 2002; Volkow et al. 2016). He proposed that, in addition to having his thyroid function checked, Tyler refrain from all cannabis use for a minimum of 90 days, noting that the half-life for cannabis is 5–13 days in chronic users, and that it might take five or more half-lives for the substance to significantly leave his body, given its storage in body fat (Ellis et al. 1985; Gunasekaran et al. 2009; Sharma et al. 2012; Smith-Kielland et al. 1999). They would then meet and reassess prior to considering pharmacological treatment for his concentration and memory symptoms.

Intrigued, and motivated to improve his job performance, Tyler agreed. His TSH level was found to be in an acceptable range, 1.3–2.5 mIU/L (Talaei et al. 2017; Wartofsky and Dickey 2005), with no measurable antibodies to his thyroid gland. Twelve weeks later, Tyler happily reported to the psychiatrist that he no longer had problems with concentration and short-term memory, an assertion the psychiatrist was able to confirm with a repeat MSE, including in-office cognitive testing (Putman 2020, pp. 53–55). They agreed that Tyler should continue his cannabis abstinence, including edibles, and reevaluate in another 3 months. Reassessment at that time confirmed that he remained symptom-free. Tyler reported that he was showing improved work performance and planned to continue to refrain from cannabis use, which he now understood had led to his reversible cognitive impairment.

A long-term working alliance with a PCP from childhood in this case led to a failure of diagnosis and treatment because the therapeutic relationship was not fully examined. Although we might not expect such exploration by nonpsychiatrists, it is a reminder that transference and countertransference can lead to interference with successful outcomes. Sociologists have shown that we are often more likely to share intimate information with relative strangers than those with whom we are closest (Kim et al. 2021; Small 2013; Small and Sukhu 2016). Telling the specialist about his cannabis use held little to no emotional risk for Tyler, compared with the loss of face he feared by disclosing his use to his childhood physician. Although it was fortuitous that the PCP made the specialist referral following treatment failure and that the conditions then favored uncovering the correct diagnosis and treatment plans, we must expect that factors may always be limiting our therapeutic alliances and take steps to look for them.

For the mental health professional, such steps must include monitoring the quality of the therapeutic alliance, addressing and repairing any ruptures in it, and always directly asking patients about essential information, such as substance use (see section "Lifestyle Factors" in Chapter 7, "Underappreciated Causes of Treatment Failure," and Chapter 9). A quality therapeutic relationship helps the patient understand the value of fuller self-disclosure and its impact on treatment outcome. Discovering the solutions to therapeutic impasses reinforces for practitioners the importance of performing consistently thorough assessments (see Chapter 5) and not presuming that referring providers have uncovered all necessary information.

In this case, the patient was willing to let go of his use of cannabis, which he described as recreational, and was fully compliant because he believed the opinion and guidance of the specialist and eventually saw the benefits himself. Although this is an actual case, we know that compliance with lifestyle recommendations, such as avoiding substance use, is not always so simple and easy. We must use our alliance to build enough trust and mutual understanding that patients attempt to follow essential steps they may find disappointing, unrealistic, objectionable, or difficult. We must also be fully prepared to provide assistance with achieving and sustaining abstinence when the patient does not find it as easy as Tyler did.

A Case of Undetected Neurological Disease

Eric (not his real name), a 17-year-old adolescent, was brought to a psychiatric hospital by his frightened single mother in 1988. A high-functioning and successful teenager, in a wheelchair because of spina bifida, he showed sudden onset of psychosis, with mood-congruent delusions and auditory hallucinations. Eric was affable and coherent, but he was largely autistic in his attention to his inner world, so he did not always give complete answers to diagnostic questions (although he did not meet criteria for catatonia). For this reason, it was difficult to ascertain whether he was also experiencing olfactory or visual hallucinations, although he did not seem to be attending to such hallucinations as he was to the auditory ones. His mother, who was so strongly devoted to him that she lacked some interpersonal boundaries, was overwhelmed with fear and anxiety, which she easily transmitted to the staff caring for her son. She declined any supportive help for herself, however.

Prior to admission, Eric had been evaluated by his PCP and neurologist, neither of whom found any underlying contributions to this abrupt onset of his first episode of psychosis. Everyone denied any prior or family psychiatric history, as well as any history of seizure, additional neurological disease, or substance abuse. Physical examination and laboratory testing at the hospital also failed to uncover any findings to help explain his acute psychiatric condition: all drug and toxicity screens were normal, and there were no abnormal muscle movements.

Treatment with oral brand-name haloperidol (Haldol) up to 10 mg/day was initiated and did not result in any improvement over a 5-day period, although it was well tolerated. Eric's mother began searching for alternative facilities to treat her child. The provider changed the haloperidol to thioridazine, up to 600 mg/day, but it was also not leading to improvement 3 days into the trial, although, again, it produced no acute adverse events. As part of his complete evaluation, the attending psychiatrist had ordered CT of the head, with contrast dye, which was confirmed by neuroradiology as noncontributory. Still suspicious that the spina bifida might be playing some role, the psychiatrist ordered an EEG, which he attended and read alongside a neurologist.

The EEG showed clear spike and wave activity in Eric's dominant temporal lobe consistent with seizure, although there remained no motor symptoms (Flor-Henry 1969; Gibbs 1951; Nadkarni et al. 2007; Shukla et al. 1979; Vinti et al. 2021; Wells 1975). Together, the psychiatrist and neurologist decided to stop the second antipsychotic and started phenytoin, which led to rapid reversal of Eric's psychosis in less than 36 hours. His mother, although very grateful for the rediagnosis and treatment, proceeded with the transfer she had been arranging to the psychiatric floor of a downtown teaching hospital, based on Eric's "treatment-refractory psychosis." The original psychiatrist was able to subsequently confirm that Eric continued his phenytoin there, tolerated it well, and remained free of psychosis without antipsychotic medication during his stay at the new facility.

Although we always wish to achieve remission of symptoms and restoration of functionality as soon as possible, it takes time for treatments to be fully expressed and to work through successive trials. The panic Eric's mother was experiencing and the pressure she placed on the staff influenced the psychiatrist to change treatments at the minimum rather than maximum time allowed for assessing response to treatment. Had the EEG been normal, this might have negatively influenced treatment outcome because effective treatments might have been discarded prematurely.

In this case, the patient was affable and passive in decisions about his care, but a therapeutic alliance also needed to be formed between his legal guardian (mother) and the psychiatrist. Although they had a working relationship and she agreed to all of the assessments and treatments, the provider and treatment team were unable to convince her to accept help addressing how she experienced this "crisis," which may have adjusted her expectations. As a result, the mother and provider were unable to share a realistic vision of the time necessary to treat her son, and this led her to move his care to an alternative facility. Interestingly, once the diagnosis was made and treatment was successful, she asked the original psychiatrist to move to the new facility with her son, which was not possible.

This case also demonstrates the importance of persistence in the face of initially negative findings. The neurological evaluation continued until completed with the EEG and was not stopped after normal neurological examination and CT scan. The psychiatrist remained alert to the possible effects of Eric's other obvious medical condition (spina bifida) and continued to believe it might explain not only his symptoms but the lack of response to traditional treatment of his psychosis (Werhagen et al. 2013; Yoshida et al. 2006). As a result, persistence of his symptoms as treatment-refractory psychosis and possible further psychiatric and neurological deterioration were avoided.

A Case of Ongoing Interference

Jessica (not her real name), a 22-year-old woman, entered the care of a psychiatrist in 2000 for the treatment of cyclical depression with psychotic features and suicidal and homicidal ideation. She lived with her parents, who had adopted her as a special needs child with fetal alcohol syndrome. Both parents were very devoted to her and involved in her treatment. In fact, when the psychiatrist at one point was able to secure placement for Jessica in a residential facility for adults with intellectual disabilities (which also offered a path to semi-independent living), her father removed her on her request, which he later regretted.

Early treatment involved frequent hospitalizations for risks of targeted violence and self-harm. Jessica often had the desire to kill her attractive female cousins and more than once obtained a knife to do so. Even more regularly, she planned to use the knife on herself. She had frequent mood-congruent noncommand auditory hallucinations and was frequently depressed and afraid. Following a comprehensive medical and psychiatric evaluation, the psychiatrist diagnosed organic affective disorder and proceeded with trials of anticonvulsant mood stabilizers, second-generation antipsychotics, and antidepressant medications. Jessica's course was often complicated by other physicians prescribing medications for her additional medical problems that interfered by provoking psychiatric symptoms or altering serum levels of her psychiatric medications.

As an example, one hospitalization in 2001 was necessary when an orthopedist prescribed propoxyphene for Jessica's chronic hip pain, without consultation. This elevated her serum carbamazepine level over 30 mcg/mL, well above the standard range of 4–12 mcg/mL. At the family's request, the carbamazepine was changed to oxcarbazepine, an alternative anticonvulsant with fewer drug-drug interactions and more stable serum levels. Although this did improve Jessica's mood cycling, she continued to have many symptomatic episodes requiring hospitalization for safety, despite trials of olanzapine, risperidone, quetiapine, valproate, clonazepam, topiramate, and paroxetine, along with family therapy and individual supportive psychotherapy. Lithium carbonate was considered contraindicated because of her cerebral injuries and visual and olfactory hallucinations. An EEG was noncontributory.

When Jessica reached age 25 with insufficient improvement of a (now chronic) affective and organic psychosis, the family accepted the psychiatrist's suggestion to file for Supplemental Security Income. It did not appear Jessica would eventually be able to find employment, and she could no longer continue treatment under her parents' insurance; the application was successful.

During an early 2003 hospital stay, Jessica and her family were willing to proceed with clozapine, as previously suggested by her psychiatrist. The medication was titrated initially to a dosage of 150 mg tid, and Jessica showed significant improvement in mood and psychotic symptoms. Because clozapine is known to lower seizure threshold even more than do most antipsychotic medications (Grover et al. 2015; Gurrera et al. 2022; Williams and Park 2015), topiramate 200 mg bid was continued in light of Jessica's visual and olfactory hallucinations. This combination was more fully effective over the next year as the dose of clozapine was increased to 300 mg tid and clonazepam was reduced to 0.5 mg qhs. Jessica showed sustained freedom from mood and psychotic symptoms, with no further thoughts of aggression or self-harm, and she was able to fully participate in activities with her extended family.

Jessica's complete blood count was monitored regularly and remained in the acceptable range; her most significant side effect was excessive salivation, necessitating shirt changes three times a day. Glycopyrrolate 0.5 mg once or twice daily, which has been reported useful for this side effect in several studies, was considered. However, because the medication also reduces diaphoresis, the family and psychiatrist did not think it would be safe for Jessica; she already had limited sweat production and poor heat tolerance and often worked outside with her father in their garden.

Jessica continued to do well until October 2004, when she again began to show signs of depressed mood with crying, which progressed over the next month to severe depression with anxiety and fear, irritability, hypersomnia up to 14 hours, and thoughts of self-harm; she had begun sleeping with her mother in order to feel safe. The family lamented that the clozapine did not appear to be working and worried they might be running out of options. However, Jessica's psychiatrist noted that another provider had prescribed lactulose syrup twice a day for constipation just prior to her decline. Although he could not find a reference to this effect, he wondered whether the lactulose might be affecting the absorption of her psychiatric medications because the timing was so suspicious. He suggested Jessica separate her doses of lactulose by 2 hours from doses of each of her psychiatric medications. The family decided to stop it instead, and Jessica's condition began to reverse immediately, returning to excellent within 2 weeks. They concluded that the lactulose had interfered with the levels of clozapine, which had been the primary reason for Jessica's clinical improvement. The family instead used apple juice effectively for her constipation.

Jessica's excellent progress continued until May 2006, when her symptoms, including depressed mood, olfactory hallucinations, command auditory hallucinations to kill herself, and moderate anxiety, again returned. Another physician, without consultation, had added atorvastatin for her lipids and risedronate for osteoporosis only weeks earlier.

At the time, statins were thought by many researchers to reduce the risk of depression, hostility, and anxiety, despite their potentially negative effects on cognition, and there were no published reports of adverse mental health effects of risedronate (Pazarlis et al. 2006; Young-Xu et al. 2003). As such, the addition of these two agents was not recognized at the time as likely reasons for the worsening of Jessica's psychiatric symptoms, nor of affecting the serum levels of her psychiatric medications; the only relevant connections were temporal. Because the psychiatrist could find no other explanation for her acute deterioration and the other physician did not wish to discontinue the new prescriptions, he concluded that the limit of benefit from the maximum dose of clozapine had been reached. In discussing options with Jessica and her family, he noted that antipsychotic medications had been more efficacious for her than antidepressants or mood stabilizers and proposed adding ziprasidone (then available only orally), first at 40 mg bid, and replacing it later with quetiapine if improvement did not occur. They all agreed, and her improvement was again quick and impressive: within a week her mood and psychotic symptoms had fully resolved.

The only problem with this effective plan developed 3 years later, when Jessica's mild depression with olfactory and auditory hallucinations returned. However, her family quickly determined that she had not taken her topiramate for a month, and when it was restarted, she regained full remission of her symptoms. Later that same year, although

Jessica's thyroid indices had previously remained within the normal range, she was diagnosed with benign thyroid nodules, had a partial thyroidectomy, and was prescribed brand-name levothyroxine (Synthroid) 75 mcg/day. As a result, her risedronate was discontinued. As long as her TSH remained at 0.3–2.5 mIU/L, she remained psychiatrically stable; her clozapine was lowered to 250 mg bid + 300 mg qhs the next year, which effectively reduced occasional daytime sedation.

In late 2014, Jessica experienced a partial complex seizure while on the same long-term treatment plan. She had been to the dentist earlier that day and received procaine. She was hospitalized, during which some doses of clozapine were missed, causing a few of her former psychiatric symptoms to return; these resolved within 24 hours when the dosing errors were corrected. Neurological consultation was obtained, but no further diagnoses or changes in treatment plan were suggested; a repeat EEG was read as normal. Although Jessica was receiving two medications that lowered her seizure threshold (clozapine itself carrying a 6% risk of tonic-clonic seizure), she was also taking two anticonvulsants and had had no prior convulsions. Seizures have been reported to follow local injection of anesthetics in dentistry, so it is possible this was a factor (Alsukhni et al. 2016).

In 2017, *N*-acetylcysteine 1,800 mg bid was added, which improved Jessica's long-term habit of picking at her skin (Grant et al. 2016; Lee and Lipner 2022). By this time, her PCP had added tolterodine for overactive bladder and alendronate for her osteoporosis; she continued taking atorvastatin. He also pressed to add a β-blocker to treat her resting tachycardia, but the psychiatrist raised considerable concern that it, as well as alendronate, might also provoke symptoms of depression and psychosis (Cojocariu et al. 2021; Coleman et al. 2004; Huffman and Stern 2007; Keshishi et al. 2021). The providers agreed to proceed with metoprolol succinate extended release 25 mg/day and to monitor Jessica's mood carefully. Four months later, she was not showing any signs of deterioration. This was her final visit with this psychiatrist, who was retiring.

Jessica obtained remission for a minimum of 14 years, after it appeared she was not showing sustained response to any combination of medical treatments for depressed mood and psychosis. Any interruptions in her remission were linked directly to interferences with the treatment plan, such as reduced absorption of clozapine due to laxative overlap or poor compliance, and did not justify a label of treatment failure or treatment resistance. Subsequent data have pointed to a number of cases of psychosis and depression linked to use of atorvastatin (Alghamdi et al. 2018; Cham et al. 2016; Peters et al. 2008; Tuccori et al. 2014), and there are new reports of psychosis, anxiety, and depression triggered by risedronate (Hirschmann et al. 2015); continued use of either may have necessitated the addition of ziprasidone for Jessica. Even if the 2006 decline was spontaneous, the treatment changes made in response sustained her remission for at least another 11 years.

Much of the treatment in psychiatry is long-term care for chronic conditions. This case points to how many factors must be considered when treatments initially or eventually disappoint: serum levels, absorption, compliance, bioavailability, contributions from the myriad other medical problems a patient may develop during chronic care that must be identified and responded to, and the constant risk of other medical treatments added by a psychiatrist or other providers, to name only a few. The task is to never give up, to never stop trying to find the answers, because they are usually there for the persistent provider to discover by reconceptualizing the problem.

A Case of Diagnostic Error

Paige (not her real name), a 25-year-old single woman, was referred for psychiatric evaluation of her anxiety. She reported that she felt anxious all the time, worried a lot, and was easily overwhelmed. She described feeling "panicky" when she had anything to accomplish and that these panic episodes were always provoked by some task she had to perform. Work had always been difficult because her anxiety was easily triggered. She had been fired on several occasions for poor performance and collected welfare payments because she had been deemed unable to work.

Paige was not assessed as depressed, and screening for bipolar disorder and psychosis was also negative. Her psychiatrist diagnosed other specified anxiety disorder and started treatment with antidepressants for her anxiety symptoms. Sertraline was prescribed initially. It was not successful, so sequential trials of escitalopram, venlafaxine, and paroxetine followed, all at standard dosages for adequate lengths of time. These selective serotonin reuptake inhibitors and the serotonin-norepinephrine reuptake inhibitor venlafaxine either did not work or worsened Paige's anxiety, even after weeks of treatment. A later trial with a benzodiazepine triggered a paradoxical reaction of agitation.

Eventually, Paige mentioned during a session that she had also experienced some academic performance anxiety while in school. This casual revelation cued the psychiatrist to begin to look for alternative diagnoses. Deeper inquiry demonstrated that Paige had also had a pattern of inattention, daydreaming, and not completing her homework on time dating back to her elementary school years. She had no history of hyperactivity and never showed increased psychomotor productivity or restlessness during sessions. The psychiatrist proceeded to assess Paige for the possibility of ADHD. He was able to determine that her anxiety was almost always triggered by cognitive tasks requiring selective or sustained attention. As an example, she was terminated from a job as a receptionist because she could not cope with the high number of calls she was receiving and was expected to screen. She had made several mistakes in directing the calls due to her difficulties in sustaining attention. The psychiatrist's new screening also revealed that Paige tended to lose keys and bank cards on a regular basis, was a chronic procrastinator, could not sustain her attention while watching a movie, and was late for many of her appointments. A diagnosis of ADHD, inattentive type, was made, and a stimulant was started. Within a week, Paige felt calmer, her attention improved markedly, and, after a few months, she was able to start a job and end her welfare supplements.

My colleague who graciously contributed this case, Giuseppe Guaiana, M.D., M.Sc., Ph.D., FRCPC (Associate Professor at Western University, Ontario, Canada, and Chief of Psychiatry at St. Thomas Elgin General Hospital), says that he learned from it that some symptoms may be described by a patient in a different way than we are expecting. He adds, and his actions illustrate, that it is important to look beyond just what patients initially report to us so that we can identify the correct diagnosis and improve their lives.

Although ADHD and generalized anxiety disorder do have a high rate of comorbidity (25%–30%; Reimherr et al. 2017), this case does not represent such an occurrence; rather it represents an alternative, single diagnosis. A symptom is not always synonymous with a diagnosis: depressed mood is not always major or bipolar depression, and anxiety is not always linked to an anxiety disorder. In fact, anxiety is the most common psychiatric symptom humans are likely to experience, and clinicians should consider many categorical and dimensional diagnoses that may lead to it (Archer et al. 2022; Bandelow and Michaelis 2015; Martín-Merino et al. 2010; Walters et al. 2012; Wittchen et al. 2002). The idea of prescribing a stimulant for what appears to be a case of anxiety may seem counterintuitive until we separate symptom from diagnosis and more fully understand what the patient is experiencing.

In this case, an assiduous physician reassessed his patient's functionality, carrying their therapeutic alliance further than would have been possible by remaining focused only on her original symptomatic complaints. We are also reminded by this case that although patients may inadvertently drop important clues at any point during our work together, thorough and broad questions about symptoms and function, early and consistently during treatment, may alert the practitioner to a correct diagnosis more quickly.

A Case of Multiple Endocrinological Diagnoses

Nancy (not her real name), a 41-year-old woman, presented to a psychiatrist in 1995 for evaluation of multiple issues, including low mood and family stress. A thorough evaluation led to a diagnosis of major depression, single episode, moderate. Nancy was treated with nefazodone 600 mg qhs and weekly individual, insight-oriented psychotherapy. In her sessions, she explored how her relationship with her parents set up dysfunctional patterns with her siblings that carried forward into present ongoing resentments on all sides. She was able to use her gains in therapy to redefine and alter her relationships with members of her family of origin and also improve interactions with her husband and daughters. Her symptoms of major depression responded well to the nefazodone. After 31 months of treatment, the psychotherapy was completed, and Nancy elected to continue her antidepressant under the care of her PCP. Both she and her psychiatrist considered her in full remission, with no residual symptoms.

In spring 2002, Nancy returned to the psychiatrist, noting a recent change in her mood symptoms. She had continued her improved interactions with family, and there appeared to be no new stresses. She had also continued the nefazodone as prescribed. During the reevaluation, she described increasing social withdrawal and feeling worse emotionally and physically. She did not want to get out of bed 3 days a week but denied hypersomnia. She was averaging 7 hours of sleep but needed a full 8 to feel rested, so she was tired throughout the day. Her appetite was lower, although her weight was steady. She reported a decline over the previous 2–3 months in her productivity at work, where she maintained a high administrative position. She also complained of poor concentration and avoiding activities of daily living, such as shopping, cooking, and cleaning. Nancy and her PCP thought reevaluation by the psychiatrist appropriate at this point.

Nancy's MSE showed depressed mood, mild to moderate anxiety, appropriate speech and affect, impaired recent memory, fair concentration, and, possibly, rapid thinking. Thought content and processing were otherwise normal; she denied active and passive suicidal and homicidal ideation, although she did have thoughts of dying. Her insight, judgment, and reliability were intact, and her intellect was estimated to be above average.

Nancy's diagnosis was changed to major depression, recurrent, moderate. She was receiving hydrocodone from her orthopedic surgeon for minor lumbar back pain and agreed to the psychiatrist's asking the surgeon to consider alternative analgesia (metaxalone 400–800 mg qid as needed), which was accomplished. One of Nancy's daughters had recently been diagnosed with bipolar disorder and was treated successfully with carbamazepine. Neither Nancy nor her psychiatrist recalled any symptoms consistent with unstable mood during their previous work together, and an extensive chart review confirmed that there had been no symptoms indicating bipolar disorder during the earlier treatment course. Noting possible rapid thinking now, however, they agreed to taper and eliminate all use of caffeine over 7 days. The psychiatrist reviewed all of the standard and promising mood stabilizers, and she chose a trial of oxcarbazepine. They both hoped it would be better tolerated than carbamazepine, with more stable serum levels, and as effective as early studies had indicated it might be (Berigan 2001); see also Chapter 9, Case Example 2. Clorazepate 3.75–7.5 mg was prescribed as needed, up to three times a day, for anxiety. The nefazodone was left at 600 mg qhs for the time being.

Two weeks later, while still titrating the oxcarbazepine, Nancy returned "on edge." Suicidal thoughts were now present most of the time, but she could distract herself from them by reading or sleeping, and there was no intent or plan. She was less nervous and agitated but still felt "fragile." Daytime anergy and poor concentration persisted, and she was now sleeping only 5 or 6 hours a night because of terminal insomnia. She decided that she had not had rapid thinking. She had been prescribed 0.9 mg conjugated estrogens tablets (Premarin) by her PCP since her hysterectomy and oophorectomy, and the psychiatrist suggested lowering the dose to 0.625 mg—the higher dose did not appear necessary, and he was uncertain about the effect it might be having on her mood (Shors and Leuner 2003). Mild headaches and nausea from initial doses of oxcarbazepine were abating, and Nancy and the psychiatrist agreed to proceed to 600 mg bid in 4 days as originally planned. They discussed the possibility that clorazepate might be lowering her mood but also considered that the reduced agitation it provided would likely reduce her suicide risk. A contract for safety, made in the previous session, was reaffirmed.

One week later, Nancy was better, with rare, brief, "inconsequential" suicidal ideation. Her mood was in the low normal range, tearfulness had abated, and she was no longer avoiding projects at work or activities of daily living. Sleep had returned to 7 or 8 hours per night, and she was rested in the morning, without daytime anergy. She felt that the new medication plan was working; she and the psychiatrist discussed her history, self-perceptions, and feelings about illness. She was now aware she might have distorted the reactions of her coworkers in the previous few months. She and the psychiatrist agreed to keep the current plan, which included avoiding caffeine, dextromethorphan, and decongestants, and to not decrease her nicotine use at the time.

Three weeks later, however, Nancy's sleep had climbed to 10–12 hours a day, unusual for her, and she now had low energy in the evenings, although she was rested during the day. She was now craving sweets and had gained 10 pounds. She was irritable and angry, and her mood was again lower, although with no suicidal ideation. Her PCP had changed her Premarin to 0.9 mg every other day, she had not been taking any clorazepate, and she denied any side effects from the oxcarbazepine at 600 mg bid. She had continued to avoid all destabilizers and depressants, including alcohol. She blamed herself for her depression and saw herself as "a failure."

Nancy was not having symptoms associated with low estrogen and, in fact, had had two recent migraines her PCP thought were associated with high estrogen levels. They agreed she would take estrogen as currently prescribed and recheck a serum level in 3 weeks. The psychiatrist thought Nancy might benefit further from a higher dose of oxcarbazepine and agreed to raise the dosage to 900 mg bid while continuing to monitor sodium levels.

Nancy's mood lability steadily decreased, and her sleep returned to 8–9 hours a night; she was rested in the morning, although she still experienced anergy later in the day. Her appetite remained high with carbohydrate craving and her weight continued to increase. She had had two drinks of alcohol while on a trip but otherwise was fully complaint with her treatment plan. Her estrogen level was in the normal range again at 166 pg/mL. Nancy and the psychiatrist discussed some feelings she was ashamed of, rediscovered her skills to handle them, and agreed to raise the oxcarbazepine dose to 900 mg in the morning and 1,200 mg in the evening, while increasing the Premarin to 0.625 mg/day.

Two weeks later, Nancy's condition had again deteriorated. She was having anxiety episodes lasting up to an hour and accompanied with lower mood if not treated, so she had resumed the clorazepate; each of these episodes occurred after awakening from a nap. The higher dose of oxcarbazepine had helped eliminate anxiety and improve mood but had not been tolerated because of dizziness. Nancy was again sleeping 5–6 hours a night. She no longer had suicidal ideation but had passive thoughts of "wanting to remove some people."

The decision was made to replace the clorazepate with clonazepam 0.25–0.5 mg tid and to replace the oxcarbazepine with topiramate, which had shown some early success with mood stability (Kusumakar et al. 1999; Letmaier et al. 2001). Nancy preferred this option to more traditional mood stabilizers. The clonazepam made her drowsy, and the topiramate impaired her concentration, so both dosages remained below target (clonazepam 0.25 mg tid and topiramate 75 mg qhs); she was more irritable, anxious, and weepy, although not suicidal. She had also slipped and fallen, resulting in torn ligaments and tendons in her right ankle and knee. Her orthopedic surgeon had given her propoxyphene and carisoprodol to take as needed. Her psychiatrist expressed concern about these medications and again reviewed potential mood stabilizers. This time she chose lithium carbonate and continued the clonazepam 0.25 mg tid.

Six weeks later, Nancy was "relatively well, a vast difference": her mood was euthymic, not labile, her appetite had significantly declined, she had lost 5 pounds without effort, and, although she had daytime anergy, she again slept 8 hours a night. The plan was to adjust the lithium serum level further and taper off the clonazepam and then eventually the nefazodone. Unfortunately, however, she misunderstood and stopped the benzodiazepine abruptly, provoking a withdrawal syndrome she mistook for lithium toxicity. She stopped the lithium as well before contacting her psychiatrist, which allowed full symptomatology and dysfunction to return.

However, once the plan had been reestablished with a serum lithium level of 1.0 mEq/L, Nancy was not much improved, showing anergy, hypersomnia up to 16 hours, anorexia, diarrhea, slow speech, word-finding problems, exaggerated body movements, and social withdrawal. Her balance was improved but still not intact, although she was not shuffling her feet as much. She had trouble holding a pen and the handbells in her church choir. Her mouth, hands, and feet moved at rest but were still under voluntary control. Her mood was depressed, and she had suicidal ideation with a plan to overdose, although she denied intent. She had no thoughts of harming others. She had resumed clonazepam 0.5 mg tid but agreed to taper and discontinue it. She agreed to an MRI of her brain, with contrast medium, and a second opinion from another psychiatrist. The MRI was read as noncontributory by both her psychiatrist and a neurologist who consulted.

Four weeks later, however, Nancy was taking sustained release lithium carbonate 300 mg bid, nefazodone 600 mg qhs, and Premarin 0.625 mg qd, and she was again much improved. Her mood was in the low normal range, and her anxiety was mild; her short-term memory was impaired, but her concentration had improved to fair, and she could read again. She no longer had a desire to harm herself or others. She told her psychiatrist she realized she had blamed the lithium for symptoms that were not related to it and asked to try another 300 mg at bedtime. She added that she had not realized how depressed she had been.

Three weeks later, Nancy was further improved, with only mild mood lability, no anxiety, and intact memory and concentration. She slept better, averaging 8 hours, but still had low energy; her appetite was strong, but her weight was stable. She and her psychiatrist thoroughly discussed the options suggested from the second opinion, but Nancy elected not to proceed with either cognitive-behavioral therapy or eye movement desensitization and reprocessing therapy suggested by the other practitioner, who had also agreed with the diagnosis. Instead, they agreed to raise her lithium dose by another 300 mg, seeking a serum level around 1.2 mEq/L. Nancy continued to show growth and retention of previous gains in psychotherapy in terms of insight and behavior. It also remained remarkable that she had shown almost none of these symptoms during their first 3 years of work together.

Getting to the slightly higher level of lithium was difficult, however. Nancy's serum level jumped to 1.5 mEq/L—a level much higher than expected by linear extrapolation from her previous measurements—with resultant side effects of toxicity. It appeared, clinically, that a serum level of at least 0.8–0.9 mEq/L would be necessary for fuller benefit, but it was also becoming clear Nancy might not be able to tolerate that. Her renal excretion appeared sluggish despite normal indices (it took 7 days to drop from a level of 1.5 mEq/L to 1.1 mEq/L following dose reduction), so a 24-hour creatine clearance was ordered, and Nancy and the psychiatrist discussed a long list of possibilities. Her remaining options for a mood stabilizer were valproate, carbamazepine, and lamotrigine. They settled on using the creatinine clearance to guide dose changes of lithium and trying 300 mg in the morning and 450 mg in the evening, targeting a serum level of 0.9 mEq/L while measuring for effectiveness and tolerability. They agreed to add lamotrigine over a 10- to 12-week titration period if necessary, retaining lithium until they were certain of the tolerability and effectiveness of this new agent.

Nancy improved as her lithium level slowly rose. Despite continued normal blood urea nitrogen and serum creatinine levels, a sluggish creatine clearance of 77 mL/min was documented, which explained the altered pharmacokinetics for lithium. The psychiatrist gave Nancy a printed copy of her creatinine clearance to evaluate further with her PCP, who diagnosed mild renal insufficiency. During the session, they discussed how to deal with the opinions of the general public about bipolar disorder and the effect of the diagnosis on her self-esteem.

Nancy continued to show some additional improvement: her attitude was different, she no longer napped daily, and although her energy remained a bit low, she was no longer oversleeping (averaging 8 hours again). She was motivated to do things in her house. Her appetite was moderate and her weight unchanged. She had a slight tremor in the morning, which did not bother her. She felt that she had reached a plateau. At this point, her psychiatrist suggested tapering the nefazodone so that it would not remain a risk for destabilizing her mood; she agreed. She did well until the dose was lowered below 300 mg, then depressed mood, unexplained anger, agitation, and weight gain (12 pounds) returned, along with cognitive impairment. The timing of this decline argued against cycling, so they agreed to resume 300 mg of the nefazodone; this combination was fully effective in eliminating symptoms and restoring functionality for 4 months.

Early in 2004, however, Nancy's mood dropped, agitation returned, short-term memory and concentration declined, sleep reverted to only 6 hours, and she was not rested in the morning, although her appetite and weight remained stable. She also reported trouble swallowing and had received recent diagnoses of esophageal spasm and irritable bowel syndrome. In late 2003, her PCP had added 50 mcg of levothyroxine sodium, although the TSH levels the psychiatrist monitored remained well within normal range (1.12–1.88 mIU/L). Her thyroid function and lithium level (1.2 mEq/L) were intact, so her nefazodone was changed to bupropion extended release because serotonin-norepinephrine reuptake inhibitors were thought to be more mood destabilizing than norepinephrine-dopamine reuptake inhibitors, and her depression had returned when discontinuation of the nefazodone had been attempted (Erfurth et al. 2002; Post et al. 2003). Nancy showed dramatic improvement in her mood and neurovegetative symptoms 10 days into the change; soon after, her lithium was changed to generic form. Nancy and the psychiatrist discussed her fears that her situation would be hopeless if her mood disorder worsened.

Shortly thereafter, the psychiatrist detected an elevated PTH level of 90 pg/mL, with normal serum calcium, on routing screening. The endocrinologist Nancy's PCP had referred her to thought this was a side effect of the lithium treatment and wanted the medication stopped, but the psychiatrist disagreed that there was sufficient indication for either conclusion (El Khoury et al. 2002). They agreed to repeat the calcium and PTH levels and obtain a bone scan. The level eventually returned to normal. In session, they explored the problems Nancy was having with her two daughters not getting along and her stress from work projects, which she was managing well. The PCP prescribed albuterol sulfate, which increased her anxiety and agitation, so its use was limited as much as possible.

In the middle of the next year, Nancy's anger returned for several months, progressing to rage for a 6-week period. She had begun drinking alcohol several times a week and on weekends, which, after strong encouragement from her psychiatrist, she agreed to taper and eliminate. They also explored new options for mood stability: although her Global Assessment of Functioning (GAF) scale score remained above 70, her symptoms could still be variable, even accounting for interference from other prescribed and over-the-counter medications. Her daughter who was being treated for bipolar disorder eventually had not responded as well to her carbamazepine as originally thought, and Nancy did not want to consider valproate because of the even more frequent necessity of laboratory work and reports about it she had heard from others.

No change was made until about a year later, however. Nancy's PTH and calcium levels had both been elevated above normal earlier that year. She began having palpitations and anxiety following a reaction to allergy desensitization injections. Her other providers wanted to treat her with an antianxiety medication, but the psychiatrist suggested she first stop her still occasional use of caffeine. Knowing that primary hyperparathyroidism could provoke symptoms of mood instability, the psychiatrist referred her for a second opinion to an alternative endocrinologist, who did find an adenoma of her parathyroid gland. A third endocrinologist was consulted who confirmed the adenoma. She also found small nodules in the right lobe of Nancy's thyroid gland (but no antibodies to her thyroid), a TSH level of 2.884 mIU/L, and normal serum vitamin D, vitamin B_{12}, and cortisol levels. About the same time, while on vacation, Nancy missed a step, fell, and hit her head on a stone floor. This did not result in loss of consciousness or amnesia but was followed by diplopia for 36 hours and dizziness for 10 days. A CT scan of her head 5 days later was read as normal, and a neurologist diagnosed concussion.

Nancy then elected to proceed with cross-taper from lithium carbonate to lamotrigine 600 mg/day while continuing bupropion 300 mg/day. She initially felt better, then returned to her more typical state of mild to moderate symptoms but good functionality. Her calcium and PTH levels remained high, and her bone density was worse; she consulted a surgeon and had the adenoma removed. Two months later, she reported, "My whole outlook is different—I'm better than I have been in two and a half years" (about the same amount of time that the elevated PTH had been observed). She was having good sleep and energy, was interested in doing things, was not anxious, was significantly less irritable, and, so far, maintained stable euthymia (no depression, hypomania, or mixed symptoms, which had become fairly common). She credited removal of her parathyroid adenoma (Weber et al. 2013). They agreed with her gynecologist that she could start a 2–3 month taper of her Premarin, and the psychiatrist, again, strongly encouraged her to never use caffeine, other stimulants, or alcohol.

From 2007 to 2013, Nancy remained euthymic, quite functional, and very satisfied. She even managed well through one of her daughter's diagnosis and treatment for breast cancer. Her lamotrigine dose was altered only slightly, in response to bioavailability differences from various generic preparations. Any minor perturbations were easily linked to use of stimulants or alcohol and were quickly corrected. One attempt to taper the bupropion was not successful, but she did well once the dosage of 300 mg/day was resumed.

In 2013, Nancy had a vestibular viral infection resulting in dizziness and was prescribed meclizine. Also that year, she began to experience feelings of impending doom and anxiety, along with tachycardia and hypertension. Her PCP and endocrinologist diagnosed a pheochromocytoma. Her dizziness continued to worsen, however, and her neurologist thought it was due to her use of lamotrigine. The psychiatrist explained to him that she had been taking essentially the same dose for years; that serum levels were referenced to seizure control, not mood stability; and that these levels also had not changed. The psychiatrist also noted to her endocrinologist, who was encouraging her to seek consultation at the Mayo Clinic, that Nancy's calcium level had again risen above normal. The dizziness was eventually diagnosed by the neurologist as silent migraines, for which she was given verapamil and diazepam. The psychiatrist expressed his concern about the latter medication potentially contributing to depressive symptoms.

Six months later, Nancy experienced another fall and closed head injury (without neurological sequelae) after tripping over a cord at a store. Almost simultaneously, she was treated for methicillin-resistant *Staphylococcus aureus* with prednisolone for a month, which adversely affected her mood. Her serum calcium levels were also high at 10.3 mg/dL. Further, her neurologist had prescribed topiramate 50 mg/day for her migraines, which resulted in panic, anxiety, and paranoia for 2 weeks. Nancy agreed to substitute clonazepam for diazepam, to be taken 0.5 mg bid, while bupropion was discontinued. As her calcium level returned to 9.3 mg/dL, the transient mood effects of the prednisolone and topiramate abated, and she returned to a euthymic state. It did seem that her mood was inversely sensitive to her calcium levels (Nagy et al. 2020; Steardo et al. 2020). In her less frequent psychotherapy sessions, she explored setting healthy boundaries with her husband and not taking responsibility for his health.

A year later, at their final visit due to the psychiatrist's retirement, Nancy continued to report sustained euthymia and a GAF score of 80; transfer to another psychiatrist had been arranged. She denied using caffeine, decongestants, dextromethorphan, alcohol, and nicotine; her dosage of clonazepam was down to 0.5 mg qd, and her dosage of lamotrigine was unchanged. Her endocrinologist was also pleased with her status.

Because her history included mood cycling caused by hyperparathyroidism, Nancy agreed to continue to work with this specialist to monitor PTH and calcium levels and thyroid function. A return of pheochromocytoma had been ruled out, but she had recently been diagnosed with diabetes mellitus, type 2.

This case illustrates not only how endocrinological disease can contribute to the difficulties in achieving and maintaining psychiatric treatment success but also how it may be responsible for many symptoms that lead to psychiatric diagnoses. The interplay between psychiatric and endocrine symptoms is highlighted: at times, it seemed that the thyroid or parathyroid gland was interfering with Nancy's treatment, and at times these organs appeared to be causing symptoms. Either way, failure to identify and respond to these endocrine contributions to the symptomatology and dysfunction of our patients is likely to result in treatment failure and an urge in some clinicians to describe the impasse as treatment resistance. It is also important to note that Nancy had four separate endocrinological conditions with differing impacts during various stages of her psychiatric treatment. Clinicians must not stop looking after the first underlying condition is identified—there may be more. Last, this case also displays how the interactions and multiple contributions, some helpful, some not, among many physicians from different specialties influence a patient's condition throughout treatment. Ongoing, active communication with these providers is essential.

A Case of Unrestrained Lifestyle Issues

Amber (not her real name), a 30-year-old woman, was referred to a psychiatrist by her PCP for evaluation of depressed mood and periodic anger outbursts, both of which occurred on a monthly basis. During these times, she also experienced increased impulsivity, spending more money than usual and shopping for items she did not need. Her anger outbursts appeared to be linked to psychosocial stressors, particularly with her husband or two children, whom she stayed home to care for. She denied any use of alcohol or recreational or illegal drugs to both physicians. She was diagnosed with persistent depressive disorder and was referred back to her PCP, with the recommendation to proceed with trials of antidepressants; paroxetine, venlafaxine, and duloxetine were suggested.

Two years later, Amber was again referred to the psychiatrist by the PCP, who reported that trials of all three of these antidepressants had failed. She had delivered her third child 1 month prior to this reconsultation, and the psychiatrist thought she was struggling with postpartum depression. At the appointment, Amber mentioned that every time she tried an antidepressant, it worked work initially, and then its benefit ceased after 3 months. The psychiatrist systematically screened her for manic and hypomanic symptoms: she endorsed several of them, including increased energy for no reason, a decreased need for sleep, increased thought production, and rapid speech. She also endorsed psychotic symptoms, particularly visual hallucinations while fully awake, independent of her mood symptoms.

Amber was referred to a neurologist, but no neurological abnormalities were found that could explain her visual hallucinations. A diagnosis of schizoaffective disorder was made. Amber was then treated serially with several mood stabilizers: lamotrigine, lithium carbonate, and valproic acid. Second-generation antipsychotic medications with indications for treating bipolar disorder were also tried: quetiapine, aripiprazole, lurasidone, and risperidone. None of these medications led to significant change, only minimally improving her mood.

Amber's psychiatrist continued to ask, many times, about alcohol or drug use, but she denied any use, and there was no evidence that she was not telling the truth. The psychiatrist also discovered that the anger outbursts were related to mood episodes. He rediagnosed these as mixed episodes because Amber reported being depressed, angry, tense, and agitated at the same time.

After a year of treatment attempts with these medications, they had made little progress. Then one day, Amber casually mentioned during a session that she felt strange after drinking her usual energy drink. The psychiatrist had never asked her about use of stimulants such as these. On further exploration, it was determined that she had been consuming three cans of energy drinks every day for several years; she did not know that energy drinks could have negative effects on her mood.

Amber agreed to gradually taper and discontinue her energy drinks over 4 weeks. Once these stimulants were discontinued, her mood started to become more stable. She was being treated with a combination of lithium carbonate and valproic acid at that time and gradually became less depressed and less angry. Her manic symptoms also markedly improved, and her schizoaffective disorder became easier to treat. Even her visual hallucinations became more manageable. She reached her longest period of stability (3–4 months), interspersed with short periods of manic, mixed, or depressed episodes.

This case (also generously contributed by my colleague Dr. Giuseppe Guaiana), illustrates the importance of systematically asking about and assessing lifestyle habits and inquiring about use of caffeine from all sources, including energy drink intake. Continued use often can have a negative impact on mood and lead to treatment failure (Casas-Gómez et al. 2018; Machado-Vieira et al. 2001); see section "Lifestyle Factors" in Chapter 7.

A Case of Misunderstanding and Inadequate Compliance

Denise (not her real name), a 42-year-old woman, consulted a psychiatrist in 2003 for "mood swings." She reported that these had begun when she was

13, about the time of her menarche, and described a series of "high highs and low lows." Her depressed phases were severe and were accompanied by hypersomnia and hyperphagia, with weight gain of 20 or 30 pounds, which were difficult to lose when her mood improved after several months (her BMI was 38.4 at initial consultation). These phases usually were followed by several more months of relative euthymia, then either a similar depressive phase or one typified by anxiety and excitability. These alternating phases also included rapid thinking and pressured speech. During all phases except euthymia, she experienced impaired cognition: poor concentration and short-term memory, misplacing objects and forgetting appointments and tasks.

Denise's PCP had treated her with bupropion for weight loss and depression, but it did not help with either problem. Over time, the mood cycles increased to approximately every 3 months, which prompted her to see the psychiatrist, who diagnosed rapid-cycling bipolar affective disorder. They reviewed possible pharmacological treatments, including the standard and promising mood stabilizers and atypical antipsychotics. Both Denise and her psychiatrist were concerned about lithium carbonate, carbamazepine, and valproate because her weight was already a significant health risk for her. Similarly, they worried about using second-generation antipsychotics, which at the time had not received indications for treating bipolar disorder. Denise asked for a trial of topiramate. Even though early reports of its benefit for mood stability had yet to be confirmed by multiple randomized controlled trials, its known effects on appetite suppression and subsequent weight loss attracted her to that option. Because the psychiatrist could find no harm in a brief trial, he agreed (see, again, Case Example 2 in Chapter 9). He also strongly advised her to avoid all caffeine, decongestants, and cough syrups, explaining that these could all worsen her mood instability (Dalton 1990; De Freitas and Schwartz 1979; Kilzieh and Akiskal 1999; Polles and Griffith 1996; Walker and Yatham 1993).

Denise's appetite was reduced; she attended Weight Watchers meetings and was able to lose weight down to a BMI of 33.0 but no lower. The topiramate was not effective for her mood, however, and she next agreed to a trial of oxcarbazepine, again, because of weight concerns. The severity of her depression and anxiety improved, but the cycles came just as often. They next agreed on a trial of lamotrigine. Denise felt calmer and her depression was milder, but her mood continued to cycle.

The psychiatrist reminded Denise at every contact to avoid all caffeine, decongestants, and cough syrups. At first, she admitted to making only a small effort to worry about this because she was much more concerned about her weight than the effects of caffeine. Eventually, however, because she did not improve, she complied fully; her mood subsequently improved but remained labile. Her sleep, appetite, memory, concentration, and anxiety still varied with her mood cycles. Her psychiatrist then prescribed lithium carbonate, followed by valproate, both of which did increase her weight and failed to improve her mood cycling. A subsequent trial of carbamazepine was better for her weight but also was ineffective, and Denise otherwise tolerated it poorly. Effective serum levels were confirmed in all three trials. The psychiatrist discussed with her the small chance that none of the medicines they were trying would work by themselves; they considered trying combinations of the mood stabilizers that had shown some partial benefit.

At her next visit, however, Denise reported to her psychiatrist that she had been sitting at her kitchen counter, languidly staring at a Slim-Fast weight loss shake canister, when suddenly it struck her that she had been drinking the chocolate-flavored form. She had been sincerely denying the use of any caffeine, including chocolate (Camandola et al. 2019), but had apparently continued it throughout their treatment efforts; she had never before thought of chocolate flavoring as chocolate. She then immediately changed to vanilla-flavored shakes.

The psychiatrist gradually returned Denise to lamotrigine 400 mg/day, and her mood cycling abated, leaving her in a euthymic state. The urge to eat was less powerful, and her BMI declined further to 26.1. Her sleep, memory, and concentration remained intact, and she no longer had rapid thoughts or speech. She remained euthymic for the next 3 years and abstained from all caffeine, at which time she transferred to another provider because of her psychiatrist's relocation.

This case is not only an additional illustration of the perhaps difficult to characterize, yet often documented, negative effects that caffeine and other stimulants can have on mood; how such use may sabotage treatment success (see section "A Case of Unrestrained Lifestyle Issues" above in this chapter) (Frigerio et al. 2021); and how interaction of the side effects of medications with a patient's other health issues may determine treatment selection and compliance. Most important, it additionally highlights the essential necessity of communicating so completely with our patients that they fully understand our concerns and recommendations and not just hear them. We must understand how patients are perceiving our guidance (see section "Perceiving and Respecting Your Patient" in Chapter 5). In this case, it was not enough to advise the patient not to use chocolate. Fuller discussion and exploration of this topic, earlier in treatment, would have been more helpful than repeating the same advice at each visit. It represents a case of treatment failure due to initially failed *shared understanding*, which, thankfully, was eventually corrected by the patient to her benefit. Flaws in a therapeutic alliance may be corrected if they are detected.

Summary

Misconceptualization, errors in problem-solving, insufficient adherence to evidence-based medicine, and inadequate initial and ongoing assessment may all lead to unsuccessful treatment efforts. Clinical success, measured by a patient's interest in improving functionality or a clinician's goal of reducing symptoms, can be found by the application of abductive reasoning and conscious efforts to avoid or uncover each of these potential missteps, often by the same practitioner who made the initial error(s).

All factors that contribute to symptoms or reduce functionality must be addressed, not just ones that the provider is most interested in or comfortable with. Even long-term working alliances with patients can distort clinical information through transference and countertransference. The clinician must monitor the therapeutic alliance and routinely ask direct questions about essential information, including lifestyle issues. Further, we must ensure that we are experiencing shared understanding with our patients and not just that they are hearing our advice; their interpretation of our recommendations will determine the accuracy of their compliance. It is also important to appreciate how interaction of the side effects of our medications with a patient's other health issues may determine their treatment selection and follow-through.

Practitioners must also remain persistent in the face of initially negative findings and still complete full assessments of systems. That is, a few negative neurological findings should not interrupt completion of a comprehensive neurological assessment. Additionally, a patient may have or develop more than one diagnosis in a system, such as multiple endocrine or gastrointestinal disorders. Effective clinicians cannot stop looking for additional diagnoses.

Much of the care provided in modern psychiatry is long-term for chronic conditions. As such, practitioners should expect that over time, there will be multiple opportunities to encounter interferences with otherwise successful treatment plans, such as changes in serum levels by alterations in absorption, compliance, or bioavailability; contributions from the many additional medical problems patients may develop during treatment; and the constant risk of new medical treatments added by a psychiatrist, other providers, or the patients themselves. Rather than quickly labeling a case as treatment failure or treatment resistance, these threats must be anticipated, investigated, and addressed, sometimes repeatedly, allowing sustained successful outcomes. Ongoing communication with other providers is important in understanding and managing these challenges and negotiating the interaction of sometimes competing treatment plans.

Patients may describe symptoms in ways that do not fit our cognitive mindsets, resulting in misdiagnosis. A symptom is not always synonymous with a diagnosis (e.g., the presence of anxiety may not result from an anxiety disorder, nor poor concentration from ADHD). Although we should be alert to inadvertently dropped clues to correct diagnoses, we may arrive at the correct solution sooner by routinely relying on thorough and broad initial and ongoing assessments. The case examples in this chapter illustrate how never-ending persistence with the effort to find solutions, rather than the quick application of meaningless labels, often leads to response and remission for our patients as well as to enhanced professional satisfaction.

Key Points

- Begin with complete, broad, comprehensive evaluations.
- Evaluate as a generalist, not a subspecialist.
- Patients seek functionality, whereas clinicians address symptom reduction.
- Symptom descriptions may not fit our mindsets.
- Allow adequate time for the full impact of treatments.
- Monitor and adjust the therapeutic alliance.
- Seek and confirm shared understanding.
- Anticipate new and multiple health problems during long-term treatment.
- Communicate and negotiate with other providers.
- Additional information and reconceptualization often can reverse treatment failure.

Self-Assessment Questions

1. Which of the following substances may have negative impacts on cognition?

   A. Statins.
   B. Cannabis.

C. A and B.

D. None of the above.

Correct answer: C. A and B.

The contributions to cognitive decline of both of these agents, along with other substance use or abuse and medications (e.g., antihistamines, anticholinergic medications, β-blockers) must always be considered and addressed for accurate diagnosis and effective treatment.

2. Which of the following may contribute to mood disorders?

A. Thyroid disorders.

B. Parathyroid disorders.

C. Stimulants.

D. All of the above.

Correct answer: D. All of the above.

Patients may develop multiple medical problems, even in the same system, which add symptoms to and interfere with treatment of psychiatric disorders. They also may not fully appreciate how to carry out our treatment recommendations.

3. Which of the following is true of a dysfunctional therapeutic alliance?

A. It may prevent adequate disclosure from patients.

B. It is always obvious to the practitioner.

C. It need not be directly addressed.

D. None of the above.

Correct answer: A. It may prevent adequate disclosure from patients.

Unless transference and countertransference are examined (even in cases with predominately psychopharmacological or somatic treatments), patients may be too embarrassed to fully disclose information that is essential to avoiding treatment failure. Threats to the alliance are not always clear, and the provider must always be monitoring and adjusting for them. Studies show that the best outcomes result from direct focus on any ruptures to the therapeutic alliance, which many authors advise should be expected during the process of treatment.

4.   Depressed mood, psychosis, and anxiety have been reported from the use of which of the following?

A. Atorvastatin.
B. Risedronate.
C. Alendronate.
D. All of the above.

Correct answer: D. All of the above.

Any appearance or worsening of symptoms temporally related to the use of medications linked by report to psychiatric symptoms should always prompt further investigation.

5.   Which of the following statements is *not* true of seizures?

A. They can occur after injection of local anesthetics.
B. They always involve a motor component.
C. Patients with seizures may present with signs of psychosis.
D. All of the above.

Correct answer: B. They always involve a motor component.

Cortical instability (and spike and wave activity confirmed by EEG) does not necessarily result in abnormal motor activity, so the absence of abnormal movement is no justification for rejecting seizure from the differential diagnosis. Seizure activity may manifest with symptoms of psychosis, including not just visual, olfactory, and tactile hallucinations, but also auditory hallucinations and delusions. Tonic-clonic seizures have been reported following the injection of local anesthetics by dentists.

Discussion Topics

1. During a routine visit with a patient you are treating for major depression, you find that her primary care internist has added a β-blocker

for hypertension and that her previous remission is less robust. She gives you permission to discuss her case with the provider, who insists that the β-blocker is the only option he is willing to prescribe for her. What further steps should you take in evaluating the changes in her condition, and how might you proceed with the patient and the internist?

2. You are the long-term provider for a man you are treating for bipolar I disorder. Although your working alliance has been helpful in terms of the prescription medication to which he has responded, he frequently starts over-the-counter supplements, including ones containing stimulants, without telling you until symptoms have been provoked. How do you examine the therapeutic alliance further, and what steps should you take to try to improve his outcome?

Additional Readings

Dewan MJ, Pies RW (eds): The Difficult-to-Treat Psychiatric Patient. Washington, DC, American Psychiatric Publishing, 2001: *An older text in terms of treatment strategies, this volume does reinforce many of the concepts in this chapter, including how therapeutic alliance, cognitive schemas, beliefs, and optimism help lead to better outcomes*

Raju NN, Naga Pavan Kumar KSVR, Nihal G: Management of medication-induced psychiatric disorders. Indian J Psychiatry 64(Suppl 2):S281–S291, 2022: *A good overview and reminder of the many syndromic symptoms that medications can provoke, interfering with diagnosis, response, and remission; tools for assessment and management are also discussed*

References

Alghamdi J, Matou-Nasri S, Alghamdi F, et al: Risk of neuropsychiatric adverse effects of lipid-lowering drugs: a Mendelian randomization study. Int J Neuropsychopharmacol 21(12):1067–1075, 2018 29986042

Alsukhni RA, Ghoubari MS, Farfouti MT, et al: Status epilepticus following local anesthesia in a previously healthy adult. BMC Res Notes 9:300, 2016 27287503

Archer C, Turner K, Kessler D, et al: Trends in the recording of anxiety in UK primary care: a multi-method approach. Soc Psychiatry Psychiatr Epidemiol 57(2):375–386, 2022 34196743

Bandelow B, Michaelis S: Epidemiology of anxiety disorders in the 21st century. Dialogues Clin Neurosci 17(3):327–335, 2015 26487813

Berigan TR: Psychiatric uses of newer anticonvulsants. Prim Care Companion J Clin Psychiatry 3(2):82–84, 2001 15014621

Bhalla RK, Butters MA, Becker JT, et al: Patterns of mild cognitive impairment after treatment of depression in the elderly. Am J Geriatr Psychiatry 17(4):308–316, 2009 19307859

Camandola S, Plick N, Mattson MP: Impact of coffee and cacao purine metabolites on neuroplasticity and neurodegenerative disease. Neurochem Res 44(1):214–227, 2019 29417473

Carlsson CM, Nondahl DM, Klein BE, et al: Increased atherogenic lipoproteins are associated with cognitive impairment: effects of statins and subclinical atherosclerosis. Alzheimer Dis Assoc Disord 23(1):11–17, 2009 19266697

Casas-Gómez C, Muñoz-Molero MJ, Guerrero-Sánchez R, et al: Mania and energy drinks. Actas Esp Psiquiatr 46(4):156–158, 2018 30079930

Cham S, Koslik HJ, Golomb BA: Mood, personality, and behavior changes during treatment with statins: a case series. Drug Saf Case Rep 3(1):1, 2016 27747681

Cojocariu SA, Maştaleru A, Sascău RA, et al: Neuropsychiatric consequences of lipophilic beta-blockers. Medicina (Kaunas) 57(2):155, 2021 33572109

Coleman CI, Perkerson KA, Lewis A: Alendronate-induced auditory hallucinations and visual disturbances. Pharmacotherapy 24(6):799–802, 2004 15222671

Dalton R: Mixed bipolar disorder precipitated by pseudoephedrine hydrochloride. South Med J 83(1):64–65, 1990 2300837

De Freitas B, Schwartz G: Effects of caffeine in chronic psychiatric patients. Am J Psychiatry 136(10):1337–1338, 1979 484737

Eijsvogel MM, Ubbink R, Dekker J, et al: Sleep position trainer versus tennis ball technique in positional obstructive sleep apnea syndrome. J Clin Sleep Med 11(2):139–147, 2015 25515276

El Khoury A, Petterson U, Kallner G, et al: Calcium homeostasis in long-term lithium-treated women with bipolar affective disorder. Prog Neuropsychopharmacol Biol Psychiatry 26(6):1063–1069, 2002 12452527

Ellis GM Jr, Mann MA, Judson BA, et al: Excretion patterns of cannabinoid metabolites after last use in a group of chronic users. Clin Pharmacol Ther 38(5):572–578, 1985 3902318

Epstein D: Range: Why Generalists Triumph in a Specialized World. New York, Riverhead Books, 2019

Erfurth A, Michael N, Stadtland C, Arolt V: Bupropion as add-on strategy in difficult-to-treat bipolar depressive patients. Neuropsychobiology 45(Suppl 1):33–36, 2002 11893875

Etgen T, Sander D, Bickel H, Förstl H: Mild cognitive impairment and dementia: the importance of modifiable risk factors. Dtsch Arztebl Int 108(44):743–750, 2011 22163250

Flor-Henry P: Psychosis and temporal lobe epilepsy. a controlled investigation. Epilepsia 10(3):363–395, 1969 5256909

Frigerio S, Strawbridge R, Young AH: The impact of caffeine consumption on clinical symptoms in patients with bipolar disorder: a systematic review. Bipolar Disord 23(3):241–251, 2021 32949106

Gibbs FA: Ictal and non-ictal psychiatric disorders in temporal lobe epilepsy. J Nerv Ment Dis 113(6):522–528, 1951 14841528

Grant JE, Chamberlain SR, Redden SA, et al: N-acetylcysteine in the treatment of excoriation disorder: a randomized clinical trial. JAMA Psychiatry 73(5):490–496, 2016 27007062

Grover S, Hazari N, Chakrabarti S, Avasthi A: Association of clozapine with seizures: a brief report involving 222 patients prescribed clozapine. East Asian Arch Psychiatry 25(2):73–78, 2015 26118746

Gruber AJ, Pope HG, Hudson JI, et al: Attributes of long-term heavy cannabis users: a case-control study. Psychol Med 33(8):1415–1422, 2003 14672250

Gunasekaran N, Long LE, Dawson BL, et al: Reintoxication: the release of fat-stored delta(9)-tetrahydrocannabinol (THC) into blood is enhanced by food deprivation or ACTH exposure. Br J Pharmacol 158(5):1330–1337, 2009 19681888

Gurrera RJ, Gearin PF, Love J, et al: Recognition and management of clozapine adverse effects: a systematic review and qualitative synthesis. Acta Psychiatr Scand 145(5):423–441, 2022 35178700

Hall W, Degenhardt L: The adverse health effects of chronic cannabis use. Drug Test Anal 6(1–2):39–45, 2014 23836598

Hartman RL, Huestis MA: Cannabis effects on driving skills. Clin Chem 59(3):478–492, 2013 23220273

Harvey MA, Sellman JD, Porter RJ, et al: The relationship between non-acute adolescent cannabis use and cognition. Drug Alcohol Rev 26(3):309–319, 2007 17454021

Hirschmann S, Gibel A, Tsvelikhovsky I, Lisker A: Late-onset psychosis and risedronate treatment for osteoporosis. Clin Schizophr Relat Psychoses 9(1):36–39, 2015 23644167

Howes OD, Thase ME, Pillinger T: Treatment resistance in psychiatry: state of the art and new directions. Mol Psychiatry 27(1):58–72, 2022 34257409

Huffman JC, Stern TA: Neuropsychiatric consequences of cardiovascular medications. Dialogues Clin Neurosci 9(1):29–45, 2007 17506224

Iraniparast M, Shi Y, Wu Y, et al: Cognitive reserve and mild cognitive impairment: predictors and rates of reversion to intact cognition vs progression to dementia. Neurology 98(11):e1114–e1123, 2022 35121669

Kang H, Zhao F, You L, et al: Pseudo-dementia: a neuropsychological review. Ann Indian Acad Neurol 17(2):147–154, 2014 25024563

Kavey NB, Gidro-Frank S, Sewitch DE: The importance of sleeping position in sleep apnea and a simple treatment technique. Sleep Res 11:152, 1982

Keshishi D, Makunts T, Abagyan R: Common osteoporosis drug associated with increased rates of depression and anxiety. Sci Rep 11(1):23956, 2021 34907232

Kilzieh N, Akiskal HS: Rapid-cycling bipolar disorder: an overview of research and clinical experience. Psychiatr Clin North Am 22(3):585–607, 1999 10550857

Kim S, Liu PJ, Min KE: Reminder avoidance: why people hesitate to disclose their insecurities to friends. J Pers Soc Psychol 121(1):59–75, 2021 32718167

King DS, Wilburn AJ, Wofford MR, et al: Cognitive impairment associated with atorvastatin and simvastatin. Pharmacotherapy 23(12):1663–1667, 2003 14695047

Kusumakar V, Lakshmi N, Yatham MB, et al: Topiramate in rapid cycling bipolar women. Paper presented at 152nd Annual Meeting of the American Psychiatric Association, Washington, DC, 1999

Lee DK, Lipner SR: The potential of N-acetylcysteine for treatment of trichotillomania, excoriation disorder, onychophagia, and onychotillomania: an updated literature review. Int J Environ Res Public Health 19(11):6370, 2022 35681955

Letmaier M, Schreinzer D, Wolf R, et al: Topiramate as a mood stabilizer. Int Clin Psychopharmacol 16(5):295–298, 2001 11552774

Machado-Vieira R, Viale CI, Kapczinski F: Mania associated with an energy drink: the possible role of caffeine, taurine, and inositol. Can J Psychiatry 46(5):454–455, 2001 11441790

Martín-Merino E, Ruigómez A, Wallander MA, et al: Prevalence, incidence, morbidity and treatment patterns in a cohort of patients diagnosed with anxiety in UK primary care. Fam Pract 27(1):9–16, 2010 19884124

Maslow AH: The Psychology of Science: A Reconnaissance. New York, Harper and Row, 1966

Messinis L, Kyprianidou A, Malefaki S, Papathanasopoulos P: Neuropsychological deficits in long-term frequent cannabis users. Neurology 66(5):737–739, 2006 16534113

Nadkarni S, Arnedo V, Devinsky O: Psychosis in epilepsy patients. Epilepsia 48(Suppl 9):17–19, 2007 18047594

Nagy L, Mangini P, Schroen C, et al: Prolonged hypercalcemia-induced psychosis. Case Rep Psychiatry 2020:6954036, 2020 32099711

Panza F, Frisardi V, Capurso C, et al: Late-life depression, mild cognitive impairment, and dementia: possible continuum? Am J Geriatr Psychiatry 18(2):98–116, 2010 20104067

Pazarlis P, Katsigiannopoulos K, Bolimou S, et al: Statins cholesterol lowering and mental health: a review. Ann Gen Psychiatry 5(Suppl 1):S251, 2006

Peters JT, Garwood CL, Lepczyk M: Behavioral changes with paranoia in an elderly woman taking atorvastatin. Am J Geriatr Pharmacother 6(1):28–32, 2008 18396246

Petker T, DeJesus J, Lee A, et al: Cannabis use, cognitive performance, and symptoms of attention deficit/hyperactivity disorder in community adults. Exp Clin Psychopharmacol 28(6):638–648, 2020 32105137

Polles A, Griffith JL: Dextromethorphan-induced mania. Psychosomatics 37(1):71–74, 1996 8600498

Post RM, Leverich GS, Nolen WA, et al: A re-evaluation of the role of antidepressants in the treatment of bipolar depression: data from the Stanley Foundation Bipolar Network. Bipolar Disord 5(6):396–406, 2003 14636363

Putman HP: Rational Psychopharmacology: A Book of Clinical Skills. Washington, DC, American Psychiatric Association Publishing, 2020

Quinlan P, Nordlund A, Lind K, et al: Thyroid hormones are associated with poorer cognition in mild cognitive impairment. Dement Geriatr Cogn Disord 30(3):205–211, 2010 20798541

Reimherr FW, Marchant BK, Gift TE, et al: ADHD and anxiety: clinical significance and treatment implications. Curr Psychiatry Rep 19(12):109, 2017 29152677

Ritchie M, Yeap BB: Thyroid hormone: influences on mood and cognition in adults. Maturitas 81(2):266–275, 2015 25896972

Rojas-Fernandez CH, Cameron JC: Is statin-associated cognitive impairment clinically relevant? A narrative review and clinical recommendations. Ann Pharmacother 46(4):549–557, 2012 22474137

Sharma P, Murthy P, Bharath MM: Chemistry, metabolism, and toxicology of cannabis: clinical implications. Iran J Psychiatry 7(4):149–156, 2012 23408483

Shors TJ, Leuner B: Estrogen-mediated effects on depression and memory formation in females. J Affect Disord 74(1):85–96, 2003 12646301

Shukla GD, Srivastava ON, Katiyar BC, et al: Psychiatric manifestations in temporal lobe epilepsy: a controlled study. Br J Psychiatry 135:411–417, 1979 120210

Small ML: Weak ties and the core discussion network: why people regularly discuss important matters with unimportant alters. Soc Networks 35(3):470–483, 2013

Small ML, Sukhu C: Because they were there: access, deliberation, and the mobilization of networks for support. Soc Networks 47:73–84, 2016

Smith-Kielland A, Skuterud B, Mørland J: Urinary excretion of 11-nor-9-carboxy-delta9-tetrahydrocannabinol and cannabinoids in frequent and infrequent drug users. J Anal Toxicol 23(5):323–332, 1999 10488918

Solowij N, Stephens RS, Roffman RA, et al: Cognitive functioning of long-term heavy cannabis users seeking treatment JAMA 287(9):1123–1131, 2002 11879109

Steardo L Jr, Luciano M, Sampogna G, et al: Clinical severity and calcium metabolism in patients with bipolar disorder. Brain Sci 10(7):417, 2020 32630307 (Correction JAMA 287(13):1651, 2002)

Talaei A, Rafee N, Rafei F, Chehrei A: TSH cut off point based on depression in hypothyroid patients. BMC Psychiatry 17(1):327, 2017 28882111

Tuccori M, Montagnani S, Mantarro S, et al: Neuropsychiatric adverse events associated with statins: epidemiology, pathophysiology, prevention and management. CNS Drugs 28(3):249–272, 2014 24435290

Vinti V, Dell'Isola GB, Tascini G, et al: Temporal lobe epilepsy and psychiatric comorbidity. Front Neurol 12:775781, 2021 34917019

Volkow ND, Swanson JM, Evins AE, et al: Effects of cannabis use on human behavior, including cognition, motivation, and psychosis: a review. JAMA Psychiatry 73(3):292–297, 2016 26842658

Walker J, Yatham LN: Benylin (dextromethorphan) abuse and mania. BMJ 306(6882):896, 1993 8490415

Walters K, Rait G, Griffin M, et al: Recent trends in the incidence of anxiety diagnoses and symptoms in primary care. PLoS One 7(8):e41670, 2012 22870242

Wartofsky L, Dickey RA: The evidence for a narrower thyrotropin reference range is compelling. J Clin Endocrinol Metab 90(9):5483–5488, 2005 16148345

Weber T, Eberle J, Messelhäuser U, et al: Parathyroidectomy, elevated depression scores, and suicidal ideation in patients with primary hyperparathyroidism: results of a prospective multicenter study. JAMA Surg 148(2):109–115, 2013 23560281

Wells CE: Transient ictal psychosis. Arch Gen Psychiatry 32(9):1201–1203, 1975 1180671

Werhagen L, Gabrielsson H, Westgren N, et al: Medical complication in adults with spina bifida. Clin Neurol Neurosurg 115(8):1226–1229, 2013 23245854

Williams AM, Park SH: Seizure associated with clozapine: incidence, etiology, and management. CNS Drugs 29(2):101–111, 2015 25537107

Wittchen HU, Kessler RC, Beesdo K, et al: Generalized anxiety and depression in primary care: prevalence, recognition, and management. J Clin Psychiatry 63(Suppl 8):24–34, 2002 12044105

Yoshida F, Morioka T, Hashiguchi K, et al: Epilepsy in patients with spina bifida in the lumbosacral region. Neurosurg Rev 29(4):327–332, 2006 16933125

Young-Xu Y, Chan KA, Liao JK, et al: Long-term statin use and psychological well-being. J Am Coll Cardiol 42(4):690–697, 2003 12932603

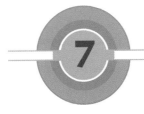

Underappreciated Causes of Treatment Failure

In Chapter 5, "Essential Assessment and Reevaluation," and Chapter 6, "Successful Outcomes," I stress the importance of anticipating and discovering unexpected factors that interfere with treatment success and lead to the illusion of treatment resistance. It should be quite clear that the list of possible sources of treatment failure is unending, as should be our search for these causes. This requires us as providers to employ our full knowledge of medicine and psychiatry, remaining current with treatment options and the broad literature.

Among patients with serious mental illnesses, 75% have been found to have at least one chronic nonpsychiatric medical problem, and 50% have two or more (Jones et al. 2004). Comorbid nonpsychiatric medical conditions may cause or exacerbate psychiatric symptoms, yet frequently they are not diagnosed (Rothbard et al. 2009). Atypical presentations of these comorbidities are frequent, and common illnesses often manifest quite differently as patients age, when the risk of comorbidity also increases (Bair 1998; Felker et al. 1996). New medications and supplements arrive frequently and may unexpectedly affect mental status or interfere with treatment. Inadequate attention to sleep hygiene, use of substances, and even diet often derails successful treatment.

We must use creativity in imagining possible impediments to remission, while also remaining alert for the more common explanations. In the following sections, I discuss contributions to clinical states that are often underappreciated.

Mild to Moderate Head Trauma

Globally, more than 27 million new cases of traumatic brain injury (TBI) were estimated to have occurred in 2016, an 8.4% increase over the previous 16 years (GBD 2016 Traumatic Brain Injury and Spinal Cord Injury Collaborators 2019). Another survey (Dewan et al. 2018) estimated 69 million, the difference likely due to disagreement on severity and definition. Dewan and colleagues found the highest incidence in North America (1,299 cases per 100,000 people) and Europe (1,012 per 100,000). In 2014, a survey found that 21.7% of all noninstitutionalized adults in Ohio had had at least one lifetime TBI with loss of consciousness (LOC), 9.1% of these occurring before age 15, and 3% having had at least one TBI that was moderate or severe (Corrigan et al. 2018). Although estimates vary, the frequency is high enough for practitioners to view some sort of head injury as common among the population (Kwentus et al. 1985).

Symptoms related to TBI may appear acutely but also decades later. Sometimes these insults permanently predispose a patient to psychiatric symptoms and disorders, including major depression and anxiety (especially panic disorder), that cannot be linked to the severity of the injury (Koponen et al. 2002) and may involve not only diffuse axonal injury but also epigenetic changes (Nagalakshmi et al. 2018). In a retrospective study, 45% of patients met DSM-IV criteria for major depression (American Psychiatric Association 1994) up to 5.5 years following TBI, and 38% met criteria for an anxiety disorder, two-thirds of which were new-onset cases and showed poor rates of resolution (Whelan-Goodinson et al. 2009). In a separate study, examination of a random sample determined that individuals who had incurred head injury with LOC or confusion demonstrated an increased risk for major depression, dysthymia, panic disorder, OCD, phobias, and drug abuse or dependence (Silver et al. 2001).

Even a decade post injury, the incidence (in decreasing order) of psychiatric symptoms remains high for depression, anxiety, sleep disorders, and panic attacks, the last reported particularly in younger patients (Hammond et al. 2019). Acute secondary psychiatric disorders have been reported to manifest many years after a TBI (Yoshino et al. 2020), and, in one study, 42% of patients experienced onset of post-TBI psychosis following a latency period of 10 years (Achté et al. 1969).

Twenty percent of patients experiencing even mild TBI (mTBI; a closed head injury, also called a concussion) experience a postconcussive syndrome (PCS), which may affect behavioral, cognitive, or affective domains. These patients display irritability, fatigue, inattention, impulsivity, and judgment problems, in addition to memory deficits, anxiety, and depression (Dunkley et al. 2015; Levin et al. 1987; Ryan and Warden 2003). Twenty percent of PCS cases are also chronic (Binder et al. 1997).

This can be a difficult area to discuss and assess, however, because many patients consider head injury to be synonymous with "brain damage" and eschew the label to avoid stigma. Even if they are open to consideration of the topic, definitions are, again, difficult to align. It is common for a patient to deny head injury two or three times but acknowledge "getting knocked out, with a concussion" when asked about LOC. Because 75% of all head injuries are characterized as mild (Dunkley et al. 2015), practitioners must be sensitive to nuance, as well as persistent, to uncover this important element of a patient's history.

As a clinician, you should always ask if there have been any "bumps" to the head, even if the patient saw them as insignificant, and request as much detail as possible. Explain that accidents and sports incidents, as well as everyday life events such as bumping one's head on a shelf or trunk, are essential for the practitioner to be made aware of. Were airbags deployed during motor vehicle incidents? Was the patient wearing a helmet during a fall involving a bicycle? Inquire as to forms of recreation (e.g., skiing, climbing) and whether the patient played any organized sports. If so, determine at what ages; to what level of competition; and whether any activities put the patient's head at risk, such as boxing, rugby, lacrosse, American and Canadian football, and headers in soccer (football). Note that recent data show that it may not be a properly performed header itself that results in TBI but rather the other hits acquired while attempting to accomplish it (Bunc et al. 2017; Mooney et al. 2020). Additionally, obtaining details of actual experiences and job duties during employment and military service may provide clues.

Falls now outnumber motor vehicle incidents as the most common cause of TBI in countries with better recordkeeping, so direct questions about such accidents should be routine (GBD 2016 Traumatic Brain Injury and Spinal Cord Injury Collaborators 2019; Peeters et al. 2015; Roozenbeek et al. 2013). Males are more likely to have experienced TBI (Corrigan et al. 2018), but although the index of suspicion might be higher with this sex or gender, all patients should be sufficiently queried.

Because 30%–50% of all new mTBIs occur under the influence of alcohol (Scheenen et al. 2016), exploration of injury may also be confirmed while taking a detailed history of substance use.

Searching for a history of even mTBI may require the patient to ask their family of origin or to help the provider obtain medical records of past assessments and treatments. Adults who suffered physical trauma as a child are sometimes "protected" by family, who may have withheld important details from them. However, most family members are usually willing to disclose this information when asked to aid assessment.

Should a history of any insult to the head be elicited, clinicians must inquire as to the nature of any previous assessments: were they performed in an emergency department (where a nonenhanced CT scan is a commonly used tool), by emergency medical services, at another location such as a physician's office, or by a team doctor or trainer on the sidelines or in the locker room? Try to determine what level of professional evaluated the injury, whether a neurological consultation was obtained, and how long after the incident additional assessment(s) and any imaging took place. A CT without contrast media in the emergency department may show nothing remarkable, whereas MRI with contrast performed 3 weeks later may show scarring, given time for inflammation processes to alter tissue. If possible, obtain copies of any assessments and imaging from the appropriate facility, the patient, or even family. Attempt to clarify whether the patient or others noticed any transient or persistent alterations following the insult.

MRI studies find 85% more intracranial lesions following TBI than do CT scans and also indicate that lesions are larger than estimations based on CT (Levin et al. 1987). Structural imaging, however, more often fails to assist in the diagnosis of TBI, and efforts are under way to develop functional imaging techniques that will better aid the clinician. The use of noninvasive magnetoencephalography (MEG) has demonstrated increased functional connectivity in the low-frequency resting state following mTBI. Areas affected include frontal, temporal, and deep gray regions and distinct networks associated with attention, anxiety, and depression (Dunkley et al. 2015). MEG is also being explored to identify neural features that can separate TBI and PTSD, two diagnoses with overlapping symptomatology, such as high levels of anxiety and depression, that are often quite difficult to distinguish clinically (Zhang et al. 2021). MEG, however, is currently a research tool. It may eventually be validated for clinical use, but so far further study is needed to confirm biomarkers for mTBI (Mayer et al. 2018; Peitz et al. 2021). For the practicing clinician, however, this highlights the value of remaining alert to the existence of distinct diagnoses that we cannot separate categorically or dimensionally, which might affect function, cause symptoms, and complicate treatment.

The review of systems is an important ally for the clinician attempting to find any current or past symptoms that may point to brain injury thwarting a patient's clinical course. Decreased taste acuity (hypogeusia), distortion of taste acuity (dysgeusia), decreased smell acuity (hyposmia), and dysosmia can occur after even mTBI and begin days to months after injury (Mehkri et al. 2022; Schechter and Henkin 1974). Visual disturbances and noise sensitivity are often reported in PCS (Ryan and Warden 2003). Even a thorough mental status examination, although insufficient alone, may help in this endeavor. Visual, olfactory, and tactile hallucinations are more likely to be associated with neurological dysfunction, although auditory hallucinations and delusions are still common after TBI (Burghaus et al. 2012; Ciurleo et al. 2020; Duarte et al. 2023; Fénelon 2013, pp. 59–83; O'Brien et al. 2020).

Any alteration or interruption of consciousness should be similarly queried and explored. Determine if there was actual LOC, or whether the patient came close to LOC, and explore antecedents, descriptions, and possible causes. Ask whether the event was observed and, if so, obtain a physical description. Determine the length of any LOC and sequelae, such as postictal depression or motor weakness. Inquire about any loss of bladder or stool control, which might occur during a seizure.

Specifically ask if the patient has ever had, or been diagnosed as having had, a seizure, describing the various types, if necessary. Learn all the surrounding details, including how many times one might have occurred. Again, inquire as to the timing and nature of any assessment and the type of professional performing it. If an electroencephalogram (EEG) was performed, ask when and how many. Were lights flashed in their eyes or electrodes put in their nose? How long did the EEG last (24- and 72-hour studies are increasingly common)? Was the patient sleep deprived? Again, was imaging performed, and, if so, what type, and was contrast used? Learn what the patient was told about the results and obtain them, if possible. Incomplete evaluations and premature conclusions about LOC, and even diagnosed seizures, are common in medicine, so the psychiatrist might be the provider who is most interested in the details.

Although to some patients inquiries such as these may appear as excessive interest in an area they deem unimportant, missing this information about TBI can lead to treatment failure and can risk complications from treatment. It is essential to investigate these possibilities until the information is complete and clear prior to the development of treatment failure or an adverse event. Fortunately, patients have experienced greater media exposure to the dangers of TBI in the past decade, so they may be open to your concern about and detection of this important clinical information.

Treating psychiatric disorders in the context of a documented or suspected TBI, even mTBI, requires an individualized, and often multidisciplinary, approach. Effort must be made to estimate function and to review diagnoses and any symptomatology that occurred prior to the first TBI. It is helpful to determine whether the damage from TBI is diffuse (as with concussion) or focal (following hematoma or contusion) (Morse and Garner 2018).

In considering syndrome-indicated psychopharmacological interventions, actual and possible neuronal damage and excessive neurotransmitter release must be taken into account because expected side effects may be magnified and lead to new symptoms that must be addressed (Shin and Dixon 2015; Silver et al. 2009). New-onset unprovoked posttraumatic seizures (PTS) have a cumulative incidence of more than 20% measured at 5 years post trauma, and new cases have been reported 30 years post injury (Ritter et al. 2016). Compared with the general population, patients with mTBI have 1.5 times the chance of having PTS in the first 5 years; those with mTBI and LOC or posttraumatic amnesia have twice the risk for 5 years; those with moderate TBI have 2.9 times the risk over 10 years; and those with severe injuries have 17 times the risk indefinitely (Annegers et al. 1998). These are the self-report rates for convulsive seizures; they may underestimate the objective incidence, and many PTS are subclinical and may manifest with a variety of psychiatric symptoms, including mood, anxiety, and transient cognitive and behavioral problems (Binnie 2003; Grzegorzewska et al. 2021; Kanner et al. 2004; Mula et al. 2010; Ritter et al. 2016; Shewmon and Erwin 1989; Vespa et al. 1999; Zangaladze et al. 2008).

Antidepressants and antipsychotic medications lower seizure thresholds. Anticonvulsant therapies, in addition to or in place of those often used for mood stability, may provide important protection from iatrogenically provoked seizure or subclinical events and symptomatology. Anticholinergic medications are likely to worsen cognition, and even the usual serum levels of prescription and over-the-counter medications and supplements may more easily provoke delirium in these patients (Arciniegas and Silver 2006; Arciniegas et al. 2005; Roberson et al. 2021).

Limited evidence moderately supports the use of blue-wavelength light therapy for the reduction of depressive symptoms following TBI, and there is preliminary support for it improving daytime drowsiness after mTBI (Srisurapanont et al. 2022). Cognitive-behavioral therapy (CBT) and online family problem-solving therapy, as part of broader rehabilitation, have been found to improve function post TBI (Lee et al. 2019; Wade et al. 2015). As with the treatment for all conditions, the patient's understanding of their injury and their condition, as well as their hopes for progress, must be ascertained and woven into treatment planning (Morse and Garner 2018); see section "Perceiving and Respecting Your Patient" in Chapter 5 and Case Example 2 and the section "Long-Term Approach" in Chapter 9, "Managing a Sustained Therapeutic Relationship During Treatment Failure."

Clinicians must retain awareness that this type of injury is common and is likely to remain an ongoing complicating factor in treatment. Failure to address it will likely allow ongoing treatment failure and the appearance of treatment resistance.

Endocrine Disorders

The functioning of the endocrine system frequently has impacts on patients with psychiatric symptoms (Mishra et al. 2022). Additionally, many patients with primary endocrine disorders can present primarily or exclusively with psychiatric symptoms (Conner and Solomon 2017). Diabetes and adrenal disorders may be as involved in a treatment failure as are thyroid and parathyroid conditions. The main psychiatric symptoms of endocrine disorders are depression, anxiety, mania, and eating disorders. Other forms of psychosis and even suicidal ideation may appear in severe cases (Salvador et al. 2019).

The thyroid gland can play a major role, often underappreciated, in the evaluation and treatment of psychiatric disorders (Gulseren et al. 2006). Hypothyroidism is a common endocrine disorder, and the second most common for women (Dunn and Turner 2016). Thyroid hormones alter serotonergic and noradrenergic function, which has an impact on affective disorder symptoms and the efficacy of antidepressants (Mason et al. 1987; Noda 2015; Whybrow and Prange 1981). A recent meta-analysis determined that in patients younger than age 60 years, subclinical hypothyroidism (see below), defined by diverse criteria, is associated with depressive symptoms measured by standard scales (Zhao et al. 2018). Patients with hypothyroidism, hyperthyroidism, or thyroiditis all may also present with psychosis (Pollak et al. 2019; Sathya et al. 2009).

Therefore, thyroid status must be determined prior to and throughout any attempts at treatment for mood and anxiety symptoms or disorders or psychosis and should be rechecked on the reversal of previously effective therapies (Bhattarai et al. 2022; Dayan and Panicker 2013; Esposito et al. 1997). In reviewing reports of failed treatment efforts, clinicians should also attempt to determine the state of thyroid function during those trials. Routine and ongoing assessment of this important gland's function can never be ignored, and practitioners must strive to remain current on the definition of the euthyroid condition, including laboratory values. Patients must be screened with a thyroid-stimulating hormone (TSH) test, not simply thyroxine (T_4) or triiodothyronine (T_3) resin uptake (T_3RU), and it is wise to also measure thyroid antibodies, particularly anti-thyroglobulin and anti–thyroid peroxidase. A patient with thyroiditis, the most common cause of hypothyroidism, may be euthyroid, hypothyroid, or hyperthyroid at any given time, and a single TSH measurement will not confirm the diagnosis (Dunn and Turner 2016).

Many laboratories have not updated their normal range for TSH since the early 1990s, when 4.6 mIU/L was considered the upper limit of normal. Since 2005, an upper limit of 2.5 mIU/L has been reported and accepted by many as normal for the average patient (Kratzsch et al. 2005; Wartofsky and Dickey 2005; Zhao et al. 2018). Certain populations may vary (euthyroid TSH levels appear to be higher in older patients and women) (Biondi 2013; Kutluturk et al. 2014), and we know that each individual has a genetically and environmentally determined level consistent with euthyroid status that is unique; clinically important variations in TSH level may occur within what is considered a normal range (Andersen et al. 2002). The evaluation of TSH levels must also take into account other conditions or pharmacological treatments that might alter them, such as a positive correlation with body mass; elevation by allopurinol and alcohol consumption; lowering by glucocorticoids and smoking; and being affected variably by exercise, pregnancy, and exposure to chemical and heavy metals (Babić Leko et al. 2021; Biondi 2013; Choi et al. 2021; Haugen 2009; Yamamoto et al. 2020).

It is also important to remember that TSH is secreted as part of a homeostatic mechanism, and single values carry insufficient information. TSH levels should always be evaluated as part of a series, at least three measurements over several months (Biondi 2013). Sustained levels above 2.5 mIU/L may, in some cases, indicate subclinical hypothyroid function that can have an impact on psychiatric symptoms and treatment (see above), and replacement may need to be cautiously considered (see below). Levels below 0.1 mIU/L are consistent with thyroid hormone excess in the presence of elevated free thyroxine (FT_4) or free triiodothyronine (FT_3) levels (Almandoz and Gharib 2012; Andersen et al. 2002; Idrose 2015; Zhao et al. 2018). Such evaluation should replace the blind addition of thyroid hormone levothyroxine or T_3 to "potentiate" antidepressant effects, as adverse events (including cardiac response, osteoporosis, and even iatrogenic psychiatric conditions) might be provoked (Verma et al. 2013). Recent recommendations advise against the addition of levothyroxine to treat hypothyroidism in patients over 65 with a TSH under 7.0 mIU/L (Biondi and Cappola 2022).

Consultation with an endocrinologist knowledgeable about the most current thyroid hormone data and accustomed to assisting psychiatrists in making these recommendations is encouraged (Calissendorff and Falhammar 2020). It is important to clarify with each case that it is the improvement of psychiatric symptoms you are targeting, not just the syndrome of hypothyroidism. Treatment for overt or subclinical hypothyroidism must be discussed and decided collaboratively with your patient, of course. If the decision is made to add levothyroxine to the treatment plan, many endocrinologists express concern about the bioavailability and bioequivalence of generic preparations, particularly when changing brands or from brand name to generic (see section "Polypharmacy and Bioavailability Complications" below) (Benvenga and Carlé 2019). Anecdotal evidence is not a valid indication for treatment planning, and the following case is included only to illustrate the type of thinking that might lead to an attempt to reverse psychiatric treatment failure with thyroid hormone.

Case Example

Megan (not her real name), a 38-year-old woman, had been in treatment with her psychiatrist for 2 years. During that time, a diagnosis of major depression, moderate, recurrent had been made, and adequate trials of a selective serotonin reuptake inhibitor (SSRI), a norepinephrine and dopamine reuptake inhibitor, and a serotonin-norepinephrine reuptake inhibitor (SNRI) had led to response but not remission. Megan's treatment also included supportive psychotherapy, with occasional focus on cognitive and behavioral techniques, as indicated. At the time of initial evaluation, and several times since, her psychiatrist had evaluated her endocrine status, including TSH and thyroid antibodies. No measurable antibodies were found, and her TSH ranged from 2.4 to 2.9 mIU/L, averaging above 2.5 mIU/L. Because her diagnosis had been frequently re-confirmed and no other explanations could found for her lack of remission despite thorough evaluation and careful monitoring of the therapeutic alliance, Megan and her psychiatrist began to consider whether her individual thyroid function, while close to adesquate for many patients, might be too low for a complete antidepressant response.

They discussed the risks of T_4 supplementation, especially cardiac and endocrine threats, and no medical contraindications could be iden-tified. Megan and the psychiatrist agreed to a 6-week trial of levothyroxine (Synthroid) 50 mcg/day. They also agreed that if the trial was successful in improving her antidepressant response to her current SNRI, she would have an endocrinologist manage the supplementation long term. Megan tolerated the thyroid supplementation well, and at the end of 6 weeks did see enough improvement in her mood and neurovegetative symptoms that she met even conservative criteria for remission. Her TSH had dropped to 1.8 mIU/L, and her previous SNRI, at the same dose, was now more fully effective. Although not every patient can expect the same out-come, awareness that thyroid indices have been updated, yet still must be individualized, may help some patients find remission if this possibil-ity is carefully considered and cautiously approached.

The parathyroid gland can also be a cause of treatment failures in psy-chiatry, and treatment of it usually reverses psychiatric symptoms rap-idly (Enyi et al. 2022). Primary hyperparathyroidism (PHPT) is the third most common endocrine disorder (Fraser 2009), and 25% of patients with PHPT exhibit psychiatric symptoms: depression, anxiety, cognitive decline, psychosis, fatigue, and sleep disorders; increased use of antide-pressants and benzodiazepines prior to surgical repair have also been de-scribed (Enyi et al. 2022; Koman et al. 2022; Serdenes et al. 2021). PHPT should be suspected in patients with these symptoms who also have fre-quent kidney stones (Bilezikian et al. 2018), and the diagnosis can be made when levels of serum calcium rise above 10.3 mg/dL and parathy-roid hormone levels are higher than 65 pg/mL. If PHPT is confirmed by nuclear imaging and endocrinology, parathyroidectomy quickly reverses the neuropsychiatric symptoms, particularly in more severely symptom-atic cases (Enyi et al. 2022; Liu et al. 2021).

Secondary hyperparathyroidism (SHPT), associated with chronic kid-ney disease and low levels of vitamin D (Cipriani et al. 2018; Messa and Alfieri 2019), may also be associated with neuropsychiatric symptoms (Diskin and Diskin 2020; Furuie et al. 2018). Chronic treatment with lith-ium also increases the chances of hypercalcemia and hyperparathyroidism (Albert et al. 2013). Treatment for SHPT, aided by endocrinologists, ap-pears to also lower the risk of resultant dementia (Mathur et al. 2022).

Management of SHPT from chronic lithium therapy, which is often necessary to address neuropsychiatric symptoms, may require discontinuation of this mood stabilizer or, alternatively, calcimimetic therapy or parathyroidectomy (Dixon et al. 2018; Enyi et al. 2022; Kovacs et al. 2022).

Patients with suboptimal control of type 1 or type 2 diabetes mellitus have twice to three times the incidence of depression, and diabetes also carries elevated comorbidities with anxiety disorders, cognitive impairment, dementia, ADHD, schizophrenia, disturbed eating behavior, bipolar disorders, and borderline personality disorder (Abrahamian et al. 2019; Bădescu et al. 2016; Park and Reynolds 2015; Tao et al. 2023). Gestational diabetes mellitus is also comorbid with antenatal and postpartum depression (Riggin 2020). In many cases, such as depression, gestational diabetes, ADHD, and schizophrenia, the relationship is bidirectional (Al-Atram 2018; Mizuki et al. 2021; Tao et al. 2023). Routine screening and appropriate intervention for this most common endocrine disorder is important to interrupt the cross-contributions with psychiatric disorder treatments and symptoms.

Patients with less common endocrinological diseases, such as primary adrenal insufficiency (Addison's disease) and hypercortisolism (Cushing's syndrome), may also present with neuropsychiatric symptoms (e.g., depression, insomnia, cognitive impairment, psychosis, catatonia) that are not responsive to standard psychiatric treatment (Bratek et al. 2015; Joersjö and Block 2019; Momayez Sanat and Mohajeri-Tehrani 2022; Puzanov et al. 2019; Santos et al. 2017, 2021). Treatment for the underlying endocrine disorder is primary but might still require additional interventions to fully reverse the neuropsychiatric consequences or symptoms emerging from treatment (Henry et al. 2021; Jyothi et al. 2016; Kundu et al. 2014). As always, alertness to the onset of new psychiatric illness, atypical features, and disappointing treatment results should alert the clinician to quickly look deeper because structural and functional alterations to the brain from these disorders may not be fully reversible if untreated for an extended period (Bratek et al. 2015; Liu et al. 2022).

Infectious Diseases

Infectious diseases may not dominate a mental health professional's thoughts while forming a differential diagnosis, but they are a possible source of psychiatric symptoms and potential treatment failure. Infectious diseases in a population may follow an acute or endemic route, and their frequency may vary from obscure to epidemic.

Rates of infectious disease in hospitalized patients with serious mental illness are higher than those found in the general population. In one U.S. state hospital population, 23.9% of patients had hepatitis B (compared with the U.S. prevalence of 5%), 21.5% had hepatitis C (vs. 1.8%), and 4%–23% had HIV (vs. 0.4%–0.6%). The same study found rates of 32%, 21%, and 10%, respectively, in a university hospital setting, with the diagnosis being missed in 95%, 50%, and 21% of cases (Rothbard et al. 2009). Infectious disease is second only to pulmonary illness as the most prevalent chronic health problem among persons with serious mental illness (Jones et al. 2004). The prevalence rates of infectious diseases in persons with psychiatric illness and the general population are given in Table 7–1.

Patients with hepatitis; febrile diseases, including malaria and brucellosis; herpes simplex virus (HSV); HIV; Lyme disease; rabies; and coronavirus disease 2019 (COVID-19), in addition to patients receiving some treatments for infectious diseases, such as mefloquine and interferon, can all display psychiatric symptoms (Erdogan and Hocaoglu 2020). Effective clinicians recall and consider the possibility of infectious disease causing or influencing psychiatric symptoms, particularly during initial assessment, with atypical presentations, and during treatment failure.

No doubt, your medical education included the maxim that syphilis and tuberculosis (TB) are the two great imitators in medicine because both can mimic a wide variety of other medical disorders; astute clinicians are wise to consider them during both evaluation and diagnosis. The incidence of syphilis varies by decade because efforts to control it are frequently inconsistent, and significant outbreaks tend to be localized to populations or geography, even within prosperous countries. Drug use; sexual behavior; and waning immunocompetence, such as that provoked by other infections such as HIV, have been cited as explanations for recent increases. Neurosyphilis (one possible manifestation of tertiary syphilis) represents 4%–9% of all syphilitic cases, can occur at any stage of infection, and may take 2–20 years to develop (Hutto 2001; Klein et al. 2020; Munjal et al. 2017).

Neurosyphilis has an insidious onset and has evolved so that it is often no longer associated with any distinguishing physical symptoms (such as the gummas you were taught to look for). Psychiatric presentation may involve mania or depression, psychosis, behavioral disturbances, emotional lability, and progressive intellectual decline into dementia, with personality changes and hallucinations (sometimes visual) being the most common symptoms. A variety of comorbid neurological symptoms may also

Table 7–1. **Infectious diseases frequently associated with psychiatric symptoms**

Agent	Estimated prevalence in psychiatric patients	Estimated prevalence in general population
Hepatitis B[a]	23.9%–32%	5%
Hepatitis C[a]	21%	1.8%
HIV[a]	4%–23%	0.5%
Coronavirus disease 2019 (COVID-19)	2.9%–5.45%[b]	3.3%[c]
Lyme disease	33% in endemic areas[d]	14.5%–19% in endemic areas[d,e]
Herpes simplex 1[f]	66%–80%	66%–80%
Herpes simplex 2[f]	13.2%	13.2%
Syphilis	1.1%–7.6%[g]	0.5%[h]
Tuberculosis	14%–30%[i]	5%[j]
Neurocysticerosis[k]	18.5% in endemic areas	1.57% in endemic areas
Prion transmissible spongiform encephalopathy (e.g., Creutzfeldt-Jacob disease)[l]	Not determined	1.2×10^{-5}

[a]Pirl et al. 2005; Rothbard et al. 2009.
[b]Taquet et al. 2021.
[c]Lee et al. 2020.
[d]Hájek et al. 2002.
[e]Dong et al. 2022.
[f]Andreou et al. 2022; Gotlieb-Stematsky et al. 1981.
[g]Campos et al. 2008; Issa et al. 2013.
[h]Rowley et al. 2016.
[i]Doherty et al. 2013.
[j]Bentley et al. 2012.
[k]Meza et al. 2005.
[l]Singh et al. 2019; Taşkapilioğlu et al. 2013.

be present, such as seizures, headaches, ataxia, paralysis, wide-based gait, slurred speech, aphasia, urinary and fecal incontinence, sensory changes, and impotence. Neuropsychiatric symptoms involved often belong to two or more syndromes, and an atypical presentation is most likely (Crozatti et al. 2015). Ophthalmic problems, particularly pupillary changes such as Argyll Robertson pupils (which constrict with accommodation or convergence but not in response to light), may provide another clue for neurosyphilis (Hutto 2001; Munjal et al. 2017). The presence of any of these comorbidities with psychiatric symptoms, or an atypical appearance of neuropsychiatric symptoms, particularly in vulnerable populations, should prompt the practitioner to test for syphilis if they are not routinely screening for it. It is also helpful to maintain an awareness of which populations have been recently or are currently most at risk for syphilis (Gonzalez et al. 2019).

Unfortunately, the task of confirming the diagnosis of neurosyphilis through the laboratory is complicated by a lack of consensus on the most accurate and helpful methods of testing. Current guidelines begin with the serum venereal disease research laboratory test (VDRL) and fluorescent treponemal antibody absorption tests (FTA-ABS), although these may not be sensitive enough. If neurological, otologic, or ophthalmic symptoms are present, cerebrospinal fluid (CSF) should be obtained through lumbar puncture and tested with VDRL, FTA-ABS, CSF cellularity, and protein levels. CSF treponemal tests can rule out neurosyphilis but not confirm it because of low sensitivity; hypercellularity (pleocytosis) (Tuddenham and Ghanem 2018; Østergaard et al. 2017) and high protein measurements support a diagnosis of neurosyphilis (Boog et al. 2021; Klein et al. 2020).

Once neurosyphilis is diagnosed, treatment should proceed, usually with aqueous crystalline penicillin G. In the case of penicillin allergy, alternative antibiotics are being studied in adults, but evidence-based conclusions have not yet been reached (Buitrago-Garcia et al. 2019; Klein et al. 2020). Anticonvulsants may also be necessary to mitigate an increased risk of seizure during treatment (Sutter et al. 2015). Depending on the location of the infection in the CNS (i.e., parenchymal vs. meningeal), improvement in psychiatric and neurological symptoms following treatment may be seen, but this depends on the degree of neuronal loss prior to treatment. More commonly, further symptomatic progression of the infection and death are avoided (Hutto 2001).

Guidance for separate treatment of the neuropsychiatric symptoms in neurosyphilis is not strong, but some authors argue convincingly for judicious targeting of the atypical psychiatric symptoms with standard psychotropic medications at the lowest possible doses and reducing these for any iatrogenic symptoms that emerge. Successful interventions might be continued for 3–6 months, after which drug holidays might be attempted (Sanchez and Zisselman 2007). Because evidence-based protocols for laboratory diagnosis and treatment of neurosyphilis are still being established, providers are cautioned to seek infectious disease consultation when neurosyphilis is suspected.

The other great imitator, TB—the leading cause of death worldwide from infectious disease prior to COVID-19 (Holmes et al. 2017; Vega et al. 2004)—is also not unknown in psychiatric populations. In one day program, 30% of patients with depression and 14% of those with psychosis tested positive for purified protein derivative of tuberculosis, as did 19% of admissions to a separate inpatient unit. Conversely, 70% of patients with TB meet criteria for depressive disorder or anxiety (Doherty et al. 2013). Additionally, heavy alcohol use (three or more drinks per day [40 g]) nearly triples the risk of developing TB (Imtiaz et al. 2017; Lönnroth et al. 2008). However, when alcohol use is controlled for, mental illness itself, especially depression and schizophrenia, has been demonstrated as an independent risk factor for active TB infection. Given the significant comorbidity, practitioners should screen appropriate populations and seek consultation for treatment of *Mycobacterium tuberculosis* (Hayward et al. 2022; Trenton and Currier 2001).

Tuberculous meningitis, the most common form of TB spread to the CNS, is rare in developed countries but more common in the very young and among those with immunodeficiency, including patients who are aging (Marx and Chan 2011). Without displaying any sign of meningitis, patients can present with psychosis or personality change prior to the appearance of altered mental status (Rahim and Ghazali 2016). As with neurosyphilis, diagnosis may be difficult: culture of the microorganism and acid-fast smear from the CSF both have low sensitivity. Again, pleocytosis and elevated protein in the CSF may support the diagnosis, but neuroimaging may also be necessary, searching for basal meningeal enhancement and hydrocephalus (Marx and Chan 2011).

There are several protocols for the treatment of pulmonary TB, often individualized to specific populations and designed to minimize antibiotic resistance (Centers for Disease Control and Prevention 2022c). Treatment of CNS TB is based on the following medications: 60 days of daily isoniazid, rifampin, pyrazinamide, and either streptomycin or ethambutol, followed by 7–10 months of isoniazid and rifampin (Thwaites et al. 2009). Given the length and complexity of many of these protocols, compliance often complicates success, so all of the elements of an effective therapeutic alliance must be called on to achieve remission (see Chapter 5, section "Perceiving and Respecting Your Patient," and Chapter 9). Patients with alcohol use disorder respond poorly to treatment (Wigger et al.

2022). The use of alcohol is more hepatotoxic with the use of isoniazid, and, although alcohol does not appear to affect the metabolism of isoniazid directly (Wilcke et al. 2004), it also invalidates its effectiveness, particularly when combined with smoking tobacco; therefore, alcohol should be avoided during treatment (Mergenhagen et al. 2020; Song et al. 2022).

Treatment of the associated psychiatric symptoms is also complex because drug-drug interactions (DDIs) may occur through the cytochrome P450 (CYP) system or isoniazid's inhibition of monoamine oxidase, which may affect tolerability and outcome. Although there is minimal to no direct evidence of toxicity, there is considerable reason to take these possibilities into account during concomitant treatment of TB and psychiatric symptoms, primary or secondary. In a meta-analysis by Wu et al. (2016), 13.2% of patients treated for multidrug-resistant TB exhibited psychiatric symptoms as side effects. Rifampicin lowers serum levels of antipsychotics, cycloserine may worsen depression, and psychosis has been reported with the use of most anti-TB antibiotics. Paroxetine has been touted as the SSRI most likely to avoid DDIs during treatment for TB (Doherty et al. 2013; Trenton and Currier 2001). Again, infectious disease consultation is essential in helping to clarify diagnosis and treatment planning.

HIV infection, with and without AIDS, may lead to psychiatric symptoms, as well as to symptoms caused by opportunistic infections (e.g., toxoplasmosis, cytomegalovirus infection, John Cunningham virus–induced progressive multifocal leukoencephalopathy, cryptococcal meningitis), secondary tumors (e.g., lymphoma), and multiple secondary endocrinological problems (e.g., thyroid and adrenal perturbations; see section "Endocrine Disorders" earlier in this chapter) (Munjal et al. 2017; Saribas et al. 2010).

The most common HIV-associated mental health symptoms and disorders are depression (35.6%), PTSD (30%), substance misuse (30%), apathy (26%), sleep disturbance (10%–50%), anxiety (13%), psychosis (8.5%), adjustment disorder (7%), and bipolar disorder (1.5%). Most of these prevalences are higher than in the general population or noninfected cohorts. Anxiety has been found to be 1.6 times more likely in patients with HIV who are not receiving antiretroviral treatment (ART; Shacham et al. 2012).

HIV-associated neurocognitive disorder (HAND) is common (a prevalence of 47%), with three levels of severity: asymptomatic neurocognitive impairment (23.5%–33%), mild neurocognitive disorder (12%–13.3%), and dementia (2%–8%). Poor episodic memory is the most common cognitive impairment associated with HIV infection. The use of ART has reduced the severity of HAND, but not the incidence, and sometimes it worsens it instead (Knights et al. 2017; Nedelcovych et al. 2017; Vastag et al. 2022). ART may also contribute to psychiatric morbidity, with interferon alfa-2a and efavirenz provoking the neuropsychiatric domain (only sometimes transiently) in more than half of treated patients, resulting in depression, suicidality, anxiety, psychosis, nightmares, and/or insomnia. Plus, because the average patient with HIV is treated with seven medications, DDIs are very possible (Munjal et al. 2017).

Despite these significant symptoms, psychiatric conditions are underidentified and undertreated in HIV-infected patients (Nedelcovych et al. 2017). This is particularly surprising because standard treatment of depressive and psychotic syndromes is effective in this patient group. Patients with HIV-associated mood disorders respond well to pharmacotherapy, CBT, and, in general, even better to the combination (Sherr et al. 2011). Lithium is contraindicated because of HIV nephropathy, as is carbamazepine because of pancytopenia and induction of ART metabolism, but valproate has been found to be effective and safe if use is carefully monitored. Antipsychotics are generally effective for secondary psychosis in this group, but side effects (e.g., tardive dyskinesia, extrapyramidal syndrome) may be more prominent. Exercise may also play a helpful role in the mental health symptoms of HIV patients (O'Brien et al. 2016). In all cases, the use of medications that have DDIs with ART or that may worsen neurocognitive functioning should generally be avoided or considered cautiously (Knights et al. 2017).

Hepatitis B virus (HBV) and hepatitis C virus (HCV) affect not only the liver but also the CNS. HCV, mentioned earlier as having an incidence more than 10 times higher in hospitalized psychiatric patients than in the general population, may manifest with cognitive impairment, particularly in attention, memory, and higher-level functioning, as well as with depression, anxiety, and fatigue (Adinolfi et al. 2015; Munjal et al. 2017; Rifai et al. 2010; Tan et al. 2022). In one study, 30.2% of HBV carriers asymptomatic for their liver disease were diagnosed with a DSM-IV psychiatric diagnosis (particularly depressive and anxiety disorders), a rate similar to that for HCV and three times higher than found in noninfected matched control subjects (Atesci et al. 2005); depressive and anxiety symptom rates approached 50% in HBV-infected patients in another report (Diagne et al. 2022). Associated cognitive impairment with HBV involves language and executive function (Tan et al. 2022).

Unfortunately, treatment for hepatitis virus with interferon alfa and ribavirin commonly leads to psychiatric symptoms (particularly depression, anxiety, mania, hypomania, and fatigue, but also agitation, apathy, anhedonia, anorexia, emotional lability, irritability, psychosis, hostility, anger, psychomotor retardation, sexual dysfunction, sleep disturbance, further cognitive impairment, suicidality, and suicide) (Huckans et al. 2015; Rifai et al. 2010). Standard psychiatric treatments, particularly for mood disorders, may be attempted and may be helpful, but they may also result in DDIs and toxicity, related sometimes to hepatic metabolism (Lotrich 2013; Rifai et al. 2010). Additionally, although reduction of the viral load may improve psychiatric symptoms, it does not often reverse infection or treatment-associated cognitive deficits, underscoring the importance of early suspicion and detection of HBV and HCV in patients with new or chronic psychiatric symptoms (Cattie et al. 2014; Gragnani et al. 2022; Schmidt et al. 2009). Consultation with gastroenterology and infectious disease colleagues is important for the mental health practitioner, and each case must be considered individually. Interferon-free treatments are being developed, which so far appear to have measurable benefit and to cause significantly fewer mental health side effects (Gragnani et al. 2022; Sackey et al. 2018; Skolnik et al. 2019).

Coronaviruses are potentially neuroinvasive, neurotropic, and neurovirulent. Severe acute respiratory syndrome coronavirus 2 (SARS-CoV-2), the virus that causes the disease COVID-19, is burned into our collective history, but it is not the first coronavirus of this century to affect large numbers of people. The severe acute respiratory syndrome coronavirus (SARS-CoV-1) outbreak from 2002–2004 and the 2012 Middle East respiratory syndrome (MERS) outbreak affected 31 and 27 countries, respectively (Sommer and Bakker 2020; World Health Organization 2015, 2023). The cumulative incidence of DSM-IV diagnoses 30 months post SARS-CoV-1 infection was 58.9%; the prevalence was 33.3%, including 25% for PTSD and 15.6% for depressive disorders (Mak et al. 2009). Acute psychiatric symptoms reported for the three coronavirus outbreaks this century (through April 2020) are led by insomnia, with an incidence of 41.9%, and followed by anxiety (35.7%), impaired memory (34.1%), acute delirium (27.9% overall but 69% for patients in the ICU), and depressed mood (26.2%). The acute incidence of steroid-induced psychosis and mania was reported at 0.7%, but other authors have provided evidence that the incidence of initial episodes of SARS-CoV-2 infection–related mania, iatrogenic or spontaneous, may be underestimated (Russo et al. 2022). The 2020 study lists a post-illness point prevalence of 32.2%

for PTSD, 14.8% for anxiety disorders, and 11.1% for depression (Rogers et al. 2020).

SARS-CoV-2 first appeared in 2019 (Roberts et al. 2021). People with a diagnosed mental disorder are at greater risk of SARS-CoV-2 infection, hospitalization, and mortality (Wang et al. 2021). Even vaccinated psychiatric patients have an increased risk for breakthrough infection (Nishimi et al. 2022). This virus crosses the blood-brain barrier, triggering an immune response linked to mood and sleep disorders (Bourmistrova et al. 2022), and investigators are determining and updating the acute and long-term neuropsychiatric sequelae of this new infectious agent (COVID-19 Mental Disorders Collaborators 2021). Fatigue may last many months post COVID-19, and cognitive and other mental symptoms may also persist. Viral damage to organs complicates symptoms, metabolism, and toxicities, making psychiatric assessment and treatment challenging. Delirium best predicts residual cognitive impairment, but persistent depression, anxiety, PTSD, amnesia, sleep disorder, and fatigue, often described as *long COVID*, appear to affect survivors of all severities of the disease (Păunescu et al. 2022; Yong 2021; Zeng et al. 2023). As always, a careful comprehensive medical history will aid the practitioner because, apparently, even mild cases of COVID-19 may contribute to residual neuropsychiatric symptoms.

Treatment for these sequelae of coronavirus infections may need to include sleep hygiene, progressive physical exercise, cognitive rehabilitation, remediation, restructuring, support groups, and brief CBT, as indicated (Krishnan et al. 2022; Rolin et al. 2022). SSRIs have been reported as effective for post-COVID-19 depression (Mazza et al. 2022), as has electroconvulsive therapy for catatonia and mania, or depression with psychosis (Austgen et al. 2022).

Other infections that may have psychiatric manifestations include Lyme disease, Creutzfeldt-Jakob disease (CJD), HSV infection, and neurocysticerosis (NCC). Lyme disease, the most common vector-borne disease in the United States, is caused by infection with the spirochete *Borrelia burgdorferi* through the bite of black-legged ticks (Centers for Disease Control and Prevention 2022a). Forty percent of infections progress to the peripheral or central nervous system, and, like syphilis, may do so quickly or after a latency period of years, resulting in neurological and/or psychiatric symptoms. Patients with this infection most often present to the mental health professional with nonspecific neuropsychiatric symptoms that often mimic major depression (26%–66%). Anxiety, irritability, and panic are also frequent symptoms, along with (less commonly) mania, psychosis, and OCD. Delirium is a common secondary complication of systemic infection, as are fatigue and cognitive impairments, including dementia from late-stage disease (Erdogan and Hocaoglu 2020; Fallon and Nields 1994; Munjal et al. 2017).

Misunderstandings have surrounded Lyme disease since its discovery in the 1970s, especially regarding its contribution to symptoms and its diagnosis and treatment. What is true is that it is not possible to diagnose this infection solely on the basis of physical or neuropsychiatric symptoms (Baker 2019). Ultimately, it is as much of an error to miss the diagnosis by neglecting to consider it as it is to conclude that Lyme disease is always responsible for every symptom. Although clinical practice guidelines from infectious disease, neurology, and rheumatology do not recommend routing testing of adult psychiatric patients for Lyme disease (Lantos et al. 2021), this should be considered when evaluating patients exposed to the areas in which Lyme disease is endemic (an ever-expanding area of the United States that currently includes Connecticut, Delaware, Maine, Maryland, Massachusetts, Minnesota, New Hampshire, New Jersey, New York, Pennsylvania, Rhode Island, Vermont, Virginia, Washington, D.C., West Virginia, and Wisconsin) (Centers for Disease Control and Prevention 2022b; Sno 2012). New *Borrelia* species have been found to be spreading in Europe (particularly in Germany, Austria, Slovenia, and Sweden), the United Kingdom, and China, although clinical presentations in humans are not identical to those of *B. burgdorferi* and are not yet fully described (Marques et al. 2021; Stone et al. 2017). Screening may be particularly important when patients present with arthritis and/or dementia (Van Hout 2018). A full evaluation to seek alternative explanations of symptoms and dysfunction is always indicated (see section "Accounting for Every Symptom of Dysfunction" in Chapter 5).

Lyme disease can be reliably diagnosed any time after the first 4–6 weeks of infection by a standard two-tier test (a quantitative sensitive enzyme-linked immunosorbent assay [ELISA] followed, if positive or equivocal, by the qualitative IgG Western blot test) or its recently modified form (two FDA-approved ELISA tests). The use of two of these methods can distinguish active infection that needs to be treated from past, inactive infection (Baker 2019; Mead et al. 2019).

Whereas standard treatment for early Lyme disease is 14–21 days of the oral antibiotic amoxicillin or doxycycline, Lyme arthritis indicates more advanced dissemination, and 28 days of treatment is recommended. In the presence of clear neurological (or psychiatric) symptoms, intravenous ceftriaxone is suggested. Disseminated cases, however, may be unresponsive to these antibiotics because of resistance or tolerance (Bobe et al. 2021). Infectious disease consultation is, again, essential.

Prion transmissible spongiform encephalopathy, a progressive and currently incurable neurodegenerative disorder, is caused by the misfolding of the cellular protein PrPC into PrPSc, which disturbs the balance between neuronal protein synthesis and degradation. Clinically, it may manifest with depressed mood or apathy and associated weight loss, insomnia, and behavioral changes, as well as cognitive decline (Cumbler et al. 2009; Sigurdson et al. 2019). Anxiety, agitation, and psychosis with both delusions and hallucinations may also result from this infection, which affects 1.2 people out of every million in the United States; 90% of these infections are diagnosed as CJD (Singh et al. 2019; Taşkapilioğlu et al. 2013). These clinical symptoms are not distinct from primary psychiatric disorders, so EEG, imaging, and laboratory testing are essential for confirming the diagnosis once the astute clinician considers the possibility, especially in older patients with no previous history of psychiatric symptoms. Cortical ribboning in the cortex and basal ganglia is usually seen on MRI, and presence of the 14-3-3 protein in the CSF is both sensitive and specific for confirming the diagnosis; tonsillar biopsy might be more helpful to diagnose a variant form (Singh et al. 2019; Munjal et al. 2017; Valente et al. 2015).

In one case during the late 1990s, a psychiatrist watched helplessly as her patient progressed steadily from depression to dementia to death, despite all efforts to treat her. Once the clinical diagnosis was made, the psychiatrist did recall her patient speaking often of her fondness for gardening. As severe neurodegeneration advanced, the doctor confirmed with the patient's spouse that she had used bone meal routinely as fertilizer for her plants. At that time, bovine spongiform encephalopathy ("mad cow disease") was particularly prominent in the United Kingdom, resulting in a new variant of CJD (vCJD) in humans (Brandel and Knight 2018). Meat and bone meal from infected animals had been demonstrated to transmit the bovine form, and avoidance of such products from the United Kingdom likely occurred too late to prevent some cases, given the long incubation period (Johnson and Gibbs 1998; Patterson and Painter 1999; Wilesmith et al. 1988). This case does illustrate how broader history taking might point to earlier answers for many patients and their families.

In this book, I have clearly stated that the terms treatment resistance and treatment failure will not be applied to conditions for which there is no known treatment because no alternative explanation exists for the clinician to discover and apply. CJD is included here, however, to stress that early diagnosis of even currently hopeless conditions is a more humane approach. Palliation may begin more promptly (see section "Enhance Clinical Reasoning" in Chapter 8, "Reducing Treatment Failure"), and the patient and family often appreciate the opportunity to deal directly with an accurate diagnosis rather than chasing dead-end treatments for nonexistent primary psychiatric conditions (Cumbler et al. 2009). That said, attempts are being made to find effective treatments for spongiform encephalopathies. As the search for effective antibiotics and neuroprotective agents continues, prion protein monoclonal antibody is also being explored (Mead et al. 2022; Miranda et al. 2022). There is hope that earlier diagnosis might allow better results if treatment is employed prior to extensive and irreversible neurodegeneration, as with neurosyphilis and TB (Watson et al. 2021).

Herpes simplex virus 1 (HSV-1) is found in a majority of the global population (66%–80%), and HSV-2 is found in 13.2% (Büttiker et al. 2022; James et al. 2020). The odds ratio for depression is 1.28 when a patient is seropositive for HSV-1 and 2.0 for HSV-2, indicating that HSV infection may be a risk factor for the symptom of depression or the diagnosis of major depression in some patients (Gale et al. 2018; Ye et al. 2020). Additionally, HSV-1 resides in the trigeminal nerve following initial infection; periodic reactivation leads to neuronal loss, inflammation, and then, possibly, to neurodegenerative disease, including cognitive deficits in schizophrenia (Doll et al. 2019; Iqbal et al. 2020; Yolken et al. 2011). Reactivation of HSV-1 and HSV-2 may trigger tau hyperphosphorylation (p-tau) with possible propagation, and secretion of amyloid beta peptide (Aβ) in genetically susceptible individuals (Devanand 2018; Fülöp et al. 2020).

Studies are under way to determine whether antiviral treatments (AVTs) such as acyclovir, penciclovir, and foscarnet can reverse some of the symptoms of dementia by reducing Aβ and p-tau (Devanand et al. 2020; Sait et al. 2021; Wozniak et al. 2011). So far, three registry and case-control studies in Scandinavia and Taiwan have shown AVT to reduce the long-term risk of developing dementia in patients who had overt symptoms of HSV infection, although a similar study in Germany failed to show a correlation (Hemmingsson et al. 2021; Kostev and Tanislav 2021; Lopatko Lindman et al. 2021; Tzeng et al. 2018). One group has reported that the AVT valacyclovir reduced impairment in visual object learning and verbal and working memory in patients with schizophrenia, although it did not improve symptoms of psychosis (Prasad et al. 2013).

It has been estimated that 90% of cases of encephalitis in non-immuno-compromised individuals result from HSV-1 (Więdłocha et al. 2015). Anxiety, depression, and PTSD psychiatric symptoms lasting a year or longer are associated with HSV encephalitis, and memory and naming ability are also often severely affected. Although these cognitive deficits may improve over time, subjective complaints of cognitive impairment, depression, and anxiety generally do not, and they may persist long term, along with emotionalism, irritability, behavioral and personality disorders, and psychosis associated with left prefrontal hypoperfusion (Büttiker et al. 2022; Caparros-Lefebvre et al. 1996; Harris et al. 2020; Więdłocha et al. 2015). An accurate neurological history is essential.

HSV infection is best diagnosed by culture from open lesions or by the detection of serum antibodies with automated multiplexed flow enzyme immunoassays, although accuracy can depend on the phase of infection. Soon, improved point-of-contact devices may allow quicker diagnosis and response (Nath et al. 2021). Given the endemic nature of HSV, clinicians may wish to remain alert to the arrival of new data concerning the impact of AVT on psychiatric symptoms.

NCC, the most common parasitic infection in Asia, Latin America, and Africa, results from infection with the swine tapeworm *Taenia solium*. Untreated, it ultimately results in chronic, irreversible brain damage, and 80% of infected patients experience seizures. A significant number (15%) of NCC-infected patients present with only psychiatric symptoms: most commonly psychosis but possibly depression or dementia. NCC should be suspected when the acute onset of these symptoms occurs in younger patients with seizures who have been exposed to areas where *T. solium* is endemic (Munjal et al. 2017). In 2005, 18.5% of inpatients with chronic psychiatric illness in Venezuela were found to be infected, compared with 1.6% of control subjects (Meza et al. 2005).

Diagnosis of NCC is confirmed with the detection of cysts in various stages by MRI or CT of the brain, along with the discovery of antibodies and antigens in the serum and CSF. Treatment is individualized but may involve anticysticercal medications such as praziquantel and albendazole along with steroids to mitigate a possible inflammatory immune response. In some cases, surgery may be attempted to remove cysts but is now more likely to be used for the placement of ventricular shunts (Munjal et al. 2017; Takayanagui and Haes 2022). As with other conditions discussed earlier, infectious disease consultation is essential.

Respiratory Disorders

Respiratory disorders, the most common nonpsychiatric medical co-morbidity for psychiatric patients, may also manifest with anxiety, sleep disorders, cognitive impairment, irritability, agitation, and depression, all of which may be exacerbated by respiratory treatments, such as bron-chodilators, steroids, and first-generation antihistamines (Bhattacharyya et al. 2022; Liu et al. 2013). Half of severely asthmatic patients have symptoms of anxiety or depression, the former mediated by dysfunctional breathing and the latter by dyspnea (Stubbs et al. 2022).

A third of patients with chronic obstructive pulmonary disease have cognitive impairment, and more than half experience anxiety or depression. Oxygen therapy, antidepressants, CBT, and mind-body or individualized exercise programs may be helpful for addressing the neuropsychiatric symptoms in these patients (Li et al. 2019; Ouellette and Lavoie 2017).

There is an increased prevalence of depression in patients with obstructive sleep apnea, particularly those with associated snoring or excessive daytime drowsiness. Evaluation for obstructive sleep apnea is encouraged for depressed patients whose treatment fails, especially those with one or both of these symptoms (Naqvi et al. 2014).

Gastrointestinal System and Disorders

There is a well-documented bidirectional association between the CNS and gastrointestinal (GI) systems that is so strong the two might be considered a single organ (Lydiard 2001; Van Oudenhove et al. 2004). Irritable bowel syndrome (IBS), which is responsive to treatment with antidepressants and is associated with hyperventilation, anxiety, and depression, particularly illustrates the link: the presence of IBS increases the risk of subsequent development of anxiety fivefold (Fadgyas-Stanculete et al. 2014; Gracie et al. 2018; Nyhlin et al. 1993). Additionally, treatment of inflammatory bowel disease (such as ulcerative colitis and regional enteritis) with immunosuppressive therapy has been found to improve symptoms of depression (Horst et al. 2015; Gracie et al. 2019).

Changes in individual microbiomes have been linked to anxiety, depression, schizophrenia, and dementia through the GI-CNS (or gut-brain) axis (Cryan et al. 2019). Bioavailability of medications (see section "Polypharmacy and Bioavailability Complications" later in this chapter) may also be altered by changes in gut microbiota. Studies of treatment options are scarce, but a recent meta-analysis found that some probiotic treatments for depressive symptoms appear effective (Socała et al. 2021;

Zagórska et al. 2020). Much more must be learned, but awareness of how GI conditions and biome changes may affect symptoms and outcomes for our patients is becoming an increasingly important tool.

Lifestyle Factors

As mentioned in Chapter 4, "The Myth of Treatment Resistance?", lifestyle behaviors can often determine the success of a prescribed treatment. The concomitant use of alcohol and/or legal and illegal recreational drugs (including edibles), even when not reaching the threshold for comorbidity, may nevertheless interfere with successful treatment outcomes of mood, anxiety, and psychotic disorders and must be properly evaluated and monitored (Guttmannova et al. 2017; Hall and Degenhardt 2014; Volkow et al. 2016; Weinstein et al. 2016). Alcohol use is often comorbid with use of other substances, particularly among youths (Karnik 2022).

Caffeine and other over-the-counter stimulants (e.g., pseudoephedrine, energy drinks) easily contribute to sleep and anxiety symptoms and disorders directly (Bergin and Kendler 2012) and risk destabilizing bipolar disorder (Baethge et al. 2009; Dalton 1990; Frigerio et al. 2021; Rizkallah et al. 2011; Stuer and Claes 2007); see case examples "A Case of Unrestrained Lifestyle Issues" and "A Case of Misunderstanding and Inadequate Compliance" in Chapter 6). Caffeine, which is metabolized largely by CYP1A2, also alters serum levels of many antidepressants (including duloxetine, imipramine, amitriptyline, fluvoxamine, and clomipramine) and the atypical antipsychotics clozapine and olanzapine. Table 7–2 provides a list of substances that interact with caffeine, and Table 7–3 lists the caffeine content of common food and drinks.

Patients may be unaware that many products they use may contain significant amounts of caffeine. Caffeine use must be monitored, or in some cases restricted, not only because of direct effects on symptoms and functionality but also because levels of it and some medications may be altered through CYP1A2.

Although smoking nicotine is not associated with treatment-resistant depression (De Carlo et al. 2016), it does have implications for successful therapy because hydrocarbons in the smoke lower levels of circulating antipsychotic medications through enzymatic induction (Ziedonis and George 1997). Further, a reduction in nicotine use may provoke mood instability in bipolar disorder (Glassman 1993; Thomson et al. 2015).

Probably one of the most important lifestyle contributions to successful treatment is routine adequate sleep. Along with the treatment of co-

Table 7–2.   Interactions between caffeine and medications

Medications whose levels are increased by caffeine

Asenapine

Theophylline

Riluzole

Clozapine

Acetaminophen

Duloxetine

Paroxetine

Imipramine

Amitriptyline

Clomipramine

Olanzapine

Clonidine

Medications and substances that increase caffeine levels

Fluvoxamine

Disulfiram

Ciprofloxacin

Verapamil

Estrogens

morbid and secondary sleep disorders, sleep hygiene is so essential that it is unlikely remission will be achieved without it (Bassetti et al. 2015; Costa e Silva 2006; Saradhadevi and Hemavathy 2022; Tufik et al. 2009).

Many patients take supplements or nutraceuticals, often without consulting their provider; practitioners may avoid interference with outcomes by maintaining current knowledge about popular supplements. Ginkgo biloba, while not effective in preventing dementia, does lower levels of valproic acid and omeprazole through induction of CYP2C19 (DeKosky et al. 2008; Di Lorenzo et al. 2015; Vellas et al. 2012; Yin et al. 2004). Ginseng in high doses, or with long-term use, may lead to insomnia and nervousness, and there are reports of it inducing mania (Bostock et al. 2018; Joshi and Faubion 2005).

Although L-methylfolate may be useful in treating depressed patients with the *MTHFR* polymorphism, its use in treatment-resistant depression in patients with normal serum folate levels has produced only modest response (Alpert et al. 2002). Measurement of folate in serum or erythrocytes, not always low at the time of depression, is also insufficient to detect

Table 7–3.   Caffeine content of commonly used substances

Product	Caffeine content, mg
Average soft drink with caffeine	30–40
Green or black tea	30–50
Coffee (8 oz)	80–100
Energy drink (8 oz)	40–250
Dark chocolate (per ounce)	5–20
Milk chocolate	3.5–6
White chocolate	Check ingredients to see if added

cerebral folate deficiency (CFD; Hyland et al. 2010; Wolfersdorf and König 1995); see section "Metabolic Factors" in Chapter 4. L-methylfolate supplementation is not effective in the treatment of CFD, and its use distorts measurements of folate in the CSF. Therefore, testing for CFD must take place prior to L-methylfolate administration (Pan et al. 2017).

S-adenosyl-L-methionine, a popular self-treatment for depression, can provoke anxiety, agitation, and insomnia in all patients, as well as hypomania and mania in patients with bipolar disorder (Sharma et al. 2017). A more detailed discussion of lifestyle contributions to effective psychiatric treatment and the role of supplements may be found in Chapters 8 and 9 of *Rational Psychopharmacology: A Book of Clinical Skills* (Putman 2020).

Polypharmacy and Bioavailability Complications

We must also remain alert for treatment failure induced through iatrogenic means. Treatment failure itself often leads to polypharmacy or combined medications, that is, the prescription of more than one psychotropic medication for each indication (Govaerts et al. 2021). At times, solid rationale may support the practice, as in the treatment of schizophrenia or schizoaffective disorder (Lähteenvuo and Tiihonen 2021; Lin 2020), and polypharmacy may appear to be necessary without clear guidelines when progress is not being made (Jaracz 2018; Jašović-Gašić 2015). Hopefully, this would occur only after thorough assessment has determined that the diagnosis is accurate and that all comorbidities have been addressed.

Regardless of the reasons for choosing polypharmacy, we as clinicians must always investigate the possible ramifications of this decision that may impede treatment success, just as we would medications prescribed by other practitioners, such as steroids, β-agonists, anticholinergics, and β-blockers (Lippi et al. 2022; Stassen et al. 2022). Although we know the side effects of our medications, we must also know or routinely investigate any possible DDIs, not only for safety but also to avoid lowered efficacy (Table 7–4). For example, carbamazepine clinically induces methylphenidate to a clinically relevant degree, lowering its efficacy (Schoretsanitis et al. 2019). Adequate serum levels of each prescribed medication must be maintained, and these levels cannot always be confirmed through the local laboratory.

Practitioners must determine the impact of possible drug-drug interactions prior to prescribing polypharmaceutical interventions. Similarly, changes in relative bioavailability, the fraction of a drug that reaches systemic circulation compared with intravenous administration, may sabotage treatment or lead to success. Bioavailability can be affected by such factors as another medication being administered at the same time, food intake (with oral administration), local pH, the size of particles, and the state of the drug (e.g., suspension, liquid, solid). For example, a patient adding a fiber supplement to his regimen may see a reduction in the absorption of a routine medication and a resultant decline in benefit (see section "A Case of Ongoing Interference" in Chapter 6). A medicine may also differ in its bioavailability when given by multiple delivery systems or when produced by more than one manufacturer, which will result in different serum levels.

In the United States, the FDA once arbitrarily decided that the bioavailability of generic medications must be measured within 80%–120% of the brand name preparation, allowing a 40% variance in strength. However, because of possible differences in active drug amounts, inactive ingredients, and delivery systems, the definition of relative bioavailability is not universally agreed on for generics, so the concept of bioequivalence has been further refined. In 1992, the FDA converted to requiring the demonstration of a narrower definition of bioequivalence, ideally determined with in vivo crossover studies showing pharmacokinetic measurements, including peak serum concentrations and time of maximum drug exposure (area under the curve), within 80%–125% of brand name preparations *with a 90% confidence level* (Andrade 2015; Pharmacy Times 2016; U.S. Food and Drug Administration 2022). Even though crossover studies are not ideal or feasible for evaluating all products and more indirect measurements are sometimes allowed, these criteria are more stringent than before (Beers and Karst 2020).

Table 7–4. Examples of drug-drug interactions mediated by cytochrome P450 (CYP) enzymes

CYP enzyme	Substrates	Inhibitors	Inducers
3A4	Alprazolam,[a] diazepam, aripiprazole, ziprasidone, zolpidem, trazodone, methylphenidate, dextromethorphan, verapamil,[a] simvastatin, clomipramine, citalopram	Fluvoxamine, norfluoxetine, verapamil, erythromycin	Carbamazepine, oxcarbazepine, modafinil, phenytoin, phenobarbital, topiramate
1A2	Caffeine, clomipramine, clozapine, duloxetine, olanzapine, zolpidem	Fluvoxamine	Carbamazepine, modafinil, cigarette smoking (polycyclic aromatic hydrocarbons)
2D6	Aripiprazole, duloxetine, venlafaxine, risperidone, amphetamine, atomoxetine, dextromethorphan	Fluvoxamine, fluoxetine, paroxetine, bupropion, sertraline, ziprasidone (weak)	Carbamazepine, modafinil
2C19	Diazepam, citalopram, clomipramine, phenytoin	Fluvoxamine, oxcarbazepine, modafinil	Carbamazepine, phenytoin, primidone
2C9	Zolpidem, ibuprofen, losartan, valproic acid, warfarin, zolpidem	Fluvoxamine, sertraline, paroxetine	Carbamazepine, St. John's wort, phenytoin
2B6	Bupropion, ketamine, methadone	Sertraline	Carbamazepine, phenytoin, phenobarbital

[a]Also a substrate of CYP3A5.

Even so, this amount of change in bioavailability may be noticeable clinically and represents the best possible situation (Benvenga and Carlé 2019; Bobo et al. 2010; Elmer and Reddy 2022). Because of the worldwide location of many generic manufacturers, stringent monitoring is not feasible, and there have been many cases of generic manufacturers not adhering to these standards (Eban 2020; Hatton et al. 2022; Yang et al. 2016). Therefore, it is still essential that practitioners carefully consider any generic preparations they are changing to or prescribing and be aware that pharmacies may change manufacturers without informing the prescriber or patient, even if a specific brand has been prescribed. This may result in clinical changes such as loss of benefit or an increase or decrease in side effects, any of which may indicate a serum level change. Clinicians should educate each patient regarding these issues so that they can partner in monitoring brand changes, which should be confirmed with the pharmacy, if necessary, and recorded by the practitioner. Any clinical changes in the months following a brand change should provoke investigation of change in bioequivalence as a possible cause (Bobo et al. 2010). Similarly, unexpected therapeutic reversals should prompt inquiry into possible brand changes, including the purchase of one manufacturer by another. Serum levels may be useful but, as noted above, are not always available or linked to clinical outcomes in psychiatry.

Psychiatrists as Generalists

A compelling and effective argument has been made that psychiatry is a primary care specialty and that psychiatrists function best as generalists, working as a team with other generalists (and specialists, when necessary) (DeGruy 2006, 2023). Psychiatrists' interest in diagnosing, if not solely managing, general medical conditions is a realistic response to the awareness that the symptoms we treat are so often the tip of the iceberg medically (Jones-Bourne and Arbuckle 2019). Missing underlying or comorbid conditions often leads to treatment failure. Accepting this as treatment resistance is abdicating our full role as physicians and providers and abandons our responsibility to the therapeutic alliance. Progress in the treatment of these nonpsychiatric medical conditions, however, may ease the burden of psychiatric symptoms for a given patient. Psychiatric outcomes can only be enhanced by the thorough diagnosis and treatment of all conditions a patient has, while also monitoring for adverse events of treatments for them that may worsen mental health symptoms and can be reversed.

Summary

More than half of psychiatric patients have at least two nonpsychiatric medical problems. These comorbidities are frequently not diagnosed because of atypical presentations and often cause or worsen psychiatric symptoms. Approaching practice as a generalist, searching for and addressing all of a patient's medical problems, often in consultation with primary care providers or specialists, not only helps avoid psychiatric treatment failure but also may lead to quicker and more complete responses to treatment for all conditions present.

More than 20% of adults have experienced head trauma with loss of consciousness, which may predispose them to psychiatric symptoms and disorders for many years. Twenty percent of patients with even mTBI suffer from postconcussive syndrome with affective, behavioral, or cognitive symptoms. The possibility of TBI must be thoroughly examined because it may also exaggerate the effects of medications. Patients post TBI are at increased risk for new-onset PTS, and antipsychotic and antidepressant medications lower seizure thresholds. Many PTS are subclinical, and patients with PTS may present with many different psychiatric symptoms.

Many primary endocrine disorders, including all types of diabetes mellitus, adrenal insufficiency, and hypercortisolism, may manifest primarily or exclusively with psychiatric symptoms, and the effects are often bidirectional. Thyroid disorders (hypothyroidism, hyperthyroidism, and the common but underdiagnosed thyroiditis) and primary and secondary hyperparathyroidism contribute to psychiatric treatment failures and are often underappreciated. Practitioners should screen for these disorders and remain current on the literature regarding diagnostic levels, not merely relying on a laboratory report.

Psychiatric patients, as a group, have a higher incidence and prevalence of infectious diseases that contribute to mood, thought, and cognitive disorders. The earlier these illnesses are diagnosed and treated, the greater the chance for full recovery. Clinicians need to remain aware of the most common infectious diseases in various populations and screen appropriately. Respiratory disorders are the most common medical comorbidity for our patients. Diagnosing and addressing these disorders often improves the outcome of psychiatric treatment as well. The GI system has a potent bidirectional association with the CNS, and treatments for IBS and inflammatory bowel disease may also have positive effects on the treatment outcomes of psychiatric disorders.

Over-the-counter and dietary stimulants often contribute to sleep, anxiety, and mood symptoms, as does the use of alcohol and recreational and illegal drugs, including edibles. Smoke from nicotine use lowers serum levels of antipsychotic medications, and reduction of nicotine use may destabilize bipolar disorder. Practitioners must remain knowledgeable about commonly used and new supplements to help guide patients and to be considered a useful source of information about them. Testing for CFD must precede any use of oral L-methylfolate.

The effects of DDIs on safety and treatment outcome must be carefully considered during any use of polypharmacy. Bioavailability, and resultant treatment effectiveness, may be altered by changes in delivery system or brand, particularly of generic preparations. Practitioners must partner with patients in monitoring for any substitutions. Our responsibility to our therapeutic alliances demands that we avoid applying the term treatment resistance in practice and never quit searching for the true and possibly multiple causes of treatment failure.

Key Points

- Medical comorbidities contribute to treatment failure and are often missed.
- Mild to moderate head trauma is common but often incorrectly minimized.
- Endocrine disorders may manifest solely with psychiatric symptoms and are often bidirectional.
- Infectious disease rates are higher among psychiatric patients than the general population and contribute to morbidity.
- Respiratory disorders are the most common comorbidity and may be undertreated.
- The GI system is bidirectionally linked with the CNS.
- Over-the-counter products may interfere with treatment and present dangers.
- Medication interactions must be determined prior to polypharmacy.
- Bioavailability is altered by delivery method and manufacturer.

- Taking responsibility for identifying all active medical problems is essential.

Self-Assessment Questions

1. Which of the following statements is true?

    A. Smoking nicotine is associated with treatment-resistant depression.
    B. Ginkgo biloba raises levels of valproic acid and omeprazole through induction of CYP2C19.
    C. A reduction in nicotine use may provoke mood instability in bipolar disorder.
    D. Caffeine has little effect on levels of antidepressant and antipsychotic medications.

    Correct answer: C. A reduction in nicotine use may provoke mood instability in bipolar disorder.

    Smoking nicotine is not associated with treatment-resistant depression, although the smoke does lower levels of antipsychotic medications. Ginkgo biloba lowers levels of valproic acid and omeprazole through induction. Caffeine alters the levels of many antidepressants and the antipsychotics clozapine and olanzapine. A reduction in nicotine may provoke mood instability in bipolar disorder; therefore, any reduction should be slow and carefully monitored.

2. Hyperparathyroidism is associated with which of the following?

    A. Serum calcium levels above 10.3 mg/dL.
    B. Parathyroid hormone levels above 65 pg/mL.
    C. Chronic treatment with lithium salts.
    D. All of the above.

    Correct answer: D. All of the above.

    These values help confirm primary hyperparathyroidism. Long-term use of lithium is linked to an increased incidence of secondary hyperparathyroidism. Both conditions may cause refractory psychiatric symptoms until treated with partial parathyroidectomy.

3.   Which of the following statements is *false*?

   A. The patient may be accurately tested for cerebral folate deficiency (CFD) following ʟ-methylfolate administration.
   B. Pseudoephedrine may easily contribute to sleep and anxiety symptoms.
   C. High-dose or long-term use of ginseng may provoke anxiety, insomnia, and mania.
   D. S-adenosyl-ʟ-methionine may induce anxiety, agitation, and insomnia.

Correct answer: A. The patient may be accurately tested for cerebral folate deficiency (CFD) following ʟ-methylfolate administration.

Cerebrospinal fluid (CSF) levels of folate are distorted by oral use of ʟ-methylfolate, which is not effective in treating CFD. Therefore, the CSF must be tested *prior to* any ʟ-methylfolate use in order to correctly diagnose and treat CFD. Patients may use over-the-counter medications or nutraceutical supplements without full knowledge or agreement of the provider, and these may interfere with treatment success. Regular exploration and discussion of this possibility will improve care.

4.   The prevalence of infectious diseases is higher in hospitalized psychiatric patients except for which of the following?

   A. Hepatitis C.
   B. Herpes simplex virus 1 (HSV-1).
   C. HIV.
   D. Hepatitis B.

Correct answer: B. Herpes simplex virus 1 (HSV-1).

HSV-1 occurs in a majority of the world population, although it may be a risk factor for depression and neurodegenerative disease. Hepatitis B and C and HIV infections have been found to have significantly elevated prevalence in both community and university hospital psychiatric admissions. These infections are also not diagnosed in 95%, 50%, and 21% of cases, respectively.

5. Which of the following statements is/are true?

    A. Lyme disease cannot be diagnosed by physical or neuropsychiatric symptoms alone.
    B. Heavy alcohol use decreases the risk of contracting TB.
    C. Long COVID appears to affect survivors of all severities of the disease.
    D. A and C.

Correct answer: D. A and C.

Lyme disease must be diagnosed by a two-tiered method with a quantitative sensitive enzyme-linked immunosorbent assay (ELISA) followed, if positive or equivocal, by the qualitative IgG Western blot test, or its recently modified form (two FDA-approved ELISA tests). Daily intake of three or more alcoholic drinks triples the risk of TB infection. Delirium best predicts residual cognitive impairment from COVID-19, but depression, anxiety, PTSD, amnesia, sleep disorder, and fatigue may persist in survivors of all severities of the infection.

Discussion Topics

1. A 68-year-old man, recently relocated from Maryland, presents to you for evaluation of depressed mood and anxiety. You learn that his current symptoms also include a recent decline in short-term memory and rare, but not new, auditory hallucinations. During the review of symptoms and past medical history you discover that he also has chronic undiagnosed headaches and was treated for an unknown sexually transmitted disease as a young man in the military, where he also experienced mild TBI with LOC during combat. He has had kidney stones treated with lithotripsy twice and complains of chronic diarrhea. He uses caffeine daily, smokes two packs per day of filtered cigarettes, and admits to heavy use of alcohol. He reports that previous attempts to improve his mood and anxiety have failed, but his sleep is currently so disturbed that he is again seeking help. What diagnoses should you consider in your differential, both psychiatric and

nonpsychiatric? What treatment recommendations should you consider making? How would you approach forming an early therapeutic alliance with this man?

2. A 34-year-old woman requests a second opinion on her pharmacological treatment for major depression prescribed by another provider in your community. She reports disappointing results with two trials of antidepressants. Her provider diagnosed her condition as treatment resistant and suggested adding L-methylfolate to her current treatment plan or considering somatic treatments, such as transcranial magnetic stimulation. The patient believes she was taking generic forms of the two antidepressants she tried, which you determine were both SSRIs. During your assessment, you learn that she was tested for thyroid disorders, although she knows neither the names nor the results of the tests. She does not smoke and quit using alcohol on initiation of treatment. On the basis of the advice of a friend, she started taking probiotics but is not sure what the results are. How would you expand your knowledge base about this patient and the attempts to treat her? What specific questions have yet to be answered?

Additional Readings

Mayer AR, Quinn DK, Master CL: The spectrum of mild traumatic brain injury: a review. Neurology 89(6):623–632, 2017: *This review, from the perspective of neurologists, reinforces the strong value of employing a probabilistic approach to diagnosing the contribution of mild TBI to our patients' conditions*

McKee J, Brahm N: Medical mimics: differential diagnostic considerations for psychiatric symptoms. Ment Health Clin 6(6):289–296, 2016: *Proposes a structured method for distinguishing secondary psychiatric conditions from primary ones and provides clinical examples*

Noordsy DL (ed): Lifestyle Psychiatry. Washington, DC, American Psychiatric Association Publishing, 2019: *Reviews exercise, meditation, diet, and other nonpharmacological treatments often overlooked in treatment failures*

Putman HP: Rational Psychopharmacology: A Book of Clinical Skills. Washington, DC, American Psychiatric Association Publishing, 2020: *Chapter 8, "Supplements: Their Role in Helping and Not Helping," reviews popular and commonly used supplements it is important to be familiar with, and Chapter 9, "Critical Lifestyle Supports to Successful Clinical Psychopharmacology," offers an expanded discussion of this topic*

Wong V, Chin K, Leontieva L: Multifactorial causes of paranoid schizophrenia with auditory-visual hallucinations in a 31-year-old male with history of traumatic brain injury and substance abuse. Cureus 14(5):e25488, 2022:

A relevant example of clinicians attempting to uncover and address the contributions of multiple medical factors in a patient with chronic psychosis

References

Abrahamian H, Kautzky-Willer A, Rießland-Seifert A, et al: Mental disorders and diabetes mellitus (update 2019). Wien Klin Wochenschr 131(Suppl 1):186–195, 2019 30980168

Achté KA, Hillbom E, Aalberg V: Psychoses following war brain injuries. Acta Psychiatr Scand 45(1):1–18, 1969 5345563

Adinolfi LE, Nevola R, Lus G, et al: Chronic hepatitis C virus infection and neurological and psychiatric disorders: an overview. World J Gastroenterol 21(8):2269–2280, 2015 25741133

Al-Atram AA: A review of the bidirectional relationship between psychiatric disorders and diabetes mellitus. Neurosciences (Riyadh) 23(2):91–96, 2018 29664448

Albert U, De Cori D, Aguglia A, et al: Lithium-associated hyperparathyroidism and hypercalcaemia: a case-control cross-sectional study. J Affect Disord 151(2):786–790, 2013 23870428

Almandoz JP, Gharib H: Hypothyroidism: etiology, diagnosis, and management. Med Clin North Am 96(2):203–221, 2012 22443971

Alpert JE, Mischoulon D, Rubenstein GE, et al: Folinic acid (Leucovorin) as an adjunctive treatment for SSRI-refractory depression. Ann Clin Psychiatry 14(1):33–38, 2002 12046638

American Psychiatric Association: Diagnostic and Statistical Manual of Mental Disorders, 4th Edition. Washington, DC, American Psychiatric Association, 1994

Andersen S, Pedersen KM, Bruun NH, et al: Narrow individual variations in serum T(4) and T(3) in normal subjects: a clue to the understanding of subclinical thyroid disease. J Clin Endocrinol Metab 87(3):1068–1072, 2002 11889165

Andrade C: Bioequivalence of generic drugs: a simple explanation for a US Food and Drug Administration requirement. J Clin Psychiatry 76(6):e742–e744, 2015 26132680

Andreou D, Jørgensen KN, Nerland S, et al: Herpes simplex virus 1 infection on grey matter and general intelligence in severe mental illness. Transl Psychiatry 12(1):276, 2022 35821107

Annegers JF, Hauser WA, Coan SP, et al: A population-based study of seizures after traumatic brain injuries. N Engl J Med 338(1):20–24, 1998 9414327

Arciniegas DB, Anderson CA, Topkoff J, et al: Mild traumatic brain injury: a neuropsychiatric approach to diagnosis, evaluation, and treatment. Neuropsychiatr Dis Treat 1(4):311–327, 2005 18568112

Arciniegas DB, Silver JM: Pharmacotherapy of posttraumatic cognitive impairments. Behav Neurol 17(1):25–42, 2006 16720958

Atesci FC, Cetin BC, Oguzhanoglu NK, et al: Psychiatric disorders and functioning in hepatitis B virus carriers. Psychosomatics 46(2):142–147, 2005 15774953

Austgen G, Meyers MS, Gordon M, et al: The use of electroconvulsive therapy in neuropsychiatric complications of Coronavirus disease 2019: a systematic literature review and case report. J Acad Consult Liaison Psychiatry 63(1):86–93, 2022 34358726

Babić Leko M, Gunjača I, Pleić N, et al: Environmental factors affecting thyroid-stimulating hormone and thyroid hormone levels. Int J Mol Sci 22(12):6521, 2021 34204586

Bădescu SV, Tătaru C, Kobylinska L, et al: The association between diabetes mellitus and depression. J Med Life 9(2):120–125, 2016 27453739

Baethge C, Tondo L, Lepri B, et al: Coffee and cigarette use: association with suicidal acts in 352 Sardinian bipolar disorder patients. Bipolar Disord 11(5):494–503, 2009 19624388

Bair BD: Frequently missed diagnosis in geriatric psychiatry. Psychiatr Clin North Am 21(4):941–971, 1998 9890132

Baker PJ: Is it possible to make a correct diagnosis of Lyme disease on symptoms alone? Review of key issues and public health implications. Am J Med 132(10):1148–1152, 2019 31028718

Bassetti CL, Ferini-Strambi L, Brown S, et al: Neurology and psychiatry: waking up to opportunities of sleep: state of the art and clinical/research priorities for the next decade. Eur J Neurol 22(10):1337–1354, 2015 26255640

Beers DO, Karst KR: Generic and Innovator Drugs: A Guide to FDA Approval Requirements, 8th Edition. New York, Wolters Kluwer, 2020

Bentley TG, Catanzaro A, Ganiats TG: Implications of the impact of prevalence on test thresholds and outcomes: lessons from tuberculosis. BMC Res Notes 5:563, 2012 23050607

Benvenga S, Carlé A: Levothyroxine formulations: pharmacological and clinical implications of generic substitution. Adv Ther 36(Suppl 2):59–71, 2019 31485974

Bergin JE, Kendler KS: Common psychiatric disorders and caffeine use, tolerance, and withdrawal: an examination of shared genetic and environmental effects. Twin Res Hum Genet 15(4):473–482, 2012 22854069

Bhattacharyya R, Gozi A, Sen A: Management of psychiatric disorders in patients with respiratory diseases. Indian J Psychiatry 64(Suppl 2):S366–S378, 2022 35602365

Bhattarai HB, Kunwar GJ, Rijal A, et al: Acute psychosis unveiling diagnosis of hypothyroidism: a case report. Ann Med Surg (Lond) 82:104565, 2022 36268381

Bilezikian JP, Bandeira L, Khan A, et al: Hyperparathyroidism. Lancet 391(10116):168–178, 2018 28923463

Binder LM, Rohling ML, Larrabee GJ: A review of mild head trauma part I: meta-analytic review of neuropsychological studies. J Clin Exp Neuropsychol 19(3):421–431, 1997 9268816

Binnie CD: Cognitive impairment during epileptiform discharges: is it ever justifiable to treat the EEG? Lancet Neurol 2(12):725–730, 2003 14636777

Biondi B: The normal TSH reference range: what has changed in the last decade? J Clin Endocrinol Metab 98(9):3584–3587, 2013 24014812

Biondi B, Cappola AR: Subclinical hypothyroidism in older individuals. Lancet Diabetes Endocrinol 10(2):129–141, 2022 34953533

Bobe JR, Jutras BL, Horn EJ, et al: Recent progress in Lyme disease and remaining challenges. Front Med (Lausanne) 8:666554, 2021 34485323

Bobo WV, Stovall JA, Knostman M, et al: Converting from brand-name to generic clozapine: a review of effectiveness and tolerability data. Am J Health Syst Pharm 67(1):27–37, 2010 20044366

Boog GHP, Lopes JVZ, Mahler JV, et al: Diagnostic tools for neurosyphilis: a systematic review. BMC Infect Dis 21(1):568, 2021 34126948

Bostock E, Kirkby K, Garry M, et al: Mania associated with herbal medicines, other than cannabis: a systematic review and quality assessment of case reports. Front Psychiatry 6(9):280, 2018 30034348

Bourmistrova NW, Solomon T, Braude P, et al: Long-term effects of COVID-19 on mental health: a systematic review. J Affect Disord 299:118–125, 2022 34798148

Brandel JP, Knight R: Variant Creutzfeldt-Jakob disease. Handb Clin Neurol 153:191–205, 2018 29887136

Bratek A, Koźmin-Burzyńska A, Górniak E, et al: Psychiatric disorders associated with Cushing's syndrome. Psychiatr Danub 27(Suppl 1):S339–S343, 2015 26417792

Buitrago-Garcia D, Martí-Carvajal AJ, Jimenez A, et al: Antibiotic therapy for adults with neurosyphilis. Cochrane Database Syst Rev 5(5):CD011399, 2019 31132142

Bunc G, Ravnik J, Velnar T: May heading in soccer result in traumatic brain injury? A review of literature. Med Arh 71(5):356–359, 2017 29284906

Burghaus L, Eggers C, Timmermann L, et al: Hallucinations in neurodegenerative diseases. CNS Neurosci Ther 18(2):149–159, 2012 21592320

Büttiker P, Stefano GB, Weissenberger S, et al: HIV, HSV, SARS-CoV-2 and Ebola share long-term neuropsychiatric sequelae. Neuropsychiatr Dis Treat 18:2229–2237, 2022 36221293

Calissendorff J, Falhammar H: To treat or not to treat subclinical hypothyroidism, what is the evidence? Medicina (Kaunas) 56(1):40, 2020 31963883

Campos LN, Guimarães MD, Carmo RA, et al: HIV, syphilis, and hepatitis B and C prevalence among patients with mental illness: a review of the literature. Cad Saude Publica 24(Suppl 4):s607–s620, 2008 18797734

Caparros-Lefebvre D, Girard-Buttaz I, Reboul S, et al: Cognitive and psychiatric impairment in herpes simplex virus encephalitis suggest involvement of the amygdalo-frontal pathways. J Neurol 243(3):248–256, 1996 8936355

Cattie JE, Letendre SL, Woods SP, et al: Persistent neurocognitive decline in a clinic sample of hepatitis C virus-infected persons receiving interferon and ribavirin treatment. J Neurovirol 20(6):561–570, 2014 25326107

Centers for Disease Control and Prevention: Lyme Disease. Atlanta, GA, Centers for Disease Control and Prevention, 2022a. Available at: www.cdc.gov/lyme/index.html#:~:text=Lyme%20disease%20is%20diagnosed%20based,a%20few%20weeks%20of%20antibiotics. Accessed February 17, 2023.

Centers for Disease Control and Prevention: Lyme disease, in Tickborne Diseases of the United States. Atlanta, GA, Centers for Disease Control and Prevention, 2022b. Available at: www.cdc.gov/ticks/tickbornediseases/lyme.html#:~:text=Lyme%20disease%20is%20most%20frequently,spread%20by%20Ixodes%20pacificus%20ticks. Accessed February 21, 2023.

Centers for Disease Control and Prevention: Treatment for TB disease, in Tuberculosis (TB). Atlanta, GA, Centers for Disease Control and Prevention, March 7, 2022c. Available at: www.cdc.gov/tb/topic/treatment/tbdisease.htm. Accessed February 14, 2023.

Choi W, Yang YS, Chang DJ, et al: Association between the use of allopurinol and risk of increased thyroid-stimulating hormone level. Sci Rep 11(1):20305, 2021 34645831

Cipriani C, Pepe J, Colangelo L, et al: Vitamin D and secondary hyperparathyroid states. Front Horm Res 50:138–148, 2018 29597237

Ciurleo R, De Salvo S, Bonanno L, et al: Parosmia and neurological disorders: a neglected association. Front Neurol 11:543275, 2020 33240192

Conner SH, Solomon SS: Psychiatric manifestations of endocrine disorders. J Hum Endocrinol 1(007), 2017

Corrigan JD, Yang J, Singichetti B, et al: Lifetime prevalence of traumatic brain injury with loss of consciousness. Inj Prev 24(6):396–404, 2018 28848057

Costa e Silva JA: Sleep disorders in psychiatry. Metabolism 55(10)(Suppl 2):S40–S44, 2006 16979426

COVID-19 Mental Disorders Collaborators: Global prevalence and burden of depressive and anxiety disorders in 204 countries and territories in 2020 due to the COVID-19 pandemic. Lancet 398(10312):1700–1712, 2021 34634250

Crozatti LL, de Brito MH, Lopes BN, et al: Atypical behavioral and psychiatric symptoms: neurosyphilis should always be considered. Autops Case Rep 5(3):43–47, 2015 26558247

Cryan JF, O'Riordan KJ, Cowan CSM, et al: The microbiota-gut-brain axis. Physiol Rev 99(4):1877–2013, 2019 31460832

Cumbler E, Furfari K, Guerrasio J: Creutzfeldt-Jacob disease presenting as severe depression: a case report. Cases J 2(1):122, 2009 19193205

Dalton R: Mixed bipolar disorder precipitated by pseudoephedrine hydrochloride. South Med J 83(1):64–65, 1990 2300837

Dayan CM, Panicker V: Hypothyroidism and depression. Eur Thyroid J 2(3):168–179, 2013 24847450

De Carlo V, Calati R, Serretti A: Socio-demographic and clinical predictors of non-response/non-remission in treatment resistant depressed patients: a systematic review. Psychiatry Res 240:421–430, 2016 27155594

DeGruy FV III: A note on the partnership between psychiatry and primary care. Am J Psychiatry 163(9):1487–1489, 2006 16946169

DeGruy FV III: Psychiatry's fit in the world of modern primary care. Honorary Fellowship Lecture presented at the American College of Psychiatrists Annual Meeting, Tucson, AZ, February 25, 2023

DeKosky ST, Williamson JD, Fitzpatrick AL, et al; Ginkgo Evaluation of Memory (GEM) Study Investigators: Ginkgo biloba for prevention of dementia: a randomized controlled trial. JAMA 300(19):2253–2262, 2008 19017911

Devanand DP: Viral hypothesis and antiviral treatment in Alzheimer's disease. Curr Neurol Neurosci Rep 18(9):55, 2018 30008124

Devanand DP, Andrews H, Kreisl WC, et al: Antiviral therapy: Valacyclovir Treatment of Alzheimer's Disease (VALAD) Trial: protocol for a randomised, double-blind,placebo-controlled, treatment trial. BMJ Open 10(2):e032112, 2020 32034019

Dewan MC, Rattani A, Gupta S, et al: Estimating the global incidence of traumatic brain injury. J Neurosurg 130(4):1080–1097, 2018 29701556

Diagne BJ, Hakima A, El Harch I, et al: Depression and anxiety in patients with hepatitis B and C in a Moroccan region: a cross-sectional study. OAlib 9:1–12, 2022

Di Lorenzo C, Ceschi A, Kupferschmidt H, et al: Adverse effects of plant food supplements and botanical preparations: a systematic review with critical evaluation of causality. Br J Clin Pharmacol 79(4):578–592, 2015 25251944

Diskin J, Diskin CJ: Mental effects of excess parathyroid hormone in hemodialysis patients: a possible role for parathyroid 2 hormone receptor? Ther Apher Dial 24(3):285–289, 2020 31423747

Dixon M, Luthra V, Todd C: Use of cinacalcet in lithium-induced hyperparathyroidism. BMJ Case Rep 2018:bcr2018225154, 2018 30158262

Doherty AM, Kelly J, McDonald C, et al: A review of the interplay between tuberculosis and mental health. Gen Hosp Psychiatry 35(4):398–406, 2013 23660587

Doll JR, Thompson RL, Sawtell NM: Infectious herpes simplex virus in the brain stem is correlated with reactivation in the trigeminal ganglia. J Virol 93(8):e02209–e02218, 2019 30728262

Dong Y, Zhou G, Cao W, et al: Global seroprevalence and sociodemographic characteristics of Borrelia burgdorferi sensu lato in human populations: a systematic review and meta-analysis. BMJ Glob Health 7(6):e007744, 2022 35697507

Duarte DC, Duarte JC, Ocampo González ÁA, et al: Psychiatric disorders in post-traumatic brain injury patients: a scoping review. Heliyon 9(1):e12905, 2023 36704272

Dunkley BT, Da Costa L, Bethune A, et al: Low-frequency connectivity is associated with mild traumatic brain injury. Neuroimage Clin 7:611–621, 2015 25844315

Dunn D, Turner C: Hypothyroidism in women. Nurs Womens Health 20(1):93–98, 2016 26902444

Eban K: Can we trust the quality of generic drugs? J Manag Care Spec Pharm 26(5):589–591, 2020 32347179

Elmer S, Reddy DS: Therapeutic basis of generic substitution of antiseizure medications. J Pharmacol Exp Ther 381(2):188–196, 2022 35241634

Enyi CO, D'Souza B, Barloon L, et al: Relation of hyperparathyroidism and hypercalcemia to bipolar and psychotic disorders. Proc Bayl Univ Med Cent 35(4):540–542, 2022 35754598

Erdogan A, Hocaoglu C: Psychiatric aspect of infectious diseases and pandemic: a review. J Clin Psychiatry 23(Suppl 1):72–80, 2020

Esposito S, Prange AJ Jr, Golden RN: The thyroid axis and mood disorders: overview and future prospects. Psychopharmacol Bull 33(2):205–217, 1997 9230632

Fadgyas-Stanculete M, Buga AM, Popa-Wagner A, Dumitrascu DL: The relationship between irritable bowel syndrome and psychiatric disorders: from molecular changes to clinical manifestations. J Mol Psychiatry 2(1):4, 2014 25408914

Fallon BA, Nields JA: Lyme disease: a neuropsychiatric illness. Am J Psychiatry 151(11):1571–1583, 1994 7943444

Felker B, Yazel JJ, Short D: Mortality and medical comorbidity among psychiatric patients: a review. Psychiatr Serv 47(12):1356–1363, 1996 9117475

Fénelon G: Hallucinations associated with neurological disorders and sensory loss, in The Neuroscience of Hallucinations. Edited by Jardri R, Cachia A, Thomas P, et al. New York, Springer, 2013, pp 59–83

Fraser WD: Hyperparathyroidism. Lancet 374(9684):145–158, 2009 19595349

Frigerio S, Strawbridge R, Young AH: The impact of caffeine consumption on clinical symptoms in patients with bipolar disorder: a systematic review. Bipolar Disord 23(3):241–251, 2021 32949106

Fülöp T, Munawara U, Larbi A, et al: Targeting infectious agents as a therapeutic strategy in Alzheimer's disease. CNS Drugs 34(7):673–695, 2020 32458360

Furuie IN, Mauro MJJ, Petruzziello S, et al: Two threshold levels of vitamin D and the prevalence of comorbidities in outpatients of a tertiary hospital. Osteoporos Int 29(2):433–440, 2018 29143130

Gale SD, Berrett AN, Erickson LD, et al: Association between virus exposure and depression in US adults. Psychiatry Res 261:73–79, 2018 29287239

GBD 2016 Traumatic Brain Injury and Spinal Cord Injury Collaborators: Global, regional, and national burden of traumatic brain injury and spinal cord injury, 1990–2016: a systematic analysis for the Global Burden of Disease Study 2016. Lancet Neurol 18(1):56–87, 2019 30497965

Glassman AH: Cigarette smoking: implications for psychiatric illness. Am J Psychiatry 150(4):546–553, 1993 8465868

Gonzalez H, Koralnik IJ, Marra CM: Neurosyphilis. Semin Neurol 39(4):448–455, 2019 31533185

Gotlieb-Stematsky T, Zonis J, Arlazoroff A, et al: Antibodies to Epstein-Barr virus, herpes simplex type 1, cytomegalovirus and measles virus in psychiatric patients. Arch Virol 67(4):333–339, 1981 6263228

Govaerts J, Boeyckens J, Lammens A, et al: Defining polypharmacy: in search of a more comprehensive determination method applied in a tertiary psychiatric hospital. Ther Adv Psychopharmacol 11:20451253211000610, 2021 33796267

Gracie DJ, Guthrie EA, Hamlin PJ, Ford AC: Bi-directionality of brain-gut interactions in patients with inflammatory bowel disease. Gastroenterology 154(6):1635–1646, 2018 29366841

Gracie DJ, Hamlin PJ, Ford AC: The influence of the brain-gut axis in inflammatory bowel disease and possible implications for treatment. Lancet Gastroenterol Hepatol 4(8):632–642, 2019 31122802

Gragnani L, Lorini S, Martini L, et al: Rapid improvement of psychiatric stigmata after IFN-free treatment in HCV patients with and without cryoglobulinemic vasculitis. Clin Rheumatol 41(1):147–157, 2022 34409558

Grzegorzewska AM, Wiglusz MS, Landowski J, et al: Multiple comorbidity profile of psychiatric disorders in epilepsy. J Clin Med 10(18):410, 2021 34575214

Gulseren S, Gulseren L, Hekimsoy Z, et al: Depression, anxiety, health-related quality of life, and disability in patients with overt and subclinical thyroid dysfunction. Arch Med Res 37(1):133–139, 2006 16314199

Guttmannova K, Kosterman R, White HR, et al: The association between regular marijuana use and adult mental health outcomes. Drug Alcohol Depend 179:109–116, 2017 28763778

Hájek T, Pasková B, Janovská D, et al: Higher prevalence of antibodies to Borrelia burgdorferi in psychiatric patients than in healthy subjects. Am J Psychiatry 159(2):297–301, 2002 11823274

Hall W, Degenhardt L: The adverse health effects of chronic cannabis use. Drug Test Anal 6(1–2):39–45, 2014 23836598

Hammond FM, Corrigan JD, Ketchum JM, et al: Prevalence of medical and psychiatric comorbidities following traumatic brain injury. J Head Trauma Rehabil 34(4):E1–E10, 2019 30608311

Harris L, Griem J, Gummery A, et al: Neuropsychological and psychiatric outcomes in encephalitis: a multi-centre case-control study. PLoS One 15(3):e0230436, 2020 32210460

Hatton RC, Leighton G, Englander L: Site-specific and country-of-origin labeling for pharmaceutical manufacturing. Ann Pharmacother 56(10):1184–1187, 2022 35023388

Haugen BR: Drugs that suppress TSH or cause central hypothyroidism. Best Pract Res Clin Endocrinol Metab 23(6):793–800, 2009 19942154

Hayward SE, Deal A, Rustage K, et al: The relationship between mental health and risk of active tuberculosis: a systematic review. BMJ Open 12(1):e048945, 2022 34992103

Hemmingsson ES, Hjelmare E, Weidung B, et al: Antiviral treatment associated with reduced risk of clinical Alzheimer's disease-A nested case-control study. Alzheimers Dement (NY) 7(1):e12187, 2021 34136638

Henry M, Thomas KGF, Ross IL: Sleep, cognition and cortisol in Addison's disease: a mechanistic relationship. Front Endocrinol (Lausanne) 12:694046, 2021 34512546

Holmes KK, Bertozzi S, Bloom BR, et al (eds): Major Infectious Diseases, 3rd Edition. Washington, DC, International Bank for Reconstruction and Development/The World Bank, 2017

Horst S, Chao A, Rosen M, et al: Treatment with immunosuppressive therapy may improve depressive symptoms in patients with inflammatory bowel disease. Dig Dis Sci 60(2):465–470, 2015 25274158

Huckans M, Fuller B, Wheaton V, et al: A longitudinal study evaluating the effects of interferon-alpha therapy on cognitive and psychiatric function in adults with chronic hepatitis C. J Psychosom Res 78(2):184–192, 2015 25219976

Hutto B: Syphilis in clinical psychiatry: a review. Psychosomatics 42(6):453–460, 2001 11815679

Hyland K, Shoffner J, Heales SJ: Cerebral folate deficiency. J Inherit Metab Dis 33(5):563–570, 2010 20668945

Idrose AM: Acute and emergency care for thyrotoxicosis and thyroid storm. Acute Med Surg 2(3):147–157, 2015 29123713

Imtiaz S, Shield KD, Roerecke M, et al: Alcohol consumption as a risk factor for tuberculosis: meta-analyses and burden of disease. Eur Respir J 50(1):1700216, 2017 28705945

Iqbal UH, Zeng E, Pasinetti GM: The use of antimicrobial and antiviral drugs in Alzheimer's disease. Int J Mol Sci 21(14):4920, 2020 32664669

Issa BA, Fadeyi A, Durotoye IA, et al: Sero-prevalence of syphilis among patients with mental illness: comparison with blood donors. West Afr J Med 32(3):210–215, 2013 24122688

James C, Harfouche M, Welton NJ, et al: Herpes simplex virus: global infection prevalence and incidence estimates, 2016. Bull World Health Organ 98(5):315–329, 2020 32514197

Jaracz J: Polypharmacy in bipolar disorder: present status and future perspectives. Ment Health Addict Res 3(4):1–3, 2018

Jašović-Gašić M: Is treatment-resistance in psychiatric disorders a trap for polypharmacy? Psychiatr Danub 27(3):308–313, 2015 26400143

Joersjö P, Block L: A challenging diagnosis that eventually results in a life-threatening condition: Addison's disease and adrenal crisis. BMJ Case Rep 12(12):e231858, 2019 31888894

Johnson RT, Gibbs CJ Jr: Creutzfeldt-Jakob disease and related transmissible spongiform encephalopathies. N Engl J Med 339(27):1994–2004, 1998 9869672

Jones DR, Macias C, Barreira PJ, et al: Prevalence, severity, and co-occurrence of chronic physical health problems of persons with serious mental illness. Psychiatr Serv 55(11):1250–1257, 2004 15534013

Jones-Bourne C, Arbuckle MR: Psychiatry residents' perspectives of primary care in the psychiatric setting. Acad Psychiatry 43(2):196–199, 2019 30560349

Joshi KG, Faubion MD: Mania and psychosis associated with St. John's wort and ginseng. Psychiatry (Edgmont) 2(9):56–61, 2005 21120109

Jyothi KS, George C, Shaji KS: A case of adrenoleukodystrophy presenting with manic symptoms in a patient on steroids for Addison's disease. Indian J Psychiatry 58(4):467–470, 2016 28197008

Kanner AM, Soto A, Gross-Kanner H: Prevalence and clinical characteristics of postictal psychiatric symptoms in partial epilepsy. Neurology 62(5):708–713, 2004 15007118

Karnik NS: The next phase of child and adolescent psychiatry assessments and treatments using digital mental health. Lecture presented at Department of Psychiatry and Behavioral Sciences Grand Rounds, Dell Medical School, University of Texas at Austin, Austin, November 29, 2022

Klein M, Angstwurm K, Esser S, et al: German guidelines on the diagnosis and treatment of neurosyphilis. Neurol Res Pract 2:33, 2020 33225223

Knights MJ, Chatziagorakis A, Kumar Buggineni S: HIV infection and its psychiatric manifestations: a clinical overview. BJPsych Adv 23(4):265–277, 2017

Koman A, Bränström R, Pernow Y, et al: Neuropsychiatric comorbidity in primary hyperparathyroidism before and after parathyroidectomy: a population study. World J Surg 46(6):1420–1430, 2022 35246714

Koponen S, Taiminen T, Portin R, et al: Axis I and II psychiatric disorders after traumatic brain injury: a 30-year follow-up study. Am J Psychiatry 159(8):1315–1321, 2002 12153823

Kostev K, Tanislav C: No association between antiviral treatment and risk of Alzheimer's disease in German outpatients. Alzheimers Dement (NY) 7(1):e12216, 2021 34869824

Kovacs Z, Vestergaard P, W Licht R, et al: Lithium induced hypercalcemia: an expert opinion and management algorithm. Int J Bipolar Disord 10(1):34, 2022 36547749

Kratzsch J, Fiedler GM, Leichtle A, et al: New reference intervals for thyrotropin and thyroid hormones based on National Academy of Clinical Biochemistry criteria and regular ultrasonography of the thyroid. Clin Chem 51(8):1480–1486, 2005 15961550

Krishnan K, Lin Y, Prewitt KM, Potter DA: Multidisciplinary approach to brain fog and related persisting symptoms post COVID-19. J Health Serv Psychol 48(1):31–38, 2022 35128461

Kundu S, Bryk J, Alam A: Resolution of suicidal ideation with corticosteroids in a patient with concurrent Addison's disease and depression. Prim Care Companion CNS Disord 16(6): 2014 25834753

Kutluturk F, Yildirim B, Ozturk B, et al: The reference intervals of thyroid stimulating hormone in healthy individuals with normal levels of serum free thyroxine and without sonographic pathologies. Endocr Res 39(2):56–60, 2014 24067097

Kwentus JA, Hart RP, Peck ET, et al: Psychiatric complications of closed head trauma. Psychosomatics 26(1):8–17, 1985 3969436

Lähteenvuo M, Tiihonen J: Antipsychotic polypharmacy for the management of schizophrenia: evidence and recommendations. Drugs 81(11):1273–1284, 2021 34196945

Lantos PM, Rumbaugh J, Bockenstedt LK, et al: Clinical practice guidelines by the Infectious Diseases Society of America, American Academy of Neurology, and American College of Rheumatology: 2020 guidelines for the prevention, diagnosis, and treatment of Lyme disease. Neurology 96(6):262–273, 2021 33257476

Lee SW, Yang JM, Moon SY, et al: Association between mental illness and COVID-19 susceptibility and clinical outcomes in South Korea: a nationwide cohort study. Lancet Psychiatry 7(12):1025–1031, 2020 32950066

Lee SY, Amatya B, Judson R, et al: Clinical practice guidelines for rehabilitation in traumatic brain injury: a critical appraisal. Brain Inj 33(10):1263–1271, 2019 31314607

Levin HS, Amparo E, Eisenberg HM, et al: Magnetic resonance imaging and computerized tomography in relation to the neurobehavioral sequelae of mild and moderate head injuries. J Neurosurg 66(5):706–713, 1987 3572497

Li Z, Liu S, Wang L, Smith L: Mind-body exercise for anxiety and depression in COPD patients: a systematic review and meta-analysis. Int J Environ Res Public Health 17(1):22, 2019 31861418

Lin SK: Antipsychotic polypharmacy: a dirty little secret or a fashion? Int J Neuropsychopharmacol 23(2):125–131, 2020 31867671

Lippi M, Fanelli G, Fabbri C, et al: The dilemma of polypharmacy in psychosis: is it worth combining partial and full dopamine modulation? Int Clin Psychopharmacol 37(6):263–275, 2022 35815937

Liu D, Ahmet A, Ward L, et al: A practical guide to the monitoring and management of the complications of systemic corticosteroid therapy. Allergy Asthma Clin Immunol 9(1):30, 2013 23947590

Liu JY, Peine BS, Mlaver E, et al: Neuropsychologic changes in primary hyperparathyroidism after parathyroidectomy from a dual-institution prospective study. Surgery 169(1):114–119, 2021 32718801

Liu YF, Pan L, Feng M: Structural and functional brain alterations in Cushing's disease: a narrative review. Front Neuroendocrinol 67:101033, 2022 36126747

Lönnroth K, Williams BG, Stadlin S, et al: Alcohol use as a risk factor for tuberculosis—a systematic review. BMC Public Health 8:289, 2008 18702821

Lopatko Lindman K, Hemmingsson ES, Weidung B, et al: Herpesvirus infections, antiviral treatment, and the risk of dementia—a registry-based cohort study in Sweden. Alzheimers Dement (NY) 7(1):e12119, 2021 33614892

Lotrich FE: Psychiatric clearance for patients started on interferon-alpha-based therapies. Am J Psychiatry 170(6):592–597, 2013 23732965

Lydiard RB: Irritable bowel syndrome, anxiety, and depression: what are the links? J Clin Psychiatry 62(Suppl 8):38–47, 2001 12108820

Mak IW, Chu CM, Pan PC, et al: Long-term psychiatric morbidities among SARS survivors. Gen Hosp Psychiatry 31(4):318–326, 2009 19555791

Marques AR, Strle F, Wormser GP: Comparison of Lyme disease in the United States and Europe. Emerg Infect Dis 27(8):2017–2024, 2021 34286689

Marx GE, Chan ED: Tuberculous meningitis: diagnosis and treatment overview. Tuberc Res Treat 2011:798764, 2011 22567269

Mason GA, Bondy SC, Nemeroff CB, et al: The effects of thyroid state on beta-adrenergic and serotonergic receptors in rat brain. Psychoneuroendocrinology 12(4):261–270, 1987 2821568

Mathur A, Ahn JB, Sutton W, et al: Secondary hyperparathyroidism (CKD-MBD) treatment and the risk of dementia. Nephrol Dial Transplant 37(11):2111–2118, 2022 35512551. (Correction Nephrol Dial Transplant 38(9):2096–2097, 2023)

Mayer AR, Kaushal M, Dodd AB, et al: Advanced biomarkers of pediatric mild traumatic brain injury: progress and perils. Neurosci Biobehav Rev 94:149–165, 2018 30098989

Mazza MG, Zanardi R, Palladini M, et al: Rapid response to selective serotonin reuptake inhibitors in post-COVID depression. Eur Neuropsychopharmacol 54:1–6, 2022 34634679

Mead P, Petersen J, Hinckley A: Updated CDC recommendation for serologic diagnosis of Lyme disease. MMWR Morb Mortal Wkly Rep 68(32):703, 2019 31415492

Mead S, Khalili-Shirazi A, Potter C, et al: Prion protein monoclonal antibody (PRN100) therapy for Creutzfeldt-Jakob disease: evaluation of a first-in-human treatment programme. Lancet Neurol 21(4):342–354, 2022 35305340

Mehkri Y, Hanna C, Sriram S, et al: Overview of neurotrauma and sensory loss. J Neurol Res Rev Rep 4(3), 2022 35692955

Mergenhagen KA, Wattengel BA, Skelly MK, et al: Fact versus fiction: a review of the evidence behind alcohol and antibiotic interactions. Antimicrob Agents Chemother 64(3):e02167–19, 2020 31871085

Messa P, Alfieri CM: Secondary and tertiary hyperparathyroidism. Front Horm Res 51:91–108, 2019 30641516

Meza NW, Rossi NE, Galeazzi TN, et al: Cysticercosis in chronic psychiatric inpatients from a Venezuelan community. Am J Trop Med Hyg 73(3):504–509, 2005 16172472

Miranda LHL, Oliveira AFPH, Carvalho DM, et al: Revisão sistemática do manejo farmacológico na doença de Creutzfeldt-Jakob: ainda sem opções? Arq Neuropsiquiatr 80(8):837–844, 2022 36252593

Mishra KK, Sawant N, Garg S: Management of psychiatric disorders in patients with endocrine disorders. Indian J Psychiatry 64(Suppl 2):S402–S413, 2022 35602375

Mizuki Y, Sakamoto S, Okahisa Y, et al: Mechanisms underlying the comorbidity of schizophrenia and type 2 diabetes mellitus. Int J Neuropsychopharmacol 24(5):367–382, 2021 33315097

Momayez Sanat Z, Mohajeri-Tehrani MR: Psychotic disorder as the first manifestation of Addison disease: a case report. Int J Endocrinol Metab 20(1):e121011, 2022 35432552

Mooney J, Self M, ReFaey K, et al: Concussion in soccer: a comprehensive review of the literature. Concussion 5(3):CNC76, 2020 33005435

Morse AM, Garner DR: Traumatic brain injury, sleep disorders, and psychiatric disorders: an underrecognized relationship. Med Sci (Basel) 6(1):15, 2018 29462866

Mula M, Jauch R, Cavanna A, et al: Interictal dysphoric disorder and periictal dysphoric symptoms in patients with epilepsy. Epilepsia 51(7):1139–1145, 2010 20059526

Munjal S, Ferrando SJ, Freyberg Z: Neuropsychiatric aspects of infectious diseases: an update. Crit Care Clin 33(3):681–712, 2017 28601141

Nagalakshmi B, Sagarkar S, Sakharkar AJ: Epigenetic mechanisms of traumatic brain injuries. Prog Mol Biol Transl Sci 157:263–298, 2018 29933953

Naqvi HA, Wang D, Glozier N, et al: Sleep-disordered breathing and psychiatric disorders. Curr Psychiatry Rep 16(12):519, 2014 25308389

Nath P, Kabir MA, Doust SK, et al: Diagnosis of herpes simplex virus: laboratory and point-of-care techniques. Infect Dis Rep 13(2):518–539, 2021 34199547

Nedelcovych MT, Manning AA, Semenova S, et al: The psychiatric impact of HIV. ACS Chem Neurosci 8(7):1432–1434, 2017 28537385

Nishimi K, Neylan TC, Bertenthal D, et al: Association of psychiatric disorders with incidence of SARS-CoV-2 breakthrough infection among vaccinated adults. JAMA Netw Open 5(4):e227287, 2022 35420660

Noda M: Possible role of glial cells in the relationship between thyroid dysfunction and mental disorders. Front Cell Neurosci 9:194, 2015 26089777

Nyhlin H, Ford MJ, Eastwood J, et al: Non-alimentary aspects of the irritable bowel syndrome. J Psychosom Res 37(2):155–162, 1993 8385215

O'Brien J, Taylor JP, Ballard C, et al: Visual hallucinations in neurological and ophthalmological disease: pathophysiology and management. J Neurol Neurosurg Psychiatry 91(5):512–519, 2020 32213570

O'Brien KK, Tynan AM, Nixon SA, et al: Effectiveness of aerobic exercise for adults living with HIV: systematic review and meta-analysis using the Cochrane Collaboration protocol. BMC Infect Dis 16:182, 2016 27112335

Østergaard AA, Sydenham TV, Nybo M, et al: Cerebrospinal fluid pleocytosis level as a diagnostic predictor? A cross-sectional study. BMC Clin Pathol 17:15, 2017 28855847

Ouellette DR, Lavoie KL: Recognition, diagnosis, and treatment of cognitive and psychiatric disorders in patients with COPD. Int J Chron Obstruct Pulmon Dis 12:639–650, 2017 28243081

Pan LA, Martin P, Zimmer T, et al: Neurometabolic disorders: potentially treatable abnormalities in patients with treatment-refractory depression and suicidal behavior. Am J Psychiatry 174(1):42–50, 2017 27523499

Park M, Reynolds CF III: Depression among older adults with diabetes mellitus. Clin Geriatr Med 31(1):117–137, 2015 25453305

Patterson WJ, Painter MJ: Bovine spongiform encephalopathy and new variant Creutzfeldt-Jakob disease: an overview. Commun Dis Public Health 2(1):5–13, 1999 10462888

Păunescu RL, Miclu Ia IV, Verişezan OR, et al: Acute and longterm psychiatric symptoms associated with COVID19 (Review). Biomed Rep 18(1):4, 2022 36544852

Peeters W, van den Brande R, Polinder S, et al: Epidemiology of traumatic brain injury in Europe. Acta Neurochir (Wien) 157(10):1683–1696, 2015 26269030

Peitz GW, Wilde EA, Grandhi R: Magnetoencephalography in the detection and characterization of brain abnormalities associated with traumatic brain injury: a comprehensive review. Med Sci (Basel) 9(1):7, 2021 33557219

Pharmacy Times: Debunking a common pharmacy myth: the 80–125% bioequivalence rule. Pharmacy Times, June 8, 2016. Available at:

www.pharmacytimes.com/view/debunking-a-common-pharmacy-myth-the-80-125-bioequivalence-rule. Accessed March 10, 2023.

Pirl WF, Greer JA, Weissgarber C, et al: Screening for infectious diseases among patients in a state psychiatric hospital. Psychiatr Serv 56(12):1614–1616, 2005 16339630

Pollak TA, Rogers JP, Nagele RG, et al: Antibodies in the diagnosis, prognosis, and prediction of psychotic disorders. Schizophr Bull 45(1):233–246, 2019 29474698

Prasad KM, Eack SM, Keshavan MS, et al: Antiherpes virus-specific treatment and cognition in schizophrenia: a test-of-concept randomized double-blind placebo-controlled trial. Schizophr Bull 39(4):857–866, 2013 22446565

Putman HP: Rational Psychopharmacology: A Book of Clinical Skills. Washington, DC, American Psychiatric Association Publishing, 2020

Puzanov M, Davis H, Holmes EG: A rare presentation of catatonia due to primary adrenal insufficiency. Psychosomatics 60(6):630–633, 2019 31000141

Rahim MJ, Ghazali WS: Psychosis secondary to tuberculosis meningitis. BMJ Case Rep 2016:bcr2015213171, 2016 26969352

Rifai MA, Gleason OC, Sabouni D: Psychiatric care of the patient with hepatitis C: a review of the literature. Prim Care Companion J Clin Psychiatry 12(6):PCC.09r00877, 2010

Riggin L: Association between gestational diabetes and mental illness. Can J Diabetes 44(6):566–571, 2020 32792108

Ritter AC, Wagner AK, Fabio A, et al: Incidence and risk factors of posttraumatic seizures following traumatic brain injury: a Traumatic Brain Injury Model Systems Study. Epilepsia 57(12):1968–1977, 2016 27739577

Rizkallah E, Bélanger M, Stavro K, et al: Could the use of energy drinks induce manic or depressive relapse among abstinent substance use disorder patients with comorbid bipolar spectrum disorder? Bipolar Disord 13(5–6):578–580, 2011 22017226

Roberson SW, Patel MB, Dabrowski W, et al: Challenges of delirium management in patients with traumatic brain injury: from pathophysiology to clinical practice. Curr Neuropharmacol 19(9):1519–1544, 2021 33463474

Roberts DL, Rossman JS, Jarić I: Dating first cases of COVID-19. PLoS Pathog 17(6):e1009620, 2021 34166465

Rogers JP, Chesney E, Oliver D, et al: Psychiatric and neuropsychiatric presentations associated with severe coronavirus infections: a systematic review and meta-analysis with comparison to the COVID-19 pandemic. Lancet Psychiatry 7(7):611–627, 2020 32437679

Rolin S, Chakales A, Verduzco-Gutierrez M: Rehabilitation strategies for cognitive and neuropsychiatric manifestations of COVID-19. Curr Phys Med Rehabil Rep 10(3):182–187, 2022 35602927

Roozenbeek B, Maas AI, Menon DK: Changing patterns in the epidemiology of traumatic brain injury. Nat Rev Neurol 9(4):231–236, 2013 23443846

Rothbard AB, Blank MB, Staab JP, et al: Previously undetected metabolic syndromes and infectious diseases among psychiatric inpatients. Psychiatr Serv 60(4):534–537, 2009 19339330

Rowley J, Hoorn SV, Korenromp E, et al: Chlamydia, gonorrhea, trichomoniasis and syphilis: global prevalence and incidence estimates, Bull World Health Organ 97(8):548–562, 2016 31384073

Russo M, Calisi D, De Rosa MA, et al: COVID-19 and first manic episodes: a systematic review. Psychiatry Res 314:114677, 2022 35716481

Ryan LM, Warden DL: Post concussion syndrome. Int Rev Psychiatry 15(4):310–316, 2003 15276952

Sackey B, Shults JG, Moore TA, et al: Evaluating psychiatric outcomes associated with direct-acting antiviral treatment in veterans with hepatitis C infection. Ment Health Clin 8(3):116–121, 2018 29955556

Sait A, Angeli C, Doig AJ, Day PJR: Viral involvement in Alzheimer's disease. ACS Chem Neurosci 12(7):1049–1060, 2021 33687205

Salvador J, Gutierrez G, Llavero M, et al: Endocrine disorders and psychiatric manifestations, in Endocrinology and Systemic Diseases. Edited by Portincasa P, Frühbeck G, Nathoe HM. Cham, Switzerland, Springer, 2019, pp 1–35

Sanchez FM, Zisselman MH: Treatment of psychiatric symptoms associated with neurosyphilis. Psychosomatics 48(5):440–445, 2007 17878505

Santos A, Resmini E, Pascual JC, et al: Psychiatric symptoms in patients with Cushing's syndrome: prevalence, diagnosis and management. Drugs 77(8):829–842, 2017 28393326

Santos A, Webb SM, Resmini E: Psychological complications of Cushing's syndrome. Curr Opin Endocrinol Diabetes Obes 28(3):325–329, 2021 33764929

Saradhadevi S, Hemavathy V: Effectiveness of sleep hygiene to reduce insomnia among persons with suffering with obsessive compulsive disorder-pilot analysis. Cardiometry 22:462–466, 2022

Saribas AS, Ozdemir A, Lam C, et al: JC virus-induced progressive multifocal leukoencephalopathy. Future Virol 5(3):313–323, 2010 21731577

Sathya A, Radhika R, Mahadevan S, et al: Mania as a presentation of primary hypothyroidism. Singapore Med J 50(2):e65–e67, 2009 19296014

Schechter PJ, Henkin RI: Abnormalities of taste and smell after head trauma. J Neurol Neurosurg Psychiatry 37(7):802–810, 1974 4850368

Scheenen ME, de Koning ME, van der Horn HJ, et al: Acute alcohol intoxication in patients with mild traumatic brain injury: characteristics, recovery, and outcome. J Neurotrauma 33(4):339–345, 2016 26230219

Schmidt F, Janssen G, Martin G, et al: Factors influencing long-term changes in mental health after interferon-alpha treatment of chronic hepatitis C. Aliment Pharmacol Ther 30(10):1049–1059, 2009 19691667

Schoretsanitis G, de Leon J, Eap CB, et al: Clinically significant drug-drug interactions with agents for attention-deficit/hyperactivity disorder. CNS Drugs 33(12):1201–1222, 2019 31776871

Serdenes R, Lewis M, Chandrasekhara S: A clinical review of the psychiatric sequelae of primary hyperparathyroidism. Cureus 13(10):e19078, 2021 34722014

Shacham E, Morgan JC, Önen NF, et al: Screening anxiety in the HIV clinic. AIDS Behav 16(8):2407–2413, 2012 22718040

Sharma A, Gerbarg P, Bottiglieri T, et al: S-adenosylmethionine (SAMe) for neuropsychiatric disorders: a clinician-oriented review of research. J Clin Psychiatry 78(6):e656–e667, 2017 28682528

Sherr L, Clucas C, Harding R, et al: HIV and depression—a systematic review of interventions. Psychol Health Med 16(5):493–527, 2011 21809936

Shewmon DA, Erwin RJ: Transient impairment of visual perception induced by single interictal occipital spikes. J Clin Exp Neuropsychol 11(5):675–691, 1989 2808657

Shin SS, Dixon CE: Alterations in cholinergic pathways and therapeutic strategies targeting cholinergic system after traumatic brain injury. J Neurotrauma 32(19):1429–1440, 2015 25646580

Sigurdson CJ, Bartz JC, Glatzel M: Cellular and molecular mechanisms of prion disease. Annu Rev Pathol 14:497–516, 2019 30355150

Silver JM, Kramer R, Greenwald S, Weissman M: The association between head injuries and psychiatric disorders: findings from the New Haven NIMH Epidemiologic Catchment Area Study. Brain Inj 15(11):935–945, 2001 11689092

Silver JM, McAllister TW, Arciniegas DB: Depression and cognitive complaints following mild traumatic brain injury. Am J Psychiatry 166(6):653–661, 2009 19487401

Singh G, Mehta S, Kumar M, Salhotra A: Creutzfeldt-Jacob disease with psychiatric presentation: Hen's Teeth in Indian subcontinent: a case report. Indian J Psychol Med 41(2):184–186, 2019 30983670

Skolnik AA, Noska A, Yakovchenko V, et al: Experiences with interferon-free hepatitis C therapies: addressing barriers to adherence and optimizing treatment outcomes. BMC Health Serv Res 19(1):91, 2019 30709352

Sno HN: Signs and significance of a tick-bite: psychiatric disorders associated with Lyme disease. Tijdschr Psychiatr 54(3):235–243, 2012 22422416

Socała K, Doboszewska U, Szopa A, et al: The role of microbiota-gut-brain axis in neuropsychiatric and neurological disorders. Pharmacol Res 172:105840, 2021 34450312

Sommer IE, Bakker PR: What can psychiatrists learn from SARS and MERS outbreaks? Lancet Psychiatry 7(7):565–566, 2020 32437680

Song WM, Li SJ, Liu JY, et al: Impact of alcohol drinking and tobacco smoking on the drug-resistance of newly diagnosed tuberculosis: a retrospective cohort study in Shandong, China, during 2004–2020. BMJ Open 12(7):e059149, 2022 35902191

Srisurapanont K, Samakarn Y, Kamklong B, et al: Efficacy and acceptability of blue-wavelength light therapy for post-TBI behavioral symptoms: A systematic review and meta-analysis of randomized controlled trials. PLoS One 17(10):e0274025, 2022 36201498

Stassen HH, Bachmann S, Bridler R, et al: Detailing the effects of polypharmacy in psychiatry: longitudinal study of 320 patients hospitalized for depression or schizophrenia. Eur Arch Psychiatry Clin Neurosci 272(4):603–619, 2022 34822007

Stone BL, Tourand Y, Brissette CA: Brave new worlds: the expanding universe of Lyme disease. Vector Borne Zoonotic Dis 17(9):619–629, 2017 28727515

Stubbs MA, Clark VL, Gibson PG, et al: Associations of symptoms of anxiety and depression with health-status, asthma control, dyspnoea, dysfunction breathing and obesity in people with severe asthma. Respir Res 23(1):341, 2022 36510255

Stuer K, Claes S: Mania following the use of a decongestant. Tijdschr Psychiatr 49(2):125–129, 2007 17290343

Sutter R, Rüegg S, Tschudin-Sutter S: Seizures as adverse events of antibiotic drugs: a systematic review. Neurology 85(15):1332–1341, 2015 26400582

Takayanagui OM, Haes TM: Update on the diagnosis and management of neurocysticercosis. Arq Neuropsiquiatr 80(5)(Suppl 1):296–306, 2022 35976305

Tan CH, Chang MC, Tsai WF, et al: Different profiles of neurocognitive impairment in patients with hepatitis B and C virus infections. Sci Rep 12(1):10625, 2022 35739162

Tao H, Fan S, Zhu T, et al: Psychiatric disorders and Type 2 diabetes mellitus: a bidirectional Mendelian randomization. Eur J Clin Invest 53(3):e13893, 2023 36259254

Taquet M, Luciano S, Geddes JR, Harrison PJ: Bidirectional associations between COVID-19 and psychiatric disorder: retrospective cohort studies of 62 354 COVID-19 cases in the USA. Lancet Psychiatry 8(2):130–140, 2021 33181098

Taşkapilioğlu Ö, Seferoğlu M, Yurtoğullari Ş, et al: Sporadic Creutzfeldt-Jacob disease: an 8-year experience from a single center in Turkey. Noro Psikiyatri Arsivi 50(4):306–311, 2013 28360562

Thomson D, Berk M, Dodd S, et al: Tobacco use in bipolar disorder. Clin Psychopharmacol Neurosci 13(1):1–11, 2015 25912533

Thwaites G, Fisher M, Hemingway C, et al: British Infection Society guidelines for the diagnosis and treatment of tuberculosis of the central nervous system in adults and children. J Infect 59(3):167–187, 2009 19643501

Trenton AJ, Currier GW: Treatment of comorbid tuberculosis and depression. Prim Care Companion J Clin Psychiatry 3(6):236–243, 2001 15014591

Tuddenham S, Ghanem KG: Neurosyphilis: knowledge gaps and controversies. Sex Transm Dis 45(3):147–151, 2018 29420441

Tufik S, Andersen ML, Bittencourt LR, Mello MT: Paradoxical sleep deprivation: neurochemical, hormonal and behavioral alterations: evidence from 30 years of research. An Acad Bras Cienc 81(3):521–538, 2009 19722021

Tzeng NS, Chung CH, Lin FH, et al: Anti-herpetic medications and reduced risk of dementia in patients with herpes simplex virus infections—a nationwide, population-based cohort study in Taiwan. Neurotherapeutics 15(2):417–429, 2018 29488144

U.S. Food and Drug Administration: Bioavailability studies submitted in NDAs or INDs—general considerations: guidance for industry. Washington, DC, U.S. Department of Health and Human Services, 2022. Available at: www.fda.gov/media/121311/download. Accessed March 10, 2023.

Valente AP, Pinho PDC, Lucato LT: Magnetic resonance imaging in the diagnosis of Creutzfeldt-Jakob disease: report of two cases. Dement Neuropsychol 9(4):424–427, 2015 29213993

Van Hout MC: The controversies, challenges and complexities of Lyme disease: a narrative review. J Pharm Pharm Sci 21(1):429–436, 2018 30458921

Van Oudenhove L, Demyttenaere K, Tack J, Aziz Q: Central nervous system involvement in functional gastrointestinal disorders. Best Pract Res Clin Gastroenterol 18(4):663–680, 2004 15324706

Vastag Z, Fira-Mladinescu O, Rosca EC: HIV-associated neurocognitive disorder (HAND): obstacles to early neuropsychological diagnosis. Int J Gen Med 15:4079–4090, 2022 35450033

Vega P, Sweetland A, Acha J, et al: Psychiatric issues in the management of patients with multidrug-resistant tuberculosis. Int J Tuberc Lung Dis 8(6):749–759, 2004 15182146

Vellas B, Coley N, Ousset PJ, et al: Long-term use of standardised ginkgo biloba extract for the prevention of Alzheimer's disease (GuidAge): a randomised placebo-controlled trial. Lancet Neurol 11(10):851–859, 2012 22959217

Verma R, Sachdeva A, Singh Y, Balhara YP: Acute mania after thyroxin supplementation in hypothyroid state. Indian J Endocrinol Metab 17(5):922–923, 2013 24083180

Vespa PM, Nuwer MR, Nenov V, et al: Increased incidence and impact of nonconvulsive and convulsive seizures after traumatic brain injury as detected by continuous electroencephalographic monitoring. J Neurosurg 91(5):750–760, 1999 10541231

Volkow ND, Swanson JM, Evins AE, et al: Effects of cannabis use on human behavior, including cognition, motivation, and psychosis: a review. JAMA Psychiatry 73(3):292–297, 2016 26842658

Wade SL, Kurowski BG, Kirkwood MW, et al: Online problem-solving therapy after traumatic brain injury: a randomized controlled trial. Pediatrics 135(2):e487–e495, 2015 25583911

Wang Q, Xu R, Volkow ND: Increased risk of COVID-19 infection and mortality in people with mental disorders: analysis from electronic health records in the United States. World Psychiatry 20(1):124–130, 2021 33026219

Wartofsky L, Dickey RA: The evidence for a narrower thyrotropin reference range is compelling. J Clin Endocrinol Metab 90(9):5483–5488, 2005 16148345

Watson N, Brandel JP, Green A, et al: The importance of ongoing international surveillance for Creutzfeldt-Jakob disease. Nat Rev Neurol 17(6):362–379, 2021 33972773

Weinstein A, Livny A, Weizman A: Brain imaging studies on the cognitive, pharmacological and neurobiological effects of cannabis in humans: evidence from studies of adult users. Curr Pharm Des 22(42):6366–6379, 2016 27549374

Whelan-Goodinson R, Ponsford J, Johnston L, Grant F: Psychiatric disorders following traumatic brain injury: their nature and frequency. J Head Trauma Rehabil 24(5):324–332, 2009 19858966

Whybrow PC, Prange AJ Jr: A hypothesis of thyroid-catecholamine-receptor interaction: its relevance to affective illness. Arch Gen Psychiatry 38(1):106–113, 1981 6257196

Więdłocha M, Marcinowicz P, Stańczykiewicz B: Psychiatric aspects of herpes simplex encephalitis, tick-borne encephalitis and herpes zoster encephalitis among immunocompetent patients. Adv Clin Exp Med 24(2):361–371, 2015 25931371

Wigger GW, Bouton TC, Jacobson KR, et al: The impact of alcohol use disorder on tuberculosis: a review of the epidemiology and potential immunologic mechanisms. Front Immunol 13:864817, 2022 35432348

Wilcke JT, Døssing M, Angelo HR, et al: Unchanged acetylation of isoniazid by alcohol intake. Int J Tuberc Lung Dis 8(11):1373–1376, 2004 15581208

Wilesmith JW, Wells GA, Cranwell MP, et al: Bovine spongiform encephalopathy: epidemiological studies. Vet Rec 123(25):638–644, 1988 3218047

Wolfersdorf M, König F: Serum folic acid and vitamin B12 in depressed inpatients: a study of serum folic acid with radioimmunoassay in 121 depressed inpatients. Psychiatr Prax 22(4):162–164, 1995 7675908

World Health Organization: Summary of probable SARS cases with onset of illness from 1 November 2002 to 31 July 2003. Geneva, Switzerland, World Health Organization, July 24, 2015. Available at: https://www.who.int/publications/m/item/summary-of-probable-sars-cases-with-onset-of-illness-from-1-november-2002-to-31-july-2003. Accessed February 16, 2023.

World Health Organization: Middle East respiratory syndrome coronavirus (MERS-CoV). Geneva, Switzerland, World Health Organization, 2023. Available at: www.who.int/health-topics/middle-east-respiratory-syndrome-coronavirus-mers#tab=tab_1. Accessed February 16, 2023.

Wozniak MA, Frost AL, Preston CM, et al: Antivirals reduce the formation of key Alzheimer's disease molecules in cell cultures acutely infected with herpes simplex virus type 1. PLoS One 6(10):e25152, 2011 22003387

Wu S, Zhang Y, Sun F, et al: Adverse events associated with the treatment of multidrug-resistant tuberculosis: a systematic review and meta-analysis. Am J Ther 23(2):e521–e530, 2016 24284652

Yamamoto JM, Metcalfe A, Nerenberg KA, et al: Thyroid function testing and management during and after pregnancy among women without thyroid disease before pregnancy. CMAJ 192(22):E596–E602, 2020 32575048

Yang YT, Nagai S, Chen BK, et al: Generic oncology drugs: are they all safe? Lancet Oncol 17(11):e493–e501, 2016 27819247

Ye J, Wen Y, Chu X, et al: Association between herpes simplex virus 1 exposure and the risk of depression in UK Biobank. Clin Transl Med 10(2):e108, 2020 32564518

Yin OQ, Tomlinson B, Waye MM, et al: Pharmacogenetics and herb-drug interactions: experience with ginkgo biloba and omeprazole. Pharmacogenetics 14(12):841–850, 2004 15608563

Yolken RH, Torrey EF, Lieberman JA, et al: Serological evidence of exposure to herpes simplex virus type 1 is associated with cognitive deficits in the CATIE schizophrenia sample. Schizophr Res 128(1–3):61–65, 2011 21353483

Yong SJ: Long COVID or post-COVID-19 syndrome: putative pathophysiology, risk factors, and treatments. Infect Dis (Lond) 53(10):737–754, 2021 34024217

Yoshino H, Aoki C, Kitamura S, et al: A case report of mania with abnormal cerebral blood flow and cognitive impairment 24 years after head trauma. Ann Gen Psychiatry 19:32, 2020 32426021

Zagórska A, Marcinkowska M, Jamrozik M, et al: From probiotics to psychobiotics—the gut-brain axis in psychiatric disorders. Benef Microbes 11(8):717–732, 2020 33191776

Zangaladze A, Nei M, Liporace JD, et al: Characteristics and clinical significance of subclinical seizures. Epilepsia 49(12):2016–2021, 2008 18503561

Zeng N, Zhao YM, Yan W, et al: A systematic review and meta-analysis of long term physical and mental sequelae of COVID-19 pandemic: call for research priority and action. Mol Psychiatry 28(1):423–433, 2023 35668159

Zhang J, Emami Z, Safar K, et al: Teasing apart trauma: neural oscillations differentiate individual cases of mild traumatic brain injury from post-traumatic stress disorder even when symptoms overlap. Transl Psychiatry 11(1):345, 2021 34088901

Zhao T, Chen BM, Zhao XM, et al: Subclinical hypothyroidism and depression: a meta-analysis. Transl Psychiatry 8(1):239, 2018 30375372

Ziedonis DM, George TP: Schizophrenia and nicotine use: report of a pilot smoking cessation program and review of neurobiological and clinical issues. Schizophr Bull 23(2):247–254, 1997 9165635

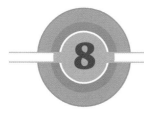

Reducing Treatment Failure

Steps to Follow

Practicing psychiatry is hard work. Much data, some difficult to obtain, must be elicited, compiled, and sorted. Patients' problems are often moving targets and must be constantly reassessed. If the assessment and treatment process ever becomes routine or automatic or contains shortcuts, the clinician will likely develop additional biases. Having one or more of such biases can lead to an unrealistic assessment of the lack of complexity in the problem, and only luck will prevent treatment failure, which many clinicians may conclude is treatment resistance. We can never allow ourselves to remain on autopilot. We must always remind ourselves to embrace the complexity of our work to provide the most value for our patients.

The previous chapters in this book focus in detail on challenging our conceptions of treatment failure and treatment resistance and finding treatment success. In this chapter, I condense these principles into broader concepts to guide our practice.

Focus on the Long Term

As reviewed in the preceding chapters, providers can address treatment failure by confirming diagnostic validity and accuracy through thorough and ongoing evaluations and monitoring, while enhancing a dynamic and flexible therapeutic alliance. Collaboration on decisions about treatment steps may not follow the exact path a provider might advise, but because acceptance and compliance on the part of the patient are essential to any successful recovery, the patient's choices must determine selection. It is of little value to identify a successful treatment that the patient will not continue. The clinician must object only when the choice is clearly inappropriate, unrealistic, or dangerous, and the practitioner should always place the patient's selection in context with other options.

Many providers, patients, families, employers, and third-party payers are highly focused on how rapidly a patient improves. Although this is indeed important, it is even more important that any improvement be as complete as possible and sustainable. This requires not only choosing the most effective treatments but also choosing interventions that fit into the patient's illness narrative and that they can accept long term, if necessary. If remission requires behavioral change in the patient, even indefinite lifestyle changes, they must be able to understand how this requirement fits with the story of them getting better before they can commit to what is sometimes a very long-term adjustment.

For this reason, it is often best, after reviewing all reasonable treatment options, putting them into perspective, and ranking them in order of expected efficacy, to openly suggest that the patient choose treatments they will be willing to endure long term. If these treatments are effective, the chances for sustained improvement are highest. Few patients continue a treatment that they find objectionable, that is poorly tolerated, or even that is expensive, particularly when they may experience periodic improvement that helps them believe continuation is not necessary.

Avoid Circular Logic

The question "What do you use to treat treatment-resistant [psychiatric disorder]?" is an oxymoron: if there is an effective treatment, the disorder is not resistant (see section "Insufficient Evidence" in Chapter 4, "The Myth of Treatment Resistance?"). If we are using the term treatment resistance to ask what the next treatment should be after one or more failed attempts, we are asking not about treatment failure but about a second or third treatment option. This is, again, an unhelpful question because there is no standard order of treatments, and the correct answer always depends on the individual case. Although treatment algorithms provide basic guidance, they cannot possibly encompass enough of the complexity in our clinical situations to provide solutions more accurate than those determined through individual assessment (Adli et al. 2006; Jašović-Gašić et al. 2013; Rutledge et al. 2019).

There is no utility in defining one treatment attempt as targeting treatment resistance and another as targeting non–treatment resistance. This is the circular logic of the failed treatment resistance concept—projecting treatment failure into a diagnosis rather than focusing on the practitioner's control over finding solutions; see sections "Implications for Clinical Practice" in Chapter 1, "Conceptualization (and Failed Concepts)," and "Insufficient Evidence" in Chapter 4. Passively accepting the concept and term *treatment resistance* abrogates our responsibility as clinicians to work tirelessly to find the right answers with our patients and so often prevents us from finding effective solutions. Manufacturers who seek an indication from the FDA to market treatments for treatment-resistant cases are using the term treatment resistance as a marketing tool rather than a rigorously defined distinction (Beers and Karst 2020; George and Post 2011; Largent et al. 2021; Ross 2007; Turner 2019); see section "Insufficient Evidence" in Chapter 4.

Record and Review

Electronic medical records (EMRs) allow practitioners to easily add or carry forward routine information and standard templates, but sometimes this threatens to obscure new details at each visit (Chivilgina et al. 2022; Dey et al. 2019; Kariotis et al. 2022). We must be careful at each patient contact to record in minute detail the symptoms, functionalities, and reactions to our treatments, along with fully explained rationales, in order to access treatment history, track progress, and help identify errors and shortcomings that may eventually be corrected (Bradshaw et al. 2014; Shah et al. 2019).

Practitioners may not always feel they have time to fully review the records of current and former patients, but this activity can provide feedback and much-needed insight into ways to improve your practice and find your way through clinical impasses. Remember, our memory apparatus was selected not for accuracy but for prediction to aid our survival. Not only are we unlikely to recall all the important details; we are likely to distort them (see sections "Implications for Medical Practice" and "Practicing and Improving Clinical Skills" in Chapter 2, "Keys to Problem-Solving"). Your routinely recorded methodical notes, not your memory, contain the correct information that you need. It is also sometimes helpful to spend sessions reading through patients' charts with them, particularly when the way forward is unclear. This gives you the opportunity to discuss observations and ideas out loud with the patient, enhancing their understanding, the therapeutic alliance, and your consideration of new options. It also offers the opportunity to make sure that you and your patient are sharing an understanding of their situation.

We have likely made errors in, misunderstood, or allowed omissions in our early assessments (see sections "Errors in Conceptualization" in Chapter 1 and "Obstacles to Problem-Solving" in Chapter 2). The data, therefore, should be substantially reviewed at each patient contact so that they can be verified and updated, if necessary. Keeping detailed notes and then devoting time to a complete review of your work, even years later, will sharpen your awareness of steps you may question and resolve to change in the future (see section "Self-Assess and Self-Correct" later in this chapter).

Enhance Clinical Reasoning

Mindfulness has recently become popular across society as a valuable tool for everyone, including our patients (Sudhir et al. 2017). The highest level of this practice has been identified as metacognition—thinking about how we think (Jankowski and Holas 2014). Metacognition can enhance the chances of compiling a useful differential diagnosis (Scordo 2014) and reduce diagnostic and treatment planning error (see Stark and Fins 2014).

Responsible clinical reasoning must be conscious, intentional, and premeditated (McCullough 2013). It should be based on rational methods, such as the abductive thinking discussed in Chapter 5, "Essential Assessment and Reevaluation" (see section "Essential Value of Bayesian Inference" in that chapter). It should also be broad, encompassing all of the data (see section "Accounting for Every Symptom or Dysfunction" in Chapter 5), and flexible because the symptoms, dysfunctions, and context of our patients' conditions are apt to change. The opportunity to reconsider our reasoning and judgment at each patient contact leads to more accurate diagnoses and treatments. The iteration of systematic assessment followed by creative thinking is the best method for improving psychiatric outcomes (Stein et al. 2022).

Good clinical reasoning should also not be limited by gaps or shortcomings in our current diagnostic systems (see section "Classification of Concepts" in Chapter 1). It is useful to consider the meaning of "treating the whole patient," a buzz phrase in psychiatry for the past several decades. Joel Yager, M.D., writes with great wisdom as he describes the important role of identifying concerns that may not relate to functionality or symptoms but nevertheless result in misery for our patients and that might yet be addressed by ourselves or others we can recruit (Yager 2021).

Similarly, the newer concept and broader definition of palliative psychiatry seeks to improve functioning as much as possible when a "cure" appears infeasible. It focuses on reducing harm and improving quality of life and personal development for the severely and chronically mentally ill, rather than limiting itself to seemingly futile and end-of-life cases. In fact, curative and palliative efforts may be carried out concurrently in psychiatry and may help lower the risk of suicide in cases of depression, psychosis, and anorexia nervosa (Trachsel et al. 2016; Westermair et al. 2022); see Case Example 2 in Chapter 9, "Managing a Sustained Therapeutic Relationship During Treatment Failure." Effective clinical reasoning individualizes care even more than we are seeking from precision medicine (see section "Anchor Translational Medicine" later in this chapter) and uses self-awareness and the complexity of a clinical situation to find answers.

Conduct Semistructured Clinical Interviews

Clinical reasoning cannot be valid if significant pieces of information are missing (Nordgaard et al. 2013). Thorough assessments are essential for providing enough data to formulate accurate diagnoses and effective treatment plans (Duckworth and Kedward 1978). Practitioners using unstructured interviews miss many more comorbidities than do those employing semistructured methods, and this eventually contributes to treatment failure (Pull et al. 2002; Zimmerman 2016; Zimmerman et al. 2008); see section "Practicing and Improving Clinical Skills" in Chapter 2. Focusing mostly on chief complaints during the time you have with a patient is insufficient; you must have some organized standard method for broadly covering systems, functionality, and symptoms (Duckworth and Kedward 1978; Zimmerman 2016); see sections "General Medical Assessment" and "Psychiatric Assessment" in Chapter 5.

Although fully structured interviews have been used by nonclinicians seeking epidemiological data and by psychiatrists doing clinical research and compiling and standardizing diagnostic schemata such as those found in DSM-III through DSM-5-TR (American Psychiatric Association 1980, 1994, 2013, 2022; Renou et al. 2004), these fixed tools are not necessary during treatment by mental health professionals, and they are often too rigid to capture the nuance and granularity necessary for success in clinical practice (Brugha et al. 1999; Nordgaard et al. 2012, 2013). However, semistructured interviews, which are often identified with research in many domains, are effective tools for patient care (Adams 2010; Lauth et al. 2008; Mestre et al. 2012). This method can ensure that all important areas are queried while still allowing flexibility in the flow of discussion, with time to explore patient concerns and pertinent areas more deeply (Nordgaard et al. 2013). The semistructured approach also assists in the development of a therapeutic alliance, while the clinician still remains responsible for how time together is used.

Numerous semistructured interviews have been proposed for use in our field, many of them focused on individual domains or diagnoses (Copeland et al. 1976; Gorlin et al. 2016; Ramos-Quiroga et al. 2019). The use of peer-reviewed scales may help in completing a thorough assessment, but, outside formal research, providers may also use their own templates and instruments or mix them as they find useful (see Chapter 5, Tables 5–1 through 5–6). For a discussion of effective methods of employing semistructured interviewing in clinical practice, see works by Fox and Gamble and by Fylan in Additional Readings at the end of this chapter.

Self-Assess and Self-Correct

Ideally, we carefully evaluate the design and data interpretation of every peer-reviewed article we read. However, who scrutinizes the steps we take in practice? Outside supervision during training, how often do we discuss cases in detail with peers, asking for oversight, and how frequently do we seek formal second opinions (see section "Ways to Give and Receive Feedback in Practice" in Chapter 2)? Psychoanalysts and other psychotherapists traditionally schedule routine supervision for themselves, but how often is this done in general practice, where pharmacological and somatic treatments so often predominate (Gold 2004)? As a model, ongoing clinical supervision is considered an important part of professional development for advanced practice mental health nurses (Hines-Martin and Robinson 2006).

The diagnostic accuracy of emergency physicians was found to be domain specific; that is, physicians tend to be more accurate with some diagnoses than others (e.g., chest disease vs. vascular disease) (Ilgen et al. 2012). Second opinions are one valuable tool to help confirm diagnoses and identify successful treatment strategies (Coulter et al. 2019). These consultations are most often requested by patients, and it appears that practitioners are more reluctant to seek them, particularly those practicing in relative isolation (Heuss et al. 2018).

There is no defensible reason why practitioners cannot initiate these outside evaluations themselves, and we should be doing so in order to practice better medicine. The era of managed care has perhaps dissipated our enthusiasm for someone looking over our shoulder, confusing it with oversight and insincere cost reduction methods. The past decade, however, has seen the development of third-party resources available to patients and busy practitioners that provide second opinions from experts they know, or know of and respect, who can provide valuable overview and feedback (Oldham 2019). Specialist services have also been developed that offer additional ideas to providers seeking successful outcomes during treatment failures (Casetta et al. 2020; Kennedy and Paykel 2004; Shepherd et al. 2009).

Eduardo Salas, Ph.D., an expert in effective team building, lists debriefing as an essential task for teams wanting to improve performance (Salas 2023). This strategy is being integrated into nursing and medical education and systems as part of a push to enhance the metacognitive strategies of practitioners (Morse et al. 2020). How do we as practitioners debrief ourselves in order to improve performance? In addition to seeking consultation and second opinions, we must train ourselves, through metacognition (see section "Enhance Clinical Reasoning"), to be an additional peer reviewer or supervisor; to be constantly evaluating, questioning, and, yes, judging our own performance, in order to consistently offer our patients the best care (Royce et al. 2019). As discussed in Chapter 2, studies have shown that feedback to providers improves clinical care. Methods for obtaining feedback from peers and patients are discussed in the sections "Ways to Receive Feedback in Practice" and "Practicing and Improving Clinical Skills" in Chapter 2.

Overconfidence in clinical decision-making is fertile ground for error and eventual and repetitive treatment failure. We must use tools that help us see deficits in our conceptualization and problem-solving because many providers are too satisfied with their below par performance, which only reinforces dysfunctional practices (Norman 2020). Nursing, dentistry, and optometry, alongside medicine, have begun to use tools that help practitioners assess their critical diagnostic and therapeutic thinking skills, often based on the Diagnostic Thinking Inventory (DTI; Bordage et al. 1990), a validated instrument for individual use in practice settings (Durning et al. 2016; Edgar et al. 2022; Owlia et al. 2022). The DTI is one of the most broadly applied self-assessment tools for clinicians. Readers are encouraged to take the 25-minute test to assess their diagnostic thinking; the DTI is available free for download through ResearchGate (www.researchgate.net/publication/263733394_DIAGNOSTIC_THINKING_INVENTORYinstrument).

In completing the DTI, practitioners should describe themselves as they actually do practice, not as they think they are supposed to practice (ideally, of course, there should be little difference between the two) (Rahayu and McAleer 2008). DTI results are given on two separate scales: Flexibility in Thinking and Structure of Memory; higher scores on each scale are associated with greater accuracy in diagnosis (Bordage et al. 1990). Through scoring the index, practitioners can learn which cognitive approaches are more successful and work to amend their method if they have been favoring the less effective strategies that are described.

Anchor Translational Medicine

As clinicians, we have three goals for improving the practice of psychiatry: 1) translate new clinical research evidence into medical practice, 2) improve the clinical reasoning power of mental health providers to make accurate diagnoses and effective treatment recommendations, and 3) enhance the skills of practitioners to implement and monitor treatments in tandem with patients. Much of this book has concerned the second (Chapters 1–5) and third (throughout, but particularly Chapter 9) goals. The first goal refers to translational medicine, which seeks more precise treatments for each patient based on evidence from basic and clinical research in genetics, genomics, and environmental influences (Machado-Vieira 2012). Clinicians represent the final leg in this journey: researchers in basic science discover information, and clinical researchers find and confirm applications, which are promulgated by educators and authors to practitioners to be put in service. If any step is incomplete, there is no translation and therefore fewer evidence-based successful treatment outcomes. Even wonderful data are not helpful to patients if clinicians do not correctly and effectively incorporate them into their treatment planning discussions.

One group studied a medium-size university hospital staff in Europe and observed that new research information resulting in changes in clinical practice by physicians was incorporated and implemented *individually* by physicians rather than by administrative leadership (Kristensen et al. 2016). Individual practitioners took the lead on adopting and sharing new science that was eventually accepted as the new norm by the group.

We must accept the initiative and seek to be that point of the arrow—both a diagnostic and a therapeutic tool, armed with the best data.

Further, it has been argued that although the purpose of medical research is to allow clinicians to apply the knowledge gained to patients' problems, the personalized approaches being developed should not just point to the most likely effective treatments but also add to a dynamic multidimensional assessment that modifies treatments, as needed, on an ongoing basis (Keck et al. 2018); see section "Enhance Clinical Reasoning" above. As clinicians, we fulfill our role in this team effort only when we detect, analyze, and reconceptualize when treatment disappoints. Rather than routinely expecting ideal outcomes, especially from increasingly personalized medicine, we should expect failures, inadequacies, and dead ends because we have insufficient knowledge from basic and clinical science, as well as our own cognitive faculties, to always correctly perceive and formulate the best solutions at the beginning.

We may not always expect full treatment failure, but we must anticipate any shortcomings in our efforts that can instruct us toward better paths. It is more effective to embrace these shortcomings than to suppress, ignore, or redefine them without utility. As discussed in Chapter 2 (sections "Best Practices for Problem-Solving" and "Implications for Medical Practice"), a treatment impasse is an opportunity to reconceptualize and discover better answers. We must not trip at the finish line, rendering the efforts and hopes of earlier team members unfulfilled.

Summary

We must always recall that the clinical tasks we face are inherently complex; routine solutions are unlikely to fit and often lead to treatment failure. Psychiatry often addresses chronic or recurrent conditions that require long-term treatment. Broad and sustained improvement is usually more important than rapid progress. It is essential to collaborate with our patients to identify successful strategies they are willing to maintain indefinitely.

Conceptualizing treatment failure as treatment resistance involves circular reasoning, adds no value to treatment planning, and abdicates our responsibility to solve clinical dilemmas with our patients. Detailed and accurate recordkeeping is essential for finding clinical solutions during treatment impasses and may be threatened by technological progress (e.g., incautious use of EMR features). Data from previous sessions should be substantially reviewed at each session and confirmed, corrected, or reappreciated as necessary. A clinician facing treatment failure will benefit from taking time to review the complete treatment record, often together with the patient. The intentional and regular use of metacognition improves diagnostic accuracy, treatment planning, and clinical outcomes in psychiatry. Clinical reasoning is best based on abductive logic with iterative and creative reassessment and requires full consideration of complete data. We must help with patient concerns that stretch beyond categorical symptoms and functionality and increase our appreciation for the value of personal growth and quality of life, particularly for the severely mentally ill.

Overconfidence breeds mediocrity and defeats clinical success. We have a duty to use tools to evaluate and improve our practice skills. Seeking regular feedback through consultation, supervision, standardized assessment instruments, second opinions, review of the record, and monitoring the therapeutic alliance enhances outcomes for patients. Many paramedical professions have already embraced these steps.

Clinicians are responsible for applying the best available evidence to treatment planning. The successful translation of basic and clinical research into patient care is most often led by individual physicians who influence their peers. We can be these leaders while remaining open to the similar guidance of colleagues. Instead of expecting ideal outcomes from initial efforts, we provide more value by anticipating roadblocks and persistently altering treatments as needed.

Key Points

- Underestimating the complexity of clinical problems leads to treatment failure.
- Treatments must be sustainable over the long term.
- The concept of treatment resistance adds no value to treatment planning.
- Maintaining and reviewing detailed records aids resolution of treatment impasses.
- Provider metacognition improves diagnostic and treatment accuracy.
- Semistructured interviews reduce treatment failure by identifying more comorbidities.

- Feedback to providers about their clinical skills and performance reduces treatment failure.
- Individual practitioners are key to useful dissemination and application of new data.

Self-Assessment Questions

1. Which of the following is true of metacognition?

    A. It is the highest level of mindfulness.
    B. It concerns thinking about how we think.
    C. It helps the clinician compile a useful differential diagnosis.
    D. All of the above.

    Correct answer: D. All of the above.

    Conscious, deliberate self-examination of our own cognition is our obligation, as well as an effective tool for better diagnosis and treatment planning.

2. Which two of the following statements are true of translational medicine?

    A. It seeks to identify personalized treatments.
    B. It establishes broad general treatment guidelines.
    C. It relies on research in genetics, genomics, and environmental influences.
    D. It solely identifies the treatments most likely to succeed.

    Correct answer: A and C.

    Translational medicine is the effort to use data gained from research in genetics, genomics, and environmental influences to identify precise treatments for individuals. It also seeks to modify treatments on the basis of dynamic ongoing multidimensional assessment.

3. Which of the following statements is *not* true?

    A. Debriefing is an essential task for those seeking to improve performance.

B. Second opinions are requested most frequently by practitioners.
C. Diagnostic accuracy may be domain specific.
D. Relatively isolated practitioners are reluctant to seek second opinions.

Correct answer: B. Second opinions are requested most frequently by practitioners.

Second opinions are commonly sought by patients and are generally avoided by more isolated providers. Debriefing is the most essential tool for improving the performance of teams and professionals. Diagnostic accuracy among emergency physicians has been documented as domain specific.

4.   "Treating the whole patient" refers to which of the following?

A. Identifying concerns that cause misery beyond symptoms and functionality.
B. Always performing our own physical examinations.
C. Assuming the role of a patient's primary care provider.
D. Identifying all of a patient's symptoms.

Correct answer: A. Identifying concerns that cause misery beyond symptoms and functionality.

As expressed by Joel Yager, M.D., this concept urges practitioners to address distressing features of a patient's situation not encompassed by traditional categorical or dimensional diagnosis ourselves or through others we can enlist. Although physical examinations are an essential part of any assessment (see section "General Medical Assessment" in Chapter 5), practitioners may arrange to share this responsibility and the knowledge gained from it with trusted colleagues. Although some authors have argued convincingly that mental health providers function effectively in a primary care setting (see section "Psychiatrists as Generalists" in Chapter 7, "Underappreciated Causes of Treatment Failure") and it is essential to identify all of a patient's symptoms and problems with functionality, these are not related to the concept in question.

5.   Which of the following is true of palliative psychiatry?

A. It is limited to treating end-of-life cases.
B. It is limited to treating futile cases.
C. It refers exclusively to consultation on oncology units.
D. It reduces harm and improves quality of life and personal development.

Correct answer: D. It reduces harm and improves quality of life and personal development.

The newer and broader definition of palliative psychiatry seeks to improve functioning when a "cure" appears unlikely. It focuses on reducing harm and improving quality of life and personal development for the severely and chronically mentally ill, rather than limiting itself to seemingly futile and end-of-life cases. Palliative psychiatry includes consultation and liaison with other specialties.

Discussion Topics

1. A woman comes to you for treatment because she believes that you significantly helped a good friend of hers. After completing a thorough evaluation and formulating a differential diagnosis, you discuss several treatment options with her. She has information on her friend's treatment and wants to follow her friend's plan, but you are aware of new research and do not see the friend's treatment as the best long-term plan for this patient. How do you proceed?
2. After practicing psychiatry for 10 years, you no longer see each case as challenging, and it seems that many patients have the same diagnoses and require similar treatments. Most of your patients seem satisfied, although many do not reach remission, and some have dropped out of treatment or transferred to other providers without discussing it with you. You are rarely asked to provide second opinions. Is anything wrong? How might you evaluate your practice?

Additional Readings

Fox J, Gamble C: Consolidating the assessment process: the semi-structured interview, in Working With Serious Mental Illness: A Manual for Clinical Practice, 2nd Edition. Edited by Gamble C, Brennan G. Amsterdam, Elsevier, 2005, pp 133–144: *This chapter describes use of a semistructured interview to develop useful treatment plans*

Fylan F: Semi-structured interviewing, in A Handbook of Research Methods for Clinical and Health Psychology. Edited by Miles J, Gilbert P. New York, Oxford University Press, 2005, pp 65–77: *Many semistructured interviews are available as psychiatric assessment tools, easily found by searching PubMed or similar search engines; this chapter, rather than detailing any single one, discusses the best practices for their application to clinical or research purposes*

Stark M, Fins JJ: The ethical imperative to think about thinking—diagnostics, metacognition, and medical professionalism. Camb Q Healthc Ethics 23(4):386–396, 2014: *A compelling apology for the application of metacognitive strategies as an essential obligation when caring for patients*

Yager J: Targeting 3 tiers of psychiatric problems in patient-focused psychiatric practice: diagnostic signs, symptoms, and impairments; specific complex subjective complaints; and contributing meta-problems. J Psychiatr Pract 27(6):472–477, 2021: *See section "Enhance Clinical Reasoning" above*

References

Adams E: The joys and challenges of semi-structured interviewing. Community Pract 83(7):18–21, 2010 20701187

Adli M, Bauer M, Rush AJ: Algorithms and collaborative-care systems for depression: are they effective and why? A systematic review. Biol Psychiatry 59(11):1029–1038, 2006 16769294

American Psychiatric Association: Diagnosis and Statistical Manual of Mental Disorders, 3rd Edition. Washington, DC, American Psychiatric Association, 1980

American Psychiatric Association: Diagnosis and Statistical Manual of Mental Disorders, 4th Edition. Washington, DC, American Psychiatric Association, 1994

American Psychiatric Association: Diagnosis and Statistical Manual of Mental Disorders, 5th Edition. Arlington, VA, American Psychiatric Association, 2013

American Psychiatric Association: Diagnosis and Statistical Manual of Mental Disorders, 5th Edition, Text Revision. Washington, DC, American Psychiatric Association, 2022

Beers DO, Karst KR: Generic and Innovator Drugs: A Guide to FDA Approval Requirements, 8th Edition. New York, Wolters Kluwer; 2020

Bordage G, Grant J, Marsden P: Quantitative assessment of diagnostic ability. Med Educ 24(5):413–425, 1990 2215294

Bradshaw KM, Donohue B, Wilks C: A review of quality assurance methods to assist professional record keeping: implications for providers of interpersonal violence treatment. Aggress Violent Behav 19(3):242–250, 2014 24976786

Brugha TS, Bebbington PE, Jenkins R: A difference that matters: comparisons of structured and semi-structured psychiatric diagnostic interviews in the general population. Psychol Med 29(5):1013–1020, 1999 10576294

Casetta C, Gaughran F, Oloyede E, et al: Real-world effectiveness of admissions to a tertiary treatment-resistant psychosis service: 2-year mirror-image study. BJPsych Open 6(5):e82, 2020 32744200

Chivilgina O, Elger BS, Benichou MM, et al: "What's the best way to document information concerning psychiatric patients? I just don't know"—A qualitative study about recording psychiatric patients notes in the era of electronic health records. PLoS One 17(3):e0264255, 2022 35239698

Copeland JR, Kelleher MJ, Kellett JM, et al: A semi-structured clinical interview for the assessment of diagnosis and mental state in the elderly: the Geriatric Mental State Schedule I: development and reliability. Psychol Med 6(3):439–449, 1976 996204

Coulter C, Baker KK, Margolis RL: Specialized consultation for suspected recent-onset schizophrenia: diagnostic clarity and the distorting impact of anxiety and reported auditory hallucinations. J Psychiatr Pract 25(2):76–81, 2019 30849055

Dey M, Buhagiar K, Jabbar F: Accuracy of prescribing documentation by UK junior doctors undertaking psychiatry placements: a multi-centre observational study. BMC Res Notes 12(1):558, 2019 31484585

Duckworth GS, Kedward HB: Man or machine in psychiatric diagnosis. Am J Psychiatry 135(1):64–68, 1978 337813

Durning SJ, Costanzo ME, Beckman TJ, et al: Functional neuroimaging correlates of thinking flexibility and knowledge structure in memory: exploring the relationships between clinical reasoning and diagnostic thinking. Med Teach 38(6):570–577, 2016 26079668

Edgar AK, Ainge L, Backhouse S, Armitage JA: A cohort study for the development and validation of a reflective inventory to quantify diagnostic reasoning skills in optometry practice. BMC Med Educ 22(1):536, 2022 35820888

George MS, Post RM: Daily left prefrontal repetitive transcranial magnetic stimulation for acute treatment of medication-resistant depression. Am J Psychiatry 168(4):356–364, 2011 21474597

Gold JH: Reflections on psychodynamic psychotherapy supervision for psychiatrists in clinical practice. J Psychiatr Pract 10(3):162–169, 2004 15330222

Gorlin EI, Dalrymple K, Chelminski I, Zimmerman M: Reliability and validity of a semi-structured DSM-based diagnostic interview module for the assessment of attention deficit hyperactivity disorder in adult psychiatric outpatients. Psychiatry Res 242:46–53, 2016 27259136

Hines-Martin V, Robinson K: Supervision as professional development for psychiatric mental health nurses. Clin Nurse Spec 20(6):293–297, 2006 17149020

Heuss SC, Schwartz BJ, Schneeberger AR: Second opinions in psychiatry: a review. J Psychiatr Pract 24(6):434–442, 2018 30395554

Ilgen JS, Humbert AJ, Kuhn G, et al: Assessing diagnostic reasoning: a consensus statement summarizing theory, practice, and future needs. Acad Emerg Med 19(12):1454–1461, 2012 23279251

Jankowski T, Holas P: Metacognitive model of mindfulness. Conscious Cogn 28:64–80, 2014 25038535

Jašović-Gašić M, Dunjic-Kostić B, Pantović M, et al: Algorithms in psychiatry: state of the art. Psychiatr Danub 25(3):280–283, 2013 24048398

Kariotis TC, Prictor M, Chang S, et al: Impact of electronic health records on information practices in mental health contexts: scoping review. J Med Internet Res 24(5):e30405, 2022 35507393

Keck ME, Kappelmann N, Kopf-Beck J: Translational research as prerequisite for personalized psychiatry. Eur Arch Psychiatry Clin Neurosci 268(3):215–217, 2018 29546658

Kennedy N, Paykel ES: Treatment and response in refractory depression: results from a specialist affective disorders service. J Affect Disord 81(1):49–53, 2004 15183599

Kristensen N, Nymann C, Konradsen H: Implementing research results in clinical practice—the experiences of healthcare professionals. BMC Health Serv Res 16:48, 2016 26860594

Largent EA, Peterson A, Lynch HF: FDA drug approval and the ethics of desperation. JAMA Intern Med 181(12):1555–1556, 2021 34694325

Lauth B, Levy SR, Júlíusdóttir G, et al: Implementing the semi-structured interview Kiddie-SADS-PL into an in-patient adolescent clinical setting: impact on frequency of diagnoses. Child Adolesc Psychiatry Ment Health 2(1):14, 2008 18597697

Machado-Vieira R: Tracking the impact of translational research in psychiatry: state of the art and perspectives. J Transl Med 10:175, 2012 22929586

McCullough LB: Critical appraisal of clinical judgment: an essential dimension of clinical ethics. J Med Philos 38(1):1–5, 2013 23334085

Mestre JI, Rossi PC, Torrens M: The assessment interview: a review of structured and semi-structured clinical interviews available for use among Hispanic clients, in Guide to Psychological Assessment With Hispanics. Edited by Benuto LT. New York, Springer, 2012 pp 33–48

Morse KJ, Fey MK, Forneris SG: Evidence-based debriefing. Annu Rev Nurs Res 39(1):129–148, 2020 33431640

Nordgaard J, Revsbech R, Sæbye D, et al: Assessing the diagnostic validity of a structured psychiatric interview in a first-admission hospital sample. World Psychiatry 11(3):181–185, 2012 23024678

Nordgaard J, Sass LA, Parnas J: The psychiatric interview: validity, structure, and subjectivity. Eur Arch Psychiatry Clin Neurosci 263(4):353–364, 2013 23001456

Norman E: Why metacognition is not always helpful. Front Psychol 11:1537, 2020 32714256

Oldham JM: Second opinions. J Psychiatr Pract 25(2):75, 2019 30849054

Owlia F, Keshmiri F, Kazemipoor M, et al: Assessment of clinical reasoning and diagnostic thinking among dental students. Int J Dent 2022:1085326, 2022 36199675

Pull CB, Cloos JM, Pull-Erpelding MC: Clinical assessment instruments in psychiatry, in Psychiatric Diagnosis and Classification. Edited by Maj M, Gaebel W, López-Ibor JJ, et al. Hoboken, NJ, Wiley, 2002, pp 177–218

Rahayu GR, McAleer S: Clinical reasoning of Indonesian medical students as measured by diagnostic thinking inventory. South-East Asian Journal of Medical Education 2(1):42–47, 2008

Ramos-Quiroga JA, Nasillo V, Richarte V, et al: Criteria and concurrent validity of DIVA 2.0: a semi-structured diagnostic interview for adult ADHD. J Atten Disord 23(10):1126–1135, 2019 27125994

Renou S, Hergueta T, Flament M, et al: Diagnostic structured interviews in child and adolescent's psychiatry. Encephale 30(2):122–134, 2004 15107714

Ross DB: The FDA and the case of Ketek. N Engl J Med 356(16):1601–1604, 2007 17442902

Royce CS, Hayes MM, Schwartzstein RM: Teaching critical thinking: a case for instruction in cognitive biases to reduce diagnostic errors and improve patient safety. Acad Med 94(2):187–194, 2019 30398993

Rutledge RB, Chekroud AM, Huys QJ: Machine learning and big data in psychiatry: toward clinical applications. Curr Opin Neurobiol 55:152–159, 2019 30999271

Salas E: Saving lives: insights from the science of teamwork. Lecture presented at the American College of Psychiatrists Annual Meeting, Tucson, AZ, February 24, 2023

Scordo KA: Differential diagnosis: correctly putting the pieces of the puzzle together. AACN Adv Crit Care 25(3):230–236, 2014 25054528

Shah AD, Quinn NJ, Chaudhry A, et al: Recording problems and diagnoses in clinical care: developing guidance for healthcare professionals and system designers. BMJ Health Care Inform 26(1):e100106, 2019 31874855

Shepherd DJ, Insole LM, McAllister-Williams RH, et al: Are specialised affective disorder services useful? Psychiatr Bull 33(2):41–43, 2009

Stark M, Fins JJ: The ethical imperative to think about thinking—diagnostics, metacognition, and medical professionalism. Camb Q Healthc Ethics 23(4):386–396, 2014

Stein DJ, Shoptaw SJ, Vigo DV, et al: Psychiatric diagnosis and treatment in the 21st century: paradigm shifts versus incremental integration. World Psychiatry 21(3):393–414, 2022 36073709

Sudhir PM, Rukmini S, Sharma MP: Combining metacognitive strategies with traditional cognitive behavior therapy in generalized anxiety disorder: a case illustration. Indian J Psychol Med 39(2):152–156, 2017 28515551

Trachsel M, Irwin SA, Biller-Andorno N, et al: Palliative psychiatry for severe persistent mental illness as a new approach to psychiatry? Definition, scope, benefits, and risks. BMC Psychiatry 16:260, 2016 27450328

Turner EH: Esketamine for treatment-resistant depression: seven concerns about efficacy and FDA approval. Lancet Psychiatry 6(12):977–979, 2019 31680014

Westermair AL, Buchman DZ, Levitt S, et al: Palliative psychiatry in a narrow and in a broad sense: a concept clarification. Aust N Z J Psychiatry 56(12):1535–1541, 2022 35999690

Yager J: Targeting 3 tiers of psychiatric problems in patient-focused psychiatric practice: diagnostic signs, symptoms, and impairments; specific complex subjective complaints; and contributing meta-problems. J Psychiatr Pract 27(6):472–477, 2021

Zimmerman M: A review of 20 years of research on overdiagnosis and underdiagnosis in the Rhode Island Methods to Improve Diagnostic Assessment and Services (MIDAS) project. Can J Psychiatry 61(2):71–79, 2016 27253697

Zimmerman M, McGlinchey JB, Chelminski I, et al: Diagnostic co-morbidity in 2300 psychiatric out-patients presenting for treatment evaluated with a semi-structured diagnostic interview. Psychol Med 38(2):199–210, 2008 17949515

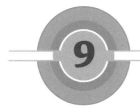

Managing a Sustained Therapeutic Relationship During Treatment Failure

Although all providers and their patients seek successful clinical outcomes from assessment and treatment, we know that as many as half of all efforts result in at least temporary treatment failure (Howes et al. 2022). A major task of the clinician is to maintain hope for and expectation of positive outcomes and to support the patient through what may be a protracted, frustrating, and difficult process. Your attention to the needs and goals of your patient prior to remission not only eases their burden but also influences the outcome.

As we approach treatment impasses, it is necessary to reconceptualize not only our diagnoses and treatment plans but also our mutual goals and measurements of success. As we consider removing symptoms and restoring or enhancing functionality, we must embrace persistent, incremental interventions that together comprise a treatment plan. This can be accomplished only by working in tandem with the patient, adopting long-term views while using short-term goals, and clearly understanding patients and their environments.

The Therapeutic Alliance

All successful treatment attempts take place in the context of a healthy therapeutic alliance: an overt, conscious agreement between patient and provider to work together solely to produce clinical benefits for the patient. This requires that the patient provide accurate information as requested, accept a mutually agreed on treatment plan, follow treatment directions, and maintain contact with the provider. The clinician must adhere to ethical standards, use a competent knowledge base and skills, provide a safe environment in which to work, and maintain access for the patient. The key essence is that both participants bring their best to the effort, and it implies that both have agreed on common goals for their work together (Daniels and Wearden 2011).

A significant relationship exists between the quality of a therapeutic alliance in psychiatry (as well as other medical and paramedical fields) and the degree of therapeutic outcome. Participation from the patient is a necessary factor. This correlation persists even across different types of therapeutic modalities, including various forms of psychotherapy and pharmacotherapy with both active and placebo agents (Arnow and Steidtmann 2014; Horvath et al. 2011; Krupnick et al. 1996; Wolfe and Goldfried 1988). Treatment concepts themselves do not play a role in psychotherapeutic outcomes (Tschuschke et al. 2020). A strong alliance, however, leads to measurably less resistance during psychotherapy sessions, fewer suicidal thoughts, and less self-harm (Daniels and Wearden 2011; Dunster-Page et al. 2017). A weak or negative alliance may contribute to treatment failure or resistance (West et al. 2022, p. 577).

Most studies indicate that a therapeutic alliance is usually stronger if it is formed early in the clinician-patient relationship (Diamond et al. 2006; Frank and Gunderson 1990; Negri et al. 2019). That said, it should also be perceived as a dynamic entity, shifting, twisting, and sometimes rupturing as it responds to different needs and challenges (from both sides) during a patient's journey toward remission or recovery (McLaughlin et al. 2014).

Threats to the Alliance

Mismatches in race and gender between patient and provider have been found to result in weaker therapeutic alliances, particularly in work with adolescents (Wintersteen et al. 2005). We must always show cultural respect and humility (West et al. 2022, p. 579); see section "Cultural Influences" in Chapter 5, "Essential Assessment and Reevaluation." In all cases, provider rigidity, uncertainty, tension, distraction, and criticism have negative impacts on the alliance, as do overstructured therapy, inappropriate self-disclosure, an excessive number of transference interpretations, and misapplied use of silence (Ackerman and Hilsenroth 2001).

Therapists' variable influence on and attention to a therapeutic alliance affect patient outcome more than do uneven contributions from the patient (Del Re et al. 2012; Eubanks et al. 2018). Maintaining a healthy and effective therapeutic alliance requires active work from the provider, who must monitor its quality throughout treatment. Investigators have found that when therapists do not begin their alliance with the perspective of the patient and continually adjust the alliance, this is correlated significantly with treatment failure (Tschuschke et al. 2020). We must understand how transference accompanies any treatment plan and manage how it fits with expectations.

Additionally, we always must be aware of and manage our countertransference, even in cases where pharmacological or somatic treatments may predominate (West et al. 2022, p. 579). It is critical that we remain aware of our own view of a patient's prognosis—when we lose the expectation of recovery, or even progress, surely the patient perceives this, and the alliance becomes less therapeutic. The patient's motivation and participation wane, and positive outcomes are even less likely.

Therapeutic Rupture and Repair

To achieve successful outcomes, providers must know how to identify and repair ruptures in a therapeutic alliance. Ruptures occur frequently, particularly during the treatment of PTSD, for example; cases in which ruptures remain unrepaired are linked to worse treatment outcomes (McLaughlin et al. 2014). Two significant types of rupture are marked by either withdrawal or confrontation on the part of the patient. Signs of deterioration include a patient pulling away, missing appointments, and no longer making an effort (West et al. 2022, pp. 575–576). Although less pleasant for a clinician than exploring expanding distance, anger toward the provider or treatment must be acknowledged and worked through to reach a satisfactory clinical outcome. Providers need to refocus from the treatment plan and highlight the rupture itself. Ignoring the problem while continuing the same technique and approach often results in further damage and disappointing outcomes (Castonguay et al. 1996; Eubanks et al. 2018; Piper et al. 1999; Safran and Muran 2000).

It is important to examine and discuss the patient's experience of a rupture and acknowledge their perspective. The practitioner should explore topics the patient is willing to discuss while comparing the situation to similar disappointments they experienced with others. Interpretation and cognitive reframing are less helpful to the repair, however, whereas helping a patient identify strategies to assist them in coping with affect and symptoms is valuable (Eubanks et al. 2018). Some researchers propose formal training in repair of therapeutic alliance rupture, whereas others have found cognitive-behavioral therapy (CBT) with supportive listening to be as effective (Newman et al. 2011).

Some authors contend that ruptures in an alliance are to be expected as providers and patients work through the steps of treatment. Weaker alliances fail, halting treatment, but stronger ones may persist and progress to response, remission, or recovery (Safran et al. 2011). Ruptures, when they occur, are key times for providers to refocus on being patient centered (see the next section) because validation trumps guidance at this stage of treatment (Eubanks et al. 2018).

Holding and Containing

When we refer to a therapeutic alliance, we often emphasize the motivation and agreement aspect—we are working together, side by side, solely for the benefit of the patient. Perhaps we do not stress enough the importance of *being with*, which, along with positive expectations by the practitioner, can help a patient develop hope and stamina—"grit," as is it is so commonly described today.

Psychotherapy in general, but particularly supportive therapy (see next section), creates a holding and containing environment that promotes stability, an important step in long-term care (Meaden and Van Marle 2008). We must remain optimistic and hopeful about our patients' chances of improvement, even if the original goals and expectations must be altered over time. We must also maintain humility about our abilities and an awareness of treatment limitations.

It is necessary for our patients to find positive meaning narratives. We must provide and carry hope when our patients cannot, offering belief that they can improve. Labeling someone "treatment resistant" is not consistent with this paradigm. We may mean something technical that we think is useful about the label, but surely it is heard as hopelessness by our patients.

Carl Rogers outlined how giving our patients "unconditional positive regard," evidenced by empathy and nonjudgmental caring, leads to self-directed growth. He called it person-centered therapy, believing that it leads to a perceptual reorganization of the self and the environment (Raskin and Rogers 2005, pp. 130–165; Rogers 1951, pp. 307–327). Supportive care from the clinician is an important intervention for a patient.

It results from a strong therapeutic alliance, helping to sustain the belief that hope is possible and appropriate (West et al. 2022, pp. 579–580). Holding hope is another way of saying, to ourselves and to our patients, that a treatment failure is not synonymous with treatment resistance.

In Doris Lessing's novel *The Making of the Representative for Planet 8* (see Additional Readings at the end of this chapter), an emissary is dispatched to a doomed planet, initially to help but eventually to witness and share the experience with those who live there. The book is a potent reminder of the action and gift of *being with*. No doubt we all hope that our patients will eventually experience much happier results, yet there is ample opportunity, prior to remission, to witness and share an understanding of their condition and their struggle while diagnosing, treating, and waiting for results.

Being there or *being with* is an action—the decision to hear, accept, and reflect understanding of a patient's internal experience during assessment and treatment. It does not automatically occur just by being in the room with a patient. To be heard, to feel understood, and to be accepted frees a patient to accept the situation and to make any possible changes, just as Rogers claimed.

Supportive Psychotherapy

Is there a distinction between being supportive and providing supportive psychotherapy? It has been said that the essential elements of supportive psychotherapy underlie all doctor-patient relationships, but there are criteria for this form of intervention (Grover et al. 2020).

The components of supportive psychotherapy include reassurance, clear validation, advice, psychoeducation, and facilitating access to community support and resources. It also includes helping a patient develop coping adaptations to enhance self-control and management, particularly when symptom resolution lags—that is, learning how to maintain successful lives with extended symptomatology (Meaden and Van Marle 2008).

Supportive psychotherapy and CBT, along with supportive counseling, psychoeducation, and family intervention, have been found to add to clinical improvement in cases of schizophrenia labeled "treatment resistant." In these studies, supportive psychotherapy (with antipsychotic medication) was found to be as, if not more, effective than CBT for symptom reduction at periods of 9 months to 2 years (Polese et al. 2019). Reassurance helps mitigate nihilistic ruminations, increasing the chances of improvement in depression labeled as "treatment resistant" (Grover et al. 2020); see section "Countertherapeutic Factors" in Chapter 4, "The Myth of Treatment Resistance?"

Yet this form of psychotherapy is often denigrated by students and trainees, who are eager to learn pithier, more intellectually stimulating paradigms that they can offer to their patients as triumphant interpretations. Hopefully, more experienced clinicians come to appreciate how supportive psychotherapy provides true value in patient care, especially during long-term alliances.

Supportive psychotherapy is an important tool, not just for the psychotherapist but for the psychopharmacologist as well. Because most psychiatric conditions are chronic, treatment often results in long-term relationships. Underappreciating the value of supportive psychotherapy (particularly during psychopharmacological treatment or for conditions such as schizophrenia that have limited outcome expectations and contraindication for many other forms of psychotherapy) denies our patients the opportunity to experience the beauty of shared understanding and acceptance.

Psychotherapy can occur without any brilliant interpretations, behavioral assignments, or cognitive linkages. Thomas E. Steele, M.D. (personal communication, July 1984) stressed that our job in psychotherapy is not to be "ardent detectives of psychopathology," but to never underestimate the value to our patients of our goodwill, undivided attention, and common sense. Supportive psychotherapy is figurative hand-holding. It is also listening, caring, and pointing the way forward for those who need hopeful guidance.

Clinical Examples

The following actual case vignettes have been selected to illustrate how a strong therapeutic alliance and holding environment can positively influence clinical outcomes, even when treatment plans disappoint, and how success may be found by allowing the goals of the patient and their family to take preference over those of the provider.

Case Example 1

In 1998, Jean (not her real name), a 52-year-old woman, was referred to a 42-year-old psychiatrist by her individual psychotherapist. Prior to the initial consultation, Jean had been treated unsuccessfully with antidepressant medications and insight-oriented psychotherapy for chronic and severe suicidality. She had made two serious attempts to kill herself by antidepressant overdose, for which she was hospitalized on both general medical and psychiatric units.

Jean also experienced chronic pain from cervical spine degeneration initiated by a motor vehicle accident (MVA) injury. She received active medical intervention, including two surgeries on her spine, both of which left her in greater pain. Her surgeons told her that the procedures carried a very low risk of worsening her condition and that she had been unfortunate twice.

Following a thorough assessment, Jean's psychiatrist diagnosed major depressive disorder, recurrent, severe. He suggested she remain in individual insight-oriented psychotherapy to address her wish to die and her anger about her pain and lack of progress in treating it, while proceeding with alternative psychopharmacological or somatic treatments. Jean and the psychiatrist were able to agree on very short-term contracts to either refrain from self-harm or notify her providers prior to such action; these agreements were renegotiated or renewed at each patient contact. Jean did adhere to the contracts, resulting in one hospitalization and several notifications to her husband, who was then able to take additional steps to support her safety, such as taking possession of her medication and providing ongoing supervision. As a result, there were no further suicide attempts, or self-harm, during Jean's work with the psychiatrist.

Because tricyclic antidepressants (TCAs) were considered too risky in overdose, prior to referral Jean had been treated solely with selective serotonin reuptake inhibitors (SSRIs) fluoxetine, paroxetine, and sertraline at adequate doses for sufficient lengths of time. At the time, monoamine oxidase inhibitors (MAOIs) were considered particularly efficacious in cases of TCA and SSRI nonresponse, so a trial of phenelzine was initiated, along with a tyramine-free diet (in order to reduce the risk of hypertensive crisis). The risks of overdose or intentional provocation of hypertensive crisis were openly discussed during treatment planning and were included in the safety contracts.

The phenelzine, at maximum dose for 12 weeks, was ineffective at treating Jean's mood and neurovegetative symptoms. An alternative MAOI, tranylcypromine, was substituted, but it was just as ineffective and quite sedating. After a literature review and consultation with senior colleagues, the psychiatrist suggested trying a return to phenelzine, combining it with cautious doses of the TCA imipramine (again, with specific discussion and acknowledgment in the safety contracts), and Jean agreed. During this treatment, serum levels of the TCA were found to be almost negligible, and Jean experienced no improvement. However, she experienced additional sedation, heat intolerance, and sweating. A secondary amine, desipramine, was substituted for its parent compound, the tertiary amine imipramine, resulting in palpitations, headaches, and lightheadedness. There was minimal improvement of Jean's depressive disorder symptoms, although she was more alert.

For the next step, the TCA was discontinued and liothyronine was added in the hope that it would potentiate the antidepressant effects of phenelzine, but Jean's mood and neurovegetative symptoms were still unchanged. Her thyroid indices remained within in the normal range. New spinal surgery was being seriously considered, so both medications were tapered and discontinued at the request of the surgeon and with Jean's agreement.

Jean was also seeing a primary care internist, a gynecologist, an orthopedic surgeon, a neurologist, a physiatrist, and a pain management specialist; her psychiatrist maintained open communication with all of these providers as well with as the psychotherapist. Jean was being prescribed methadone and hydrocodone for her chronic, intractable pain. Because the psychiatrist maintained a concern about the effects of hydrocodone on Jean's mood, the team of specialists agreed to gradually increase her methadone in an attempt to limit the necessity of her using the shorter-acting opioid. Jean's neurologist added gabapentin 400 mg qid, which eventually was raised to 600 mg qid. Jean was also prescribed a transcutaneous electrical nerve stimulation unit and a bone growth stimulator. Celecoxib was later prescribed for pain, which did help her sleep to some degree (she had been waking with pain after every 2 hours of sleep).

All treatment planning between Jean and the psychiatrist was collaborative. When further surgery was delayed, the psychiatrist next suggested a trial of the serotonin-norepinephrine reuptake inhibitor venlafaxine, which at the time was a new and safer way to approach the treatment than were full doses of a TCA. Jean agreed. The dosage was titrated from 150 to 300 mg/day, but the results were again unsatisfactory. After further literature review and consultation with colleagues, the psychiatrist returned the dosage to 150 mg/day and added 30 mg of the atypical antidepressant mirtazapine (later increased to 60 mg), but this combination was not well tolerated. The mirtazapine was discontinued, the venlafaxine was tapered, and the tetracyclic maprotiline was begun. The response was still muted.

About this time, Jean suffered additional orthopedic injury: stress fractures in her left hip, foot, and ankle. This was extremely frustrating and demoralizing for her because she had made no progress in treating the pain in her cervical spine, and now she had additional pain in her lower extremity that further limited her ambulation. Her suicidality, while never absent, was again heightened. She reluctantly agreed to surgery, expressing her hope of dying from the anesthesia. After the surgery, her ankle healed slowly but the hip never did, despite regular physical and pool therapy. She continued to refuse the additional MRI requested by her orthopedist because previous imaging had been too traumatic because of her claustrophobia. She continued to suffer, as well, from somatic memories of her MVA.

Jean's psychotherapist moved out of town in 2002; her psychiatrist explored alternative therapists for her, but she never contacted them.

Her primary psychotherapy from that point became that which the psychiatrist could provide during their (usually) once every 3- to 4-week appointments, all the time encouraging her to begin with a new therapist. The type of psychotherapy provided by her psychiatrist while discussing her medical conditions and pharmacological or somatic treatments contained some elements of insight but was mostly supportive, with occasional behavioral or cognitive elements. In 2005, Jean quit seeing her neurologist because she felt he was condescending and not paying attention to her. Her psychiatrist briefly tried to explore her possible transference to the neurologist and expanded their sessions to 50 minutes in order to have time to provide a broader level of care. Although the issue of finding a new psychotherapist came up several times during their long work together, she never made the appointments.

The 225 mg of daily maprotiline appeared to provide about 20% improvement—not enough to be termed response, let alone remission. Also in 2005, Jean's internist changed her gabapentin to topiramate, and the results were essentially the same: a bit better for pain but no benefit for mood. She refused to try fluoxetine supplemented with olanzapine, despite encouraging case reports and open-label and randomized controlled trials. Like many patients, she feared that even a less than 5% annual risk of tardive dyskinesia was too much: she had already suffered similarly unlikely outcomes twice from surgery and felt that permanent involuntary muscle movements would be absolutely intolerable.

Jean and her psychiatrist continued to look at standard and emerging somatic treatments. Electroconvulsive therapy was contraindicated because of her cervical spine condition, and she could not afford transcranial magnetic stimulation, which at the time was also less available and not fully proven. The data for vagus nerve stimulation (VNS) were encouraging, but Jean's pain management physician was strongly encouraging her to have a morphine pump implanted, which was also contraindicated with VNS. She had no interest in trying the new MAOI patch. Deep brain stimulation and other somatic treatments were also not available for her diagnosis at the time.

Jean continued to sleep in 2- to 3-hour intervals, and when the new zolpidem her primary care provider (PCP) prescribed was not effective, he ordered a sleep study. This eventually confirmed severe obstructive sleep apnea, for which continuous positive airway pressure was prescribed. This treatment was not helpful and was changed to bilevel positive airway pressure. As a result, Jean's sleep intervals expanded to 3.5 hours, resulting in a further reduction in hydrocodone use and less daytime drowsiness.

Throughout most of her treatment, Jean showed an avoidance of proceeding with further evaluations, consultations, and interventions for her medical conditions that approached passive-aggressive behavior. This included never having the morphine pump implanted, never consulting a neurosurgeon, and delaying the MRI of her spine and head for many years, despite the pleas and expressed concerns of the physicians treating her. Her psychiatrist attempted to identify and work through this resistance, to no avail. Jean did maintain contact with most of her providers and accepted treatment for fairly frequent pneumonia, sepsis, and urinary tract infections.

Jean's relationship and work with her psychiatrist were mostly supportive, outside the medical interventions he tried to provide. In addition to contracting for and maintaining her safety, together they were able to identify and acknowledge her generalized anger, and they identified that her mood was generally lower during periods of increased physical pain. Although Jean's husband was involved with and supportive of her and her treatment throughout, early in the course Jean experienced significant conflicts with her 17-year-old daughter, who expressed anger toward her.

Jean isolated herself from family and social contacts for many years, tired of feeling that everyone else was competing with her for who had the most problems. Feeling a lack of empathy from others, she had no ability to feel any for them. She gave up important activities, such as attending church, and remained socially withdrawn, irritable, and depressed. She initially sought, then canceled, religious counseling. She did feel an obligation to care for her aging and ill parents, neither of whom was able to acknowledge her own suffering. Many times she expressed that even if she did not kill herself sooner, she would probably do so after both of them died. She stated that her life "lacked meaning."

Jean and her psychiatrist maintained her treatment with maprotiline because it had produced the best measurable, if insufficient, response, but they never stopped discussing and considering alternatives to her current medical and psychiatric treatments, particularly new or pending options. The term *treatment resistance* was of no value and was never used—Jean knew her psychiatrist's optimistic expectations had yet to be met. And yet, her provider was able to model hope and enthusiasm for continuing to believe in the value of treatment. They worked on decision-making, particularly small, short-term steps that she could identify and shoot for. They identified short trips she might like to try. Together, they looked at her discouragement and how she could borrow the hope and faith of others when hers waned. Her daughter asked her to sew something for her, and Jean realized that she was asking her to act "as if" she could be helpful to her.

In the first years of Jean's work with the psychiatrist, her Global Assessment of Functioning (GAF) score (used in DSM-IV) (American Psychiatric Association 1994, p. 32; Smith et al. 2011; Tungström et al. 2005) seldom reached above 45, representing serious symptoms and major to serious impairment in several areas, including work, family relations, judgment, thinking, and mood. By 2007, 9 years into her work with the psychiatrist, Jean no longer had suicidal ideation. Although she continued only the minimally effective maprotiline and sessions were held about every 4 weeks, she began to ask for more intimacy with her siblings. She admitted that her daughter was no longer angry with her and that she had refused to acknowledge this for some time. By 2009, her psychiatrist rated her GAF as high as 70 during some sessions, indicating that she was generally functioning pretty well with some significant interpersonal relationships and that some mild symptoms may have been present but might be transient and expected reactions to stresses (American Psychiatric Association 1994, p. 32). Her mother, father, and a close friend died and she tolerated these losses well. Her daughter gave birth to twins.

In 2009, Jean also experienced another orthopedic setback: a fall that resulted in a fractured femur and ankle. She told her psychiatrist, "I didn't scream, cry, or act angry. This is something I can get over." Despite this setback and persistent hip pain, her GAF remained at 70. She eventually became more frustrated with her limitations than her disability. In 2011, with her GAF recorded at 75 (no more than slight impairment) and a notable decline in her neurovegetative symptoms, Jean traveled to the Grand Canyon with her daughter, husband, son-in-law, and grandchildren; had lunch with a friend; and attended a graduation party. She pushed herself to go shopping and was frustrated only with becoming tired and having to stop. She was doing dishes despite pain and was able to engage in more activities of daily living. She told her psychiatrist, "I have come a long way" and indicated that her daughter agreed.

In 2012, Jean joined a Bible study, a book group, and a genealogical society. Also that year, the psychiatrist agreed with her other providers to a cautious trial of prednisolone for a persistent rash. She was able to manage the mild sadness and crying that resulted, saying, "I'm not completely bad." By 2013, her motivation to change moved from external to internal. She worked with her psychiatrist, now every 6 weeks, on more open communication with her husband and attended his family reunion. She sought out more people for social relationships. Late that year, her pain specialist tapered her off the topiramate he was using for pain relief. She closed out that year by telling her psychiatrist, "Things usually do fall into place."

By 2015, Jean and the psychiatrist were meeting every 3 months. In 2016, she was averaging 6 hours of uninterrupted sleep each night. During 2017, Jean was still taking 225 mg maprotiline per day. She was unhappy about a new musculoskeletal problem limiting use of her left leg but worked readily and closely with a neurosurgeon to find solutions. She underwent spinal surgery, and her mood never dropped. As her psychiatrist worked with her on transitioning to a colleague because of his retirement at the year's end, she told him, "Family is the most important thing in my life and my reason for living."

Whether this case illustrates spontaneous remission of a mood disorder or slow and gradual response to psychotherapy, it certainly does illustrate how important the clinical relationship is, long term, between a provider and patient. Clinicians can "hold" patients within their own perception of hope and optimism and support small choices for patients to keep going and take risks that are necessary to change. While doing this, providers also demonstrate that they can identify and tolerate the feelings of their patients: the fear, uncertainty, and anger that threaten acceptance and resolution of symptoms and restoration of functionality.

Case Example 2

In 2005, Walter (not his real name), a 48-year-old man, was referred by his PCP to a 49-year-old psychiatrist to continue psychiatric care because his current psychiatrist had become a hospitalist. He reported the onset of depressed mood, delusions, and auditory hallucinations at age 11, followed by the first of two suicide attempts by overdose at age 13. By age 23 he was experiencing severe mood cycling, but he received no psychiatric treatment until after a partial colectomy and chemotherapy for colon carcinoma in 1991, when he was 35.

Diagnoses from Walter's previous four psychiatrists included bipolar disorder, schizophrenia, and paranoid disorder. He was given sertraline by a PCP in 1992, which worsened his mood and also led to hypersomnia, anergy, and heavy weight gain. He was treated with clozapine for 6 months, after which he tapered himself off and felt normal; he reported that the clozapine helped and was well tolerated. He also remembered a good response to haloperidol in 1997. Tegretol, initiated sometime between 1992 and 1994, worked well for mood stability, but Walter discontinued it in 1999 when he thought it might be causing arthritis. Olanzapine, begun in 2001, produced weight gain and was not helpful. In 2003 Walter was prescribed oral ziprasidone, which caused vertigo and insomnia. Zolpidem had been tried for persistent insomnia and was not effective. He had also taken lorazepam at some point, but there were no details of this trial in his memory or record. He had never been treated with psychotherapy.

Walter's current medications were Wellbutrin SR (sustained-release bupropion) 200 mg in the morning and 100 mg in the evening, Seroquel (quetiapine) 300 mg qhs, AcipHex (rabeprazole) 20 mg bid, and methotrexate 2.5 mg 4 days a week. He also took ibuprofen and Excedrin, two tablets each twice a day; folic acid; and fish oil twice a day. Neurontin (gabapentin) 300 mg tid had been tried as an add-on the previous year. This did result in deeper sleep for 14 hours a day, but his previous psychiatrist thought it was ineffective, and Walter felt no other differences with or without it.

In addition to his history of survival from colon carcinoma, Walter had a history of tracheal collapse. A gastroenterologist monitored his colon condition and treated him for Barrett's esophagus. He saw a rheumatologist for genetically linked rheumatoid arthritis and L5 spondylolysis. He did not have a history of head injury or seizure, although he had sustained a fever of 107 degrees Fahrenheit at age 17 years and received no medical care for it. His thyroid function had never been tested. He kept regular 6-month checkups with his PCP. He drank one serving of alcoholic beverage once a year and denied any use of illegal or recreational drugs or tobacco. He consumed nine doses a day of caffeine between Excedrin and soft drinks.

Walter reported normal early development, despite emotional neglect from both parents. There was a significant history of depressed mood on his father's side of the family, including suicide, and unexplained "oddness" on his mother's. Walter was diagnosed with a learning disorder in school and was given speech therapy through the fifth grade. He was unable to complete college work but did obtain an associate's degree. He had been married more than 27 years and had two sons, a 17-year-old at home and a 20-year-old away at college. His wife, Linda, taught early education. Because Walter experienced social and performance anxiety, he was currently unemployed, his most recent job being too stressful.

Walter's current complaints to the psychiatrist included labile mood with rapid thoughts, and he reported visual hallucinations over the preceding 6 years, seeing people who were not there. This kept him from driving a vehicle because he would stop abruptly in traffic to keep from running over nonexistent persons in the road. He also experienced auditory hallucinations of whispering but at the time denied olfactory hallucinations. He reported delusions of a tiger stalking him and frequently believed doppelgangers were present. His appetite was variable, sometimes voracious, and he had gained 10 pounds over the past year (his BMI was 28.5). His sleep also varied from initial or terminal insomnia to hypersomnia.

On mental status examination, Walter was appropriately dressed and groomed, with good eye contact and somewhat pressured speech. He reported impaired short-term memory and cognition, again with rapid thoughts. He showed labile mood and affect and mild to moderate anxiety. His thought processing was within normal limits, with hallucinations and delusions as described, and he evidenced suicidality: in this case, suicidal ideation with no current plan or intent, indicating "it is always in the back of my mind." He was cooperative, made a good effort, and appeared to have fair insight into his condition and good judgment as to how he responded to the presence of his symptoms. His intellect appeared to be in the average range.

As for further risk assessment, Walter's second suicide attempt (driving off a cliff) was interrupted by Linda. The week prior to this initial evaluation, he did admit intent to kill himself: he planned to overdose on ziprasidone but was never left alone. Walter denied ever mutilating himself and was never violent toward others, nor ever wished to be. His only violence had been hitting walls or tables.

The psychiatrist considered affective psychosis, schizoaffective disorder, and organic affective disorder in his differential diagnosis. He discussed his assessment with Walter and offered to refer him for a second opinion, which was declined. Together, they agreed on goals for their work together: stable euthymia, minimized suicidality and risk, improved treatment plan compliance, normal sleeping and eating, and the elimination of anxiety.

The psychiatrist recommended laboratory testing of Walter's thyroid-stimulating hormone and free thyroxine levels, along with measurement of antithyroglobulin and anti–thyroid peroxidase antibodies, to screen for thyroid disorders and obtaining a copy of his reportedly normal electroencephalogram (EEG) from 2001. He also recommended that Walter cut his use of all caffeine by half for 1 week, then completely discontinue it. He was also told to avoid dextromethorphan and decongestants. Also suggested was a trial of oxcarbazepine, given Walter's previous response to carbamazepine, returning to the latter if unsuccessful. The oxcarbazepine would be titrated over 4 weeks to 600 mg bid, and sodium levels would be monitored. The provider suggested raising the quetiapine dose to 400 mg nightly for 2 weeks before resuming the 300-mg dose. Walter agreed to this plan and to a contract for his safety: he agreed to refrain from any self-harm without giving adequate advance notice to his new psychiatrist.

Four weeks later, Walter denied suicidal ideation and racing thoughts, was sleeping 7–8 hours, and was experiencing only mildly low mood. His family had also noticed improvement, but he was still talking "too much, for too long." As treatment progressed, Walter's thyroid, electrolytes, lipids, and most other laboratory values were found to be in the normal range, and the EEG report was confirmed. Chronic postchemotherapy anemia persisted. Attempts were made to lower his dose of quetiapine to as low as 50 mg nightly, but this resulted in terminal insomnia (awakening after 3–4 hours, unable to return to sleep) and an increase in visual hallucinations, such as a woman in his apartment asking to take a shower.

After 6 months of treatment, Walter's mood was better but remained labile. He revealed to his psychiatrist that although his mood had improved, he had withheld some of his symptoms and their severity from his psychiatrist because he was pleased with his improvement and did not want to lose it. The psychiatrist acknowledged the disclosure and affirmed that Walter's trust in him must be growing. At the psychiatrist's suggestion, they agreed to involve Linda in the second half of their treatment sessions so that she could support Walter by providing her objective observations for both of them to consider. This consent was given in writing, and this practice continued throughout their work together.

They all agreed that Walter was unable to work, and he applied for and received Social Security Disability Insurance. Walter continued to not drive. He accepted the psychiatrist's opinion that there were many organic (neurological) features of his symptoms, particularly visual, olfactory, and tactile hallucinations. He continued to have painfully fearful delusions, such as a dark and scary force in his apartment he felt their cat also sensed. Hypersomnia, rapid cycling mood, and visual and tactile hallucinations persisted. Quetiapine, then at 600–800 mg qhs, was not effective for these symptoms or for sleep, so a change to risperidone 2 mg qhs was made. Walter had cut his oxcarbazepine by half for 3 weeks because his supply was running low, and his rheumatologist had increased his methotrexate to six doses per week. Walter agreed to resume 600 mg of oxcarbazepine bid and move to clozapine or higher doses of risperidone if this was not sufficient. His GAF had dropped to 45.

Walter bit his tongue shortly thereafter and was treated by his PCP with clindamycin, which produced adverse reactions of emotional and cognitive worsening. On his own, Walter lowered his dosage of risperidone to 1 mg qhs. His Abnormal Involuntary Movement Scale (AIMS) score was 0, although he and his psychiatrist were both fully aware of his risk of tardive dyskinesia and acute dystonic reactions (ADRs) from his antipsychotic medications. The tongue biting did not appear to be from tardive dyskinesia; some ADRs might have been involved, but none was found on examination. Anticholinergic medications were discouraged in order to avoid further cognitive impairment and not increase his chances of developing tardive dyskinesia. In session, Walter and Linda agreed he would resume 2 mg qhs of risperidone and watch for further ADRs; the psychiatrist agreed to lower the oxcarbazepine dosage to 600 mg qam and 900 mg qpm because of dizziness. After these actions, Walter's visual hallucinations decreased, but he bit his tongue again and felt too withdrawn and tranquilized, along with additional cognitive slowing. They all agreed to lower the risperidone dosage to 1.5 mg qhs, with the psychiatrist suggesting they consider replacing it with haloperidol or clozapine because both had been reported as effective previously. However, both Walter and Linda wanted to stay with the risperidone to avoid the additional side effects the other two options might cause.

After this change, about a year into their work together, Walter saw himself as "much better than before I started seeing you, much better; the best I have been in a long time." He and Linda both reported decreased paranoia and minimal delusions. He was calm and euthymic and denied rapid thoughts. He was averaging 13 hours sleep, his AIMS remained at 0, and there had been no further tongue biting or ADRs. He was still occasionally perceiving doppelgangers, saw other imaginary/fantasy friends, and still had mild sadness, along with dizziness. However, Walter requested to discontinue the risperidone because he felt tranquilized and too distant from his family. In fact, he had reduced his dosage to 1 mg qhs 4 days prior to the visit and was already mildly agitated. He and Linda continued to resist a change to either clozapine or haloperidol. The psychiatrist reluctantly agreed to a slow and cautious taper of the risperidone, by 0.5 mg/day every 4–6 weeks.

Four weeks later, while taking 1 mg risperidone qhs, Walter reported feeling better 1 week after his previous visit, consistent with a new, lower steady-state serum level of the antipsychotic. He could stay awake after 8 hours of sleep and no longer had a sense of being stalked; visual hallucinations were reduced, and he now perceived auditory hallucinations as symptoms. He felt less tranquilized and not sedated. Recognizing that this could be cycling as much as true improvement, Walter and the psychiatrist agreed to maintain the current medications and doses.

Two months later, Walter's symptoms remained improved, allowing progress in his family interactions. Linda was supervising his medications, per their agreement, so no changes had been made. They were now using a password between them to help him with the doppelganger symptom. He had become slightly hypomanic after briefly using caffeine, but the symptoms abated when he discontinued the caffeine. His delusions and hallucinations were unchanged, and he reported a recent conversation with a ghost. Walter was much more involved with his family, however: his two sons were talking to him more, a sign he used to monitor his progress, and he was agreeable to a niece renting a room from them for several months. There remained no sign of tardive dyskinesia or ADRs.

At this point, Linda was very pleased and was surprised that although Walter knew he was better, he did not really see the totality of his improvement. In exploration, the psychiatrist discovered that Walter saw his increased interactions with others as "overreacting," whereas Linda interpreted this as him becoming "more capable." On further discussion, Walter accepted her viewpoint, and together they requested the psychiatrist help them find some type of sheltered work environment for him. A referral was made to the state agency that provided such opportunities. Several months later, however, Walter's hypersomnia returned, leading him and Linda to reduce his risperidone to 0.5 mg qhs. This also allowed his delusions and hallucinations to again worsen, preventing him from completing the state evaluations and attempting the sheltered work.

Later that year, Walter's sleep improved. He and Linda agreed to again raise his risperidone to 1 mg qhs to target his delusions and hallucinations, and the higher dosage helped. Walter was given a new infusion for his spondylosis by his rheumatologist, who hoped it could replace his methotrexate. He told his psychiatrist and family, "In the daytime things are pretty good. I'm positive because I realize I have [perceptual distortions] that are not real. This is so much better." Linda concurred.

The beginning of 2008 was met with a serious threat to Walter's progress: he and his family had opted for a new, cheaper supplemental insurance policy that imposed severe restrictions on his medication reimbursement. Unfortunately, the psychiatrist had not been aware they were considering such a change, nor had he been contacted by the pharmacy. As was typical for the time, pill counts were more important to the plan than doses, and generic preparations were mandated, even if they were proven ineffective for a patient. Walter arrived at his January appointment already affected by these changes: his oxcarbazepine had been changed from brand name Trileptal to the generic form and reduced from seven 300-mg tablets a day (three in the morning and four in the evening) to the maximally allowed three capsules a day. He was still taking brand-name bupropion (Wellbutrin SR), but this would not be continued.

Clinically, Walter was disoriented and had not recognized Linda the previous day. His condition had reverted to pretreatment levels: severe auditory, olfactory, tactile, and visual hallucinations; severe delusions;

rapid thinking; excessive energy; racing thoughts; and cognitive impairment. He appeared manic and slept only 4–5 hours a day. The psychiatrist attempted to reestablish the treatment plan that had led to Walter's improvement. He changed the 300-mg capsules of oxcarbazepine to 600 mg and prescribed one and a half capsules in the morning and two in the evening, hoping that the variation in bioequivalence allowed by the FDA among generic manufacturers would still allow a sufficient steady-state serum level for response (see section "Polypharmacy and Bioavailability Complications" in Chapter 7, "Underappreciated Causes of Treatment Failure"). In fact, over the next several months, with the differences in bioequivalence of the generic preparations, which changed often because of various manufacturing practices and frequent pharmacy substitutions, increases in Walter's symptoms and side effects were marked.

That January, the psychiatrist attempted to intercede for Walter with managed care staff, the secondary insurance company, and Medicare itself. Ultimately, he logged more than 8 hours of phone conversations, not including the time he spent writing letters to each entity on Walter's behalf. Two separate staff members of Medicare Part D told him, "Put the patient in the hospital and let Part A pay for it." The psychiatrist was unable to obtain any relaxation of the new company's restrictions. He again suggested to Walter alternative medications, particularly other mood stabilizers, anticonvulsants, and antipsychotics that they could try, but both Walter and Linda insisted this was still the best he had done, and they would not agree to the change.

Ultimately, the psychiatrist, Walter, and Linda responded by adhering as closely to the restrictions as they thought medically safe, which allowed very little change. The family agreed to pay the difference between what was medically necessary and what was covered—a burden, but one they could manage until they could opt for a new supplemental plan the next year, which they did. Walter and Linda were impressed and grateful for the strong effort the psychiatrist had made to try to help them with these new restrictions and offered to pay for the extra time he expended. Because the cost based on his hourly rate would have been high, the psychiatrist expressed appreciation but declined, feeling that he had made the effort as much as a general response to such external management as he had for one patient. Privately, he felt good about his actions in response to this issue, although he lamented the outcome. Ultimately, the experience deepened an already strong therapeutic alliance.

As part of these adjustments, the risperidone dosage was changed to 0.5 mg qod, alternating with 1 mg qod. Later that year, Walter learned that he had been exposed to lead in drinking water 30 years earlier, about the time of a significant decline. His lead levels were tested, found to be not elevated, and although no conclusions could be drawn about Walter's suspicion that this contributed to his condition, the fact that his concern was taken seriously was important to him.

No formal psychotherapy sessions were ever held, and time assessing Walter, conferring with Linda, and discussing treatment plans usually took no longer than 30 minutes. Walter's sons never participated. This still allowed time for discussion of family interactions, such as how the family might use information about Walter's gating problems (inability to fully separate irrelevant stimuli from meaningful ones) (Boutros et al. 1999; Judd et al. 1992) and how his improving insight was also changing these problems to some degree. By the end of 2008, Walter continued to feel more comfortable: "This is nice." Linda saw him continuing to progress, and he was now helping her organize her classroom.

During 2009, at Walter's request, the dosage of sustained-release bupropion was lowered to 100 mg bid, but when Walter became too sad, 200 mg qam + 100 mg qpm was resumed. The risperidone dose remained alternatively 0.5 mg and 1.0 mg, and no tongue problem reoccurred. In early 2010, at a BMI of 26.4 and GAF of 68, Walter told his psychiatrist, "I'd be quite happy if I could stay like this," and Linda agreed. Later that year, in consultation, his rheumatologist proceeded with a cautious 2-week trial of adalimumab and prednisolone. The medication destabilized Walter's mood slightly and briefly, but the problem resolved without need to alter his psychiatric medication. Temporary mood destabilization recurred some months later when he again used Excedrin (caffeine) by mistake. He continued a weight loss diet approved by his PCP, gastroenterologist, and psychiatrist and was gradually losing weight in the face of a more stable appetite, one of his original goals.

By the end of 2010, at age 54, 5 years into his work with the new psychiatrist, Walter remained symptomatic, but he was assessed as having achieved his maximum level of improvement, given the current treatment options. Neither Walter nor Linda and their children, however, considered this to be treatment failure. In August 2011, Walter stated in a session, "I can live with the way I am now." He had not had any suicidal ideation since June 2008, the last time he would experience it during this treatment course. Obvious mood instability and psychotic symptoms persisted. He still experienced some dizziness and balance problems, but his sodium levels, checked in tandem by his PCP and psychiatrist, remained normal. All agreed that they had found an acceptable compromise between symptoms and side effects and, significantly, that Walter's functionality, while still limited, had notably improved within his family setting.

Having just celebrated his 55th birthday, however, Walter became bothered by a delusion that he would not survive to age 56. He was adamant that he had no intention of killing himself but had a nagging suspicion that he would die for an unknown reason, although he no longer experienced other examples of paranoia. He expressed a desire to live, saying," I like gray better than black." Reluctant to delve too deeply into insight-oriented therapy, the psychiatrist did suggest that maybe this new fear reflected the change in Walter's attitude about life, now that he valued his existence more and did not wish to lose it. Despite this attempt at reframing, Walter continued to worry throughout the year and was greatly relieved to celebrate his 56th birthday, after which he no longer thought his death was imminent. Shortly afterward, he reported, "I haven't been doing bad [sic] at all. I still have some [visual and auditory] hallucinations at times, but nothing terrifying, no black or depressive mood. Though not perfect, I can live with that."

In 2013, Linda reported that Walter was very supportive of her own stress from graduate school, work, and their son's engagement. Months later, he was able to be sociable at the wedding. Still, his psychiatrist continued to look for ways to improve his condition without risking the gains Walter and his family so valued. For example, it did not appear possible to improve Walter's concentration without making his mood more unstable, just as it was also not possible to make it more stable. Walter maintained, as he had during their initial meeting, that low anxiety was his highest priority, so he did not wish to alter the current treatment plan: "I like the current combination and don't want anything to change." Linda agreed with him. The psychiatrist had to accept that this was likely a very functional decision, because anxiety is linked to suicide more than any other symptom (Nepon et al. 2010; Weissman et al. 1989).

Walter and the psychiatrist did continue to discuss and attempt to reframe his ideas and delusions of reference, again without deep interpretation. Although he was calmer overall, he continued to experience moderate social withdrawal related to lack of interest and the awkwardness of his perceptions. He had greatly improved his ability to participate (more comfortably for everyone) in larger family events but remained most comfortable with Linda.

In December 2013, Walter appeared to experience a partial motor seizure. He and Linda declined neurological consultation, but the psychiatrist gave them the referral information anyway. They agreed to consult the specialist if he experienced any further symptoms of this type. To the psychiatrist's knowledge, these symptoms did not return. However, he reminded Walter and Linda of the relative risks of and protection from seizure by his current medication plan: risperidone alternating between 0.5 and 1 mg qhs, oxcarbazepine 600 mg qam + 900 mg qpm, and sustained-release bupropion 200 mg qam + 100 mg qpm. Linda continued to supervise his medications.

In 2014, Walter and Linda adopted a dog, and walking it helped Walter leave his house more. He tolerated his son's move to Japan well. He and Linda tried lowering his dose of risperidone for 4 weeks to try to improve his sex life (erectile dysfunction), but this was not successful. They resumed his 1-mg dose, and his PCP prescribed tadalafil, which was effective and well tolerated. By the end of the year, Walter was more active in general, and Linda completed her master's degree. In mid-2015, Walter asked to raise his risperidone back to 1 mg nightly because of a recent increase in auditory hallucinations. He also stopped his methotrexate on his own but resumed it within 6 months. Zolpidem was retried at his request; 10 mg did appear helpful for sleep and was continued. Walter's BMI dropped as low as 22.6 in June 2016 but rebounded to 23.7, where it remained through 2017. He told his psychiatrist, "I want to live longer."

The psychiatrist wrote a letter excusing Walter from jury duty, as he had in 2007, and they prepared for the termination of their work together because of the psychiatrist's planned retirement at the end of 2017. Transfer to another psychiatrist was arranged and accepted. At their final appointment in October 2017, Walter reported that he was "really good, no changes, sleeping 7 hours with no naps." He felt rested in the morning, then experienced anergy in the afternoon; he no longer experienced excessive energy. He had not needed zolpidem in more than a month. Linda reported that his mood was stable. Walter continued to feel more secure when Linda worked at home, and he still had the same degree of social withdrawal, but family visits were going very well. He never drove. He denied pervasive anhedonia, rapid thinking was rare (once a week), and no one had observed loud or rapid speech from him. He was able to stay on tasks for up to 1 hour, complete them, and redirect within 30 minutes if interrupted. He still experienced occasional olfactory, tactile, and peripheral visual hallucinations or illusions, with hypnogogic, but not command, auditory hallucinations. He denied delusions and paranoia. His GAF was estimated at 68 (some mild symptoms or some difficulty in social, occupational, or school functioning, but generally functioning pretty well; has some meaningful interpersonal relationships).

By categorical and symptomatic standards (see section "Return to the Biopsychosocial Model" in Chapter 5), this case may represent treatment failure. By considering functionality, particularly within Walter's family system, it could also be considered moderately successful by any clinician. Walter's treatment was considered significantly successful by him and his family: he wanted to live, no longer had paralyzing fear or anxiety, and was able to enjoy and interact with his family. At each visit, Walter and the psychiatrist had looked at what could be accomplished and decided together whether he wanted to risk any changes. The term *treatment resistance* was never applied. They spoke not of failure but of incremental efforts to achieve goals.

It is significant that Walter and Linda altered his medication dosages for even short-term goals either of them felt was important but resisted such risks to achieve greater treatment progress suggested by the psychiatrist. This illustrates that the mindset and goals of patients, backed by their support network, have a stronger influence on treatment planning, compliance, and treatment results than the ideas and plans of the clinician, no matter how well articulated they are. To build and sustain a productive therapeutic alliance, the clinician must anticipate, allow for, and tolerate patient goals, as long as safety is maintained. An objectively successful result may look very different from what the patient and their supporters have in mind. Our "failure" may be their success.

Long-Term Approach

No one is certain during an initial consultation how long the clinician and patient will be working together. The best outcomes, however, come from establishing a successful therapeutic relationship as early as possible, with the idea that it will continue indefinitely. Treatment efforts should also persist indeterminately, guided by the alliance and patient goals, not merely by diagnosis. This can often lead to unexpected successes: perhaps not always the original mutually agreed on goals, but still satisfactory outcomes for patients.

Psychoanalysts deride the concept of "our goals for the patient" (Benjamin C. Riggs, M.D., personal communication, February 1985). Although treatment teams often proceed as though the goal of every treatment is total self-actualization, we need to listen so we can hear what the patient is actually seeking, rather than superimposing static, general frameworks on everyone. When these frameworks do not fit, we are tempted to consider this to be failure (or resistance).

When we label a case as treatment resistant, we are essentially objectifying our patient, distancing ourselves from our failure and effectively abandoning the patient, along with a sense of hope we should be sharing. We must consciously continue to practice in a mindful manner in order to remain patient centered, respecting the patient as a person with a problem who seeks to get better in the ways they imagine; we must *be with* them through the difficulties of reaching that goal.

Hopefully, this mindset can be adopted by the practitioner, other providers, the patient, and any significant others involved in care because together they tackle short- and long-term goals that can benefit the patient. Treatment failure must be carefully defined and agreed on; any consideration of this label must prompt reconsideration and perhaps reconceptualization of the goals of treatment: symptomatic (categorical), functional (dimensional), or both. Standards and expectations will not be lowered, but goals may evolve as we better understand the patient and their environment.

Summary

Any attempt at treatment must occur in the milieu of a therapeutic alliance, a mutually respectful and open professional relationship in which both provider and patient contribute an honest and complete effort, aimed only at benefiting the patient. The quality of this relationship is linked to the likelihood of clinical success. Because half of treatments may fall short of early expectations, clinicians must be prepared to accept delays in remission. As we sustain and deepen our alliance, however, we may better understand the perhaps evolving goals and opportunities important to the patient. Being blinded by our own expectations may cause us to miss what the patient values most.

Even when the clinician's and patient's goals are fully commensurate, we must create and sustain a holding environment that communicates caring, while sharing a sense of hope that the patient may not be capable of sustaining. More important than the therapeutic modality employed, therapeutic alliances are stronger if formed early in the clinical relationship. These are likely to be dynamic relationships that will be tested by the process of treatment. If the clinician can continually adapt this alliance to the viewpoint of the patient, inevitable ruptures, such as withdrawal or anger, may be successfully negotiated and result in improved clinical outcomes. It is the therapist's contribution, more than the patient's, that is linked to clinical success.

Mismatches in gender, race, age, and ethnicity may weaken a therapeutic alliance, as do provider rigidity (particularly in treatment approach), overinterpretation, overdisclosure, tension, distraction, and criticism. Respect and humility must be shown. Most important, we must never lose hope of eventual improvement or stop trying to obtain it. Our patients will detect this sense of pessimism, which we codify by applying the label *treatment resistant*, even when technically employed and well meaning. We must expect long-term relationships with patients because we so often tackle chronic conditions that require many evolving approaches or sustained treatment.

The elements of supportive psychotherapy are present in any healthy clinician-patient relationship. In addition to providing reassurance, advice, validation, psychoeducation, and direction toward appropriate community or online resources, this technique teaches and models self-control and management of perhaps extended symptomatology or dysfunction. It offers hopeful guidance, based on goodwill, undivided attention, shared understanding, and acceptance. This empowers our patients to keep going and to take necessary risks. We must never forget that it is the perspective of our patients, within their environment, that has the stronger influence on treatment planning, compliance, and outcome, and we must ultimately define success through their eyes.

Key Points

- Prepare for long-term patient relationships.
- Clinicians must sustain the hope of eventual improvement.
- Efforts to provide clinical progress must continue.
- Clinical success must be defined by the patient.
- Therapeutic alliances are dynamic and will be tested during treatment.
- Clinicians must refocus on repair of therapeutic alliance ruptures.
- Supportive psychotherapy is a powerful and necessary tool.
- Labeling cases as treatment resistant may demoralize and distance us from a patient.

Self-Assessment Questions

1. At treatment impasses, it is important to reconceptualize which of the following?

   A. Diagnoses.
   B. Goals of treatment.
   C. Measurement of progress.
   D. All of the above.

   Correct answer: D. All of the above.

   Impasses, or treatment failures, indicate that the problem and the clinical approach to it may need to be reconceptualized. This includes definitions of success.

2. Components of supportive psychotherapy include which of the following?

   A. Clear validation.
   B. Interpretation.
   C. Psychoeducation.
   D. A and C.

   Correct answer: D. A and C.

Although any elements of psychotherapy might be used briefly during supportive therapy, interpretation usually is reserved for insight-oriented therapies and discouraged during ruptures of a therapeutic alliance. Validation is essential, and psychoeducation, when indicated, can be of value to the patient and the therapeutic alliance.

3.   Which of the following is *not* true of therapeutic alliances?

    A. They are most effective when formed early in clinical relationships.
    B. They are dependent on the therapeutic modality.
    C. They are more difficult to build and sustain when race or gender mismatches occur.
    D. They are most effective when the provider contributes consistently.

Correct answer: B. They are dependent on the therapeutic modality.

An effective therapeutic alliance transcends the type of therapeutic modalities employed. It is most effective when formed early in a therapeutic relationship. This is made more difficult with race, age, gender, or cultural mismatches between provider and patient, which require respect, humility, and as much cultural sensitivity and competence as possible (see section "Cultural Influences" in Chapter 5). The provider's contribution to the therapeutic alliance is the largest determinant of treatment success.

4.   A rupture in a therapeutic alliance is best repaired by which of the following?

    A. Persisting with the original treatment modality.
    B. Cognitive reframing.
    C. Refocusing directly on the rupture.
    D. Formal training.

Correct answer: C. Refocusing directly on the rupture.

Refocusing on the rupture and hearing what the patient is willing to talk about is the most important step. Studies show that formal training in this technique is not necessary if active listening is employed. Ignoring the rupture, continuing with the original treatment plan, and attempting to cognitively restructure or offer interpretation are much less effective.

5.   Which statement is *not* true?

     A. Advice is never given in supportive psychotherapy.
     B. Strong therapeutic alliances may result in less suicidal ideation and less self-harm.
     C. Weak or negative therapeutic alliances may result in treatment failure.
     D. Strong therapeutic alliances result in less resistance during psychotherapy.

     Correct answer: A. Advice is never given in supportive psychotherapy.

     Advice, psychoeducation, and direction to resources may be types of guidance offered in supportive psychotherapy.

Discussion Topics

1. During an initial evaluation, a potential patient describes at length her anger and despair at being repeatedly passed over for promotion by her longtime employer. Younger and, she feels, less competent coworkers are repeatedly advanced over her to positions to which she feels entitled. The psychiatrist asks whether she has ever considered leaving the firm for a different employer. At this point, the woman becomes enraged with the provider, incensed that he would even suggest that she should make a change when the fault is with the organization she works for. She shouts at him, verbally attacking him for being offensive and insensitive. Has the clinician made an error? How might he have proceeded differently? How might he continue with this potential patient following this outburst?

2. You treat a 33-year-old man with bipolar disorder, a history of substance abuse, and a closed head injury from an MVA, which resulted in seizures. After failed treatments by several other providers, you have found moderate success with doses of antipsychotic, anticonvulsant, mood-stabilizing, and antianxiety medications that have ended

the patient's suicidal ideation, paranoid delusions, visual and auditory hallucinations, and depressed mood. He lives with his mother and is disabled because he is rather somnolent during the day. Any efforts to address this somnolence through alternative medications or dosages have led quickly to a return of all of his previous symptoms. He volunteers at his mother's place of employment; they have settled into a functional pattern of life together and are both quite grateful for his improvement and that he is alive. Five years into treatment, an aunt visits and is unhappy with the patient's condition. She begins to attend sessions with the patient and his mother and pushes for changes in his medication to make him fully functional again. How do you proceed?

Additional Readings

Lessing D: The Making of the Representative for Planet 8. New York, Knopf, 1982: *An excellent example of "being with"*

Lippert CN, Roberts LW, Winston A, Goldstein M: Theory of individual supportive psychotherapy, in Gabbard's Textbook of Psychotherapeutic Treatments. Edited by Gabbard GO, Crisp-Han H. Washington, DC, American Psychiatric Association Publishing, 2022, pp 331–351: *The section on the therapeutic relationship, pp. 340–342, is particularly germane*

Novalis PN, Singer V, Peele R: Clinical Manual of Supportive Psychotherapy, 2nd Edition. Washington, DC, American Psychiatric Association Publishing, 2020: *A comprehensive clinical guide to the principles and techniques of this important form of psychotherapy*

Westermair AL, Buchman DZ, Levitt S, et al: Palliative psychiatry in a narrow and in a broad sense: a concept clarification. Aust N Z J Psychiatry 56(12):1535–1541, 2022: *Discusses how helping patients grow and develop, despite persistent symptoms, can improve their overall condition*

References

Ackerman SJ, Hilsenroth MJ: A review of therapist characteristics and techniques negatively impacting the therapeutic alliance. Psychotherapy (Chic) 38(2):171–185, 2001

American Psychiatric Association: Diagnostic and Statistical Manual of Mental Disorders, 4th Edition. Washington, DC, American Psychiatric Association Publishing, 1994

Arnow BA, Steidtmann D: Harnessing the potential of the therapeutic alliance. World Psychiatry 13(3):238–240, 2014 25273288

Boutros NN, Belger A, Campbell D, et al: Comparison of four components of sensory gating in schizophrenia and normal subjects: a preliminary report. Psychiatry Res 88(2):119–130, 1999 10622348

Castonguay LG, Goldfried MR, Wiser S, et al: Predicting the effect of cognitive therapy for depression: a study of unique and common factors. J Consult Clin Psychol 64(3):497–504, 1996 8698942

Daniels J, Wearden AJ: Socialization to the model: the active component in the therapeutic alliance? A preliminary study. Behav Cogn Psychother 39(2):221–227, 2011 21092360

Del Re AC, Flückiger C, Horvath AO, et al: Therapist effects in the therapeutic alliance-outcome relationship: a restricted-maximum likelihood meta-analysis. Clin Psychol Rev 32(7):642–649, 2012 22922705

Diamond GS, Liddle HA, Wintersteen MB, et al: Early therapeutic alliance as a predictor of treatment outcome for adolescent cannabis users in outpatient treatment. Am J Addict 15(Suppl 1):26–33, 2006 17182417

Dunster-Page C, Haddock G, Wainwright L, et al: The relationship between therapeutic alliance and patient's suicidal thoughts, self-harming behaviours and suicide attempts: a systematic review. J Affect Disord 223:165–174, 2017 28755624

Eubanks CF, Burckell LA, Goldfried MR: Clinical consensus strategies to repair ruptures in the therapeutic alliance. J Psychother Integration 28(1):60–76, 2018 29805243

Frank AF, Gunderson JG: The role of the therapeutic alliance in the treatment of schizophrenia. Relationship to course and outcome. Arch Gen Psychiatry 47(3):228–236, 1990 1968329

Grover S, Avasthi A, Jagiwala M: Clinical practice guidelines for practice of supportive psychotherapy. Indian J Psychiatry 62(Suppl 2):S173–S182, 2020 32055060

Horvath AO, Del Re AC, Flückiger C, Symonds D: Alliance in individual psychotherapy. Psychotherapy (Chic) 48(1):9–16, 2011 21401269

Howes OD, Thase ME, Pillinger T: Treatment resistance in psychiatry: state of the art and new directions. Mol Psychiatry 27(1):58–72, 2022 34257409

Judd LL, McAdams L, Budnick B, Braff DL: Sensory gating deficits in schizophrenia: new results. Am J Psychiatry 149(4):488–493, 1992 1554034

Krupnick JL, Sotsky SM, Simmens S, et al: The role of the therapeutic alliance in psychotherapy and pharmacotherapy outcome: findings in the National Institute of Mental Health Treatment of Depression Collaborative Research Program. J Consult Clin Psychol 64(3):532–539, 1996 8698947

McLaughlin AA, Keller SM, Feeny NC, et al: Patterns of therapeutic alliance: rupture-repair episodes in prolonged exposure for posttraumatic stress disorder. J Consult Clin Psychol 82(1):112–121, 2014 24188510

Meaden A, Van Marle S: When the going gets tougher: the importance of long-term supportive psychotherapy in psychosis. Adv Psychiatr Treat 14(1):42–49, 2008

Negri A, Christian C, Mariani R, et al: Linguistic features of the therapeutic alliance in the first session: a psychotherapy process study. Res Psychother 22(1):374, 2019 32913786

Nepon J, Belik SL, Bolton J, et al: The relationship between anxiety disorders and suicide attempts: findings from the National Epidemiologic Survey on Alcohol and Related Conditions. Depress Anxiety 27(9):791–798, 2010 20217852

Newman MG, Castonguay LG, Borkovec TD, et al: A randomized controlled trial of cognitive-behavioral therapy for generalized anxiety disorder with integrated techniques from emotion-focused and interpersonal therapies. J Consult Clin Psychol 79(2):171–181, 2011 21443321

Piper WE, Ogrodniczuk JS, Joyce AS, et al: Prediction of dropping out in time-limited, interpretive individual psychotherapy. Psychotherapy (Chic) 36:114–122, 1999

Polese D, Fornaro M, Palermo M, et al: Treatment-resistant to antipsychotics: a resistance to everything? Psychotherapy in treatment-resistant schizophrenia and nonaffective psychosis: a 25-year systematic review and exploratory meta-analysis. Front Psychiatry 10:210, 2019 31057434

Raskin NJ, Rogers CR: Person-centered therapy, in Current Psychotherapies, 7th Edition. Edited by Corsini RJ, Wedding D. Pacific Grove, CA, Thomson Brooks/Cole, 2005, pp 130–165

Rogers CR: Perceptual reorganization in client-centered therapy, in Perception: An Approach to Personality. Edited by Blake RR, Ramsey GV. New York, Ronald Press, 1951, pp 307–327

Safran JD, Muran JC: Negotiating the Therapeutic Alliance: A Relational Treatment Guide. New York, Guilford, 2000

Safran JD, Muran JC, Eubanks-Carter C: Repairing alliance ruptures. Psychotherapy (Chic) 48(1):80–87, 2011 21401278

Smith GN, Ehmann TS, Flynn SW, et al: The assessment of symptom severity and functional impairment with DSM-IV axis V. Psychiatr Serv 62(4):411–417, 2011 21459993

Tschuschke V, Koemeda-Lutz M, von Wyl A, et al: The impact of patients' and therapists' views of the therapeutic alliance on treatment outcome in psychotherapy. J Nerv Ment Dis 208(1):56–64, 2020 31688492

Tungström S, Söderberg P, Armelius BA: Relationship between the Global Assessment of Functioning and other DSM axes in routine clinical work. Psychiatr Serv 56(4):439–443, 2005 15812094

Weissman MM, Klerman GL, Markowitz JS, et al: Suicidal ideation and suicide attempts in panic disorder and attacks. N Engl J Med 321(18):1209–1214, 1989 2797086

West JC, Vance MC, Ursano RJ: Maintaining motivation and preserving the therapeutic alliance as tools to overcome treatment-resistant depression, in Managing Treatment-Resistant Depression: Road to Novel Therapeutics.

Edited by Quevedo J, Riva-Posse P, Bobo WV. Cambridge, MA, Academic Press, 2022, pp 575–582.

Wintersteen MB, Mensinger JL, Diamond GS: Do gender and racial differences between patient and therapist affect therapeutic alliance and treatment retention in adolescents? Prof Psychol Res Pr 36(4):400–408, 2005

Wolfe BE, Goldfried MR: Research on psychotherapy integration: recommendations and conclusions from an NIMH workshop. J Consult Clin Psychol 56(3):448–451, 1988 2899579

Index